HEART FUNCTION AND METABOLISM

DEVELOPMENTS IN CARDIOVASCULAR MEDICINE

Morganroth, Joel, Moore, E.N., eds.: Sudden cardiac death and congestive heart failure: Diagnosis and treatment. 1983. ISBN 0-89838-580-6.
Perry, H.M., ed.: Lifelong management of hypertension. ISBN 0-89838-582-2.
Jaffe, E.A., ed.: Biology of endothelial cells. ISBN 0-89838-587-3.
Surawicz, B., Reddy, C.P., Prystowsky, E.N., eds.: Tachycardias. 1984. ISBN 0-89838-588-1.
Spencer, M.P., ed.: Cardiac doppler diagnosis. ISBN 0-89838-591-1.
Villareal, H.V., Sambhi, M.P., eds.: Topics in pathophysiology of hypertension. ISBN 0-89838-595-4.
Messerli, F.H., ed.: Cardiovascular disease in the elderly. 1984. ISBN 0-89838-596-2.
Simoons, M.L., Reiber, J.H.C., eds.: Nuclear imaging in clinical cardiology. ISBN 0-89838-599-7.
Ter Keurs, H.E.D.J., Schipperheym, J.J., eds.: Cardiac left ventricular hypertrophy. ISBN 0-89838-612-8.
Sperelakis, N., ed.: Physiology and pathophysiology of the heart. ISBN 0-89838-615-2.
Messerli, F.H., ed.: Kidney in essential hypertension. 1983. ISBN 0-89838-616-0.
Sambhi, M.P., ed.: Fundamental fault in hypertension. ISBN 0-89838-638-1.
Marchesi, D., ed.: Ambulatory monitoring: Cardiovascular system and allied applications. ISBN 0-89838-642-X.
Kupper, W., Macalpin, R.N., Bleifeld, W., eds.: Coronary tone in ischemic heart disease. ISBN 0-89838-646-2.
Sperelakis, N., Caulfield, J.B., eds.: Calcium antagonists: Mechanisms of action on cardiac muscle and vascular smooth muscle. ISBN 0-89838-655-1.
Godfraind, T., Herman, A.S., Wellens, D., eds.: Entry blockers in cardiovascular and cerebral dysfunctions. ISBN 0-89838-658-6.
Morganroth, J., Moore, E.N., eds.: Interventions in the acute phase of myocardial infarction. ISBN 0-89838-659-4.
Abel, F.L., Newman, W.H., eds.: Functional aspects of the normal, hypertrophied, and failing heart. ISBN 0-89838-665-9.
Sideman, S., and Beyar, R., eds.: Simulation and imaging of the cardiac system. ISBN 0-89838-687-X.
van de Wall, E., Lie, K.I., eds.: Recent views on hypertrophic cardiomyopathy. ISBN 0-89838-694-2.
Beamish, R.E., Singal, P.K., Dhalla, N.S., eds.: Stress and heart disease. ISBN 089838-709-4.
Beamish, R.E., Panagia, V., Dhalla, N.S., eds.: Pathogenesis of stress-induced heart disease. ISBN 0-89838-710-8.
Morganroth, J., Moore, E.N., eds., Cardiac arrhythmias: New therapeutic drugs and devices. ISBN 0-89838-716-7.
Mathes, P., ed.: Secondary prevention in coronary artery disease and myocardial infarction. ISBN 0-89838-736-1.
Stone, H. Lowell, Weglicki, W.B., eds., Pathology of cardiovascular injury. ISBN 0-89838-743-4.
Meyer, J., Erbel, R., Rupprecht, H.J., eds., Improvement of myocardial perfusion. ISBN 0-89838-748-5.
Reiber, J.H.C., Serruys, P.W., Slager, C.J.: Quantitative coronary and left ventricular cineangiography. ISBN 0-89838-760-4.
Fagard, R.H., Bekaert, I.E., eds., Sports cardiology. ISBN 0-89838-782-5.
Reiber, J.H.C., Serruys, P.W., eds., State of the art in quantitative coronary arteriography. ISBN 0-89838-804-X.
Roelandt, J., ed.: Color doppler flow imaging. ISBN 0-89838-806-6.
van de Wall, E.E., ed.: Noninvasive imaging of cardiac metabolism. ISBN 0-89838-812-0.
Liebman, J., Plonsey, R., Rudy, Y., eds., Pediatric and fundamental electrocardiography. ISBN 0-89838-815-5.
Higler, H., Hombach, V., eds., Invasive cardiovascular therapy. ISBN 0-89838-818-X.
Serruys, P.W., Meester, G.T., eds., Coronary angioplasty: a controlled model for ischemia. ISBN 0-89838-819-8.
Tooke, J.E., Smaje, L.H., eds.: Clinical investigation of the microcirculation. ISBN 0-89838-833-3.
van Dam, Th., van Oosterom, A., eds.: Electrocardiographic body surface mapping. ISBN 0-89838-834-1.
Spencer, M.P., ed.: Ultrasonic diagnosis of cerebrovascular disease. ISBN 0-89838-836-8.
Legato, M.J., ed.: The stressed heart. ISBN 0-89838-849-X.
Safar, M.E., ed.: Arterial and venous systems in essential hypertension. ISBN 0-89838-857-0.
Roelandt, J., ed.: Digital techniques in echocardiography. ISBN 0-89838-861-9.
Dhalla, N.S., Singal, P.K., Beamish, R.E., eds.: Pathophysiology of heart disease. ISBN 0-89838-864-3.

This book is a volume in the series, "Advances in Myocardiology" (N.S. Dhalla, Series Editor). "Advances in Myocardiology" is a subseries within "Developments in Cardiovascular Medicine".

HEART FUNCTION AND METABOLISM

Proceedings of the Symposium held at the Eighth
Annual Meeting of the American Section of the
International Society for Heart Research,
July 8–11, 1986, Winnipeg, Canada

edited by

Naranjan S. Dhalla
Grant N. Pierce
Robert E. Beamish
*Youville Research Institute, St. Boniface General
Hospital, and University of Manitoba, Department of
Physiology, Winnipeg, Canada*

Martinus Nijhoff Publishing
a member of the Kluwer Academic Publishers Group
Boston/Dordrecht/Lancaster

Distributors

for North America: Kluwer Academic Publishers, 101 Philip Drive, Assinippi Park,
Norwell, MA 02061, USA

for the UK and Ireland: Kluwer Academic Publishers, MTP Press Limited,
Falcon House, Queen Square, Lancaster LA1 1RN, UK

for all other countries: Kluwer Academic Publishers Group,
Distribution Centre, Post Office Box 322, 3300 AH Dordrecht,
The Netherlands

Library of Congress Cataloging-in-Publication Data

Heart function and metabolism

  (Developments in cardiovascular medicine)
  1. Heart—Congresses.   2. Heart—Muscle—Congresses.
3. Sarcolemma—Congresses.   4. Sarcoplasmic reticulum—Congresses.
5. Metabolism.
I. Dhalla, Naranjan S.   II. Pierce, Grant N.   III. Beamish,
Robert E.   IV. International Society For Heart Research. American
Section. Meeting (8th : 1986 : Winnipeg, Man.) V. Series.
[DNLM: 1. Heart—metabolism—congresses.   2. Heart—physiology—
congresses. W1 DE997VME /
WG 202 H4365 1986]
QP111.2.H43   1987   612′.17   86-33107
ISBN 0-89838-865-1

CONTENTS

ix

In the course of the last two decades, it has become increasingly
evident that the sarcolemmal, sarcoplasmic reticular and mitochondrial
membrane systems play an important role in determining the status of heart
function in health and disease. These organelles have been shown to be
intimately involved in the regulation of cation movements during the
contraction-relaxation cycle. Various proteins imbedded in the phospholipid
bilayers of these membranes control Ca^{2+}, Na^+, Cl^-, K^+ and H^+ concentrations
within the cytoplasm by indirect or direct means. Cationic channels, Na^+,
K^+-ATPase, Ca^{2+}/Mg^{2+} ATPase, Ca^{2+} pump, Na^+-Ca^{2+} exchanger, Na^+-H^+ exchanger
and adenylate cyclase affect myocardial function and viability through their
role as regulators of specific ion movements. However, proteins are not the
only important constituents of the membrane. Any disturbance in the
interaction between proteins and phospholipids in the membrane has been
suggested to alter the function of the organelles, upset ionic homeostasis
and precipitate the development of abnormalities in cardiac performance. It
is, therefore, crucial to understand the factors which regulate membrane
function in their totality if we are to comprehend the nature of heart
performance in healthy subjects. Similarly, the study of membrane
dysfunction in a wide variety of experimental models of heart disease at
various stages of failure is essential if we are to fully understand the
pathogenesis of heart dysfunction and improve its treatment. However, study
of only the membrane systems would be short-sighted indeed. The contractile
proteins which ultimately transform subcellular events into the physical
reaction of contractile force in muscle are certainly worthy of
investigation. The nature of their interactions during force development
and the molecular factors which determine the characteristics of the
individual contractile proteins are lines of investigation which provide us
with valuable insight into the mechanisms of the contractile process in the
heart. Of course, the critical denominator of cellular energy cannot be
overlooked in any assessment of factors important to myocardial function and
viability. The more that we can understand about the close interaction of
energy-producing and energy utilizing systems within the cell, the better we
will be able to treat and possibly prevent energy imbalance within the
myocardial cell. Thus in view of the preponderance of cellular factors
which may affect cardiac performance in health and disease, it should be

obvious that a multidisciplinary approach to cardiac research would be most successful. This volume of research investigations from some of the most distinguished scientists from across the world represents an embodiment of such a philosophy. It is hoped that the electrophysiological, morphological, metabolic, electrochemical and biochemical approaches employed by these investigators will offer the advantage of providing the reader with a global picture for defining cardiac function in health and disease.

Naranjan S. Dhalla, Ph.D.
Grant N. Pierce, Ph.D.
Robert E. Beamish, M.D.

<u>Acknowledgements</u>

We are grateful to the following Agencies and Foundations for their generous financial support of the Symposium, which formed the basis of this book.

A. <u>Major Contributors</u>:

1. Manitoba Heart Foundation
2. Sterling-Winthrop Research Institute
3. Squibb Canada, Inc.
4. St. Boniface Hospital Research Foundation
5. Manitoba Medical Service Foundation, Inc.
6. Health Sciences Centre Research Foundation
7. International Society for Heart Research - American Section
8. Knoll Pharmaceuticals Canada Inc.
9. Section of Cardiology - St. Boniface General Hospital
10. Section of Cardiology - Health Sciences Centre
11. Children's Hospital of Winnipeg Research Foundation Inc.
12. Medical Research Council of Canada

B. <u>Contributors</u>:

1. Ayerst Laboratories (U.S.A.)
2. Bayer AG/Miles
3. Beckman Instrument, Inc.
4. Boehringer Ingelheim (Canada) Ltd.
5. Canadian Heart Foundation
6. ICI Pharma, Canada
7. Merck Frosst Canada Inc.
8. Merrell Dow Pharmaceutical Ltd. (U.K.)
9. Nordic Laboratories Canada Inc.
10. Rhone-Poulenc Pharma Inc.
11. Sandoz Canada Inc.
12. Schering Corporation (U.S.A.)
13. Smith Kline & French Laboratories (U.S.A.)
14. Syntex International Ltd. (U.S.A.)
15. The Upjohn Company (U.S.A.)
16. Rorer Canada, Inc.

C. <u>Supporters</u>:

1. American Critical Care (U.S.A.)
2. Marion Laboratories, Inc. (U.S.A.)

xiv

3. Merck Sharp & Dohme (U.S.A.)
4. Medtronic of Canada Ltd.
5. A.H. Robins Canada Inc.
6. G.D. Searle and Co. (U.S.A.)
7. G.D. Searle and Co. (Canada)
8. NOVOPHARM Ltd., Canada

We are thankful to Mrs. Susie Petrychko and the editorial staff of Martinus Nijhoff for their valuable assistance in the preparation of this book. Special thanks are due to the members of the Symposium Organization Committee, Session Chairmen, participants and all those who helped in so many ways to make this Symposium an outstanding scientific and social event. We are indebted to Dr. Arnold Naimark, President, University of Manitoba, Dr. John Wade, Dean, Faculty of Medicine, and Dr. Henry Friesen, Head, Department of Physiology for their continued interest and encouragement.

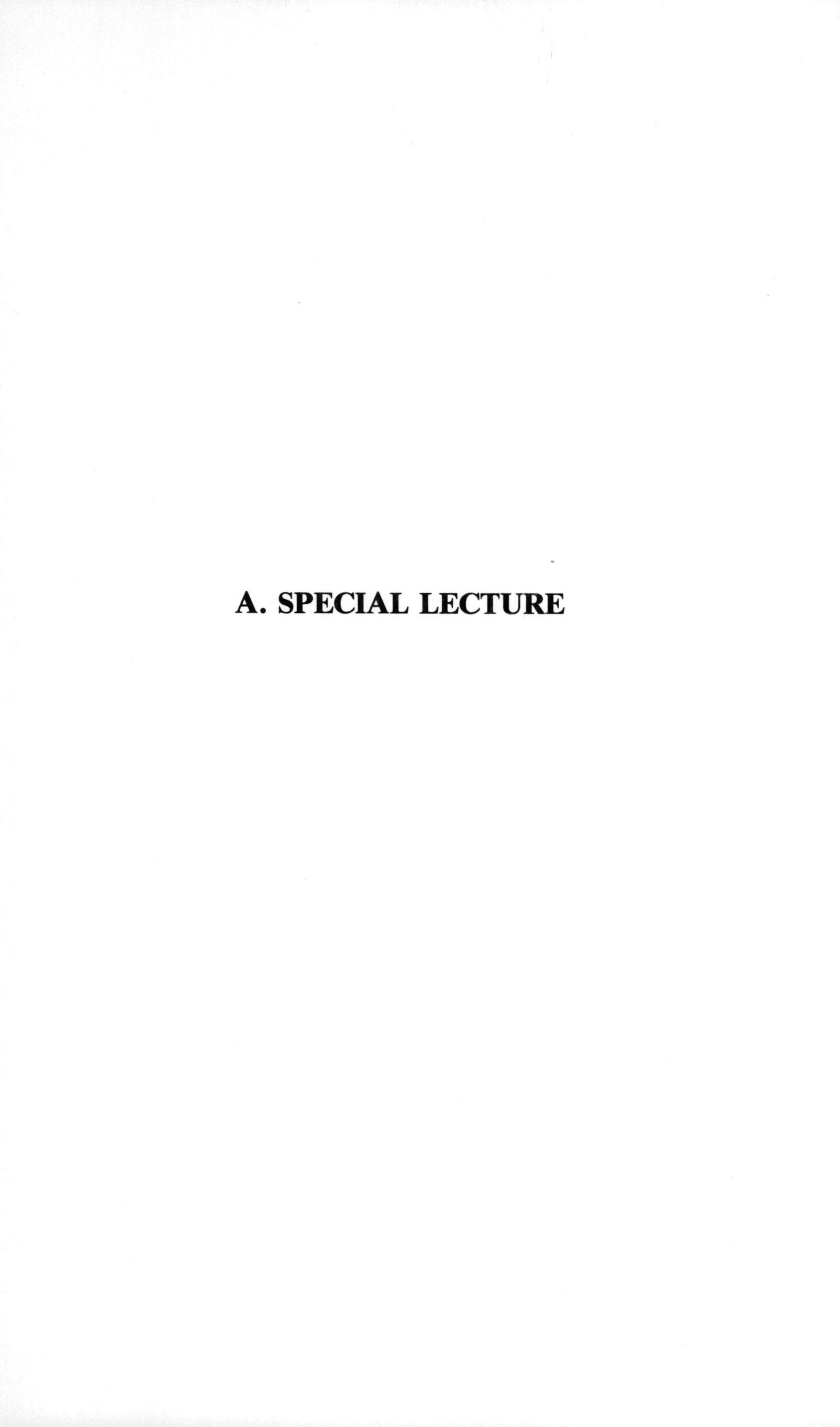

A. SPECIAL LECTURE

1

MOLECULAR BIOLOGY AND CARDIAC FUNCTION, PAST, PRESENT AND FUTURE

Richard J. Bing, Maythem Saeed, Andreas Hartmann, Gabor Sutsch, Marianne Z. Metz and Ricardo Navas

Huntington Medical Research Institutes, Pasadena, California 91105   USA

INTRODUCTION

Molecular biology is the outgrowth of the ascendence of biology, chemistry and physics. Medicine has been the beneficiary of this development. While during the last 40 years physics has changed our understanding of the universe, molecular biology has altered our ideas of the function of primitive and advanced organisms. Molecular biology has opened new vistas to the recognition and treatment of a number of diseases. The ascendence of molecular biology is influencing our life, our health, and our ideas on evolution. Molecular biology is defined here as life processes at the cellular level, that is at a level so small (molecular) that they cannot be perceived or measured by classical chemical or anatomical means. Consequently, molecular biology originated simultaneously with our ability to perform measurements and structural observation at the "molecular" level.

In order to relate molecular biology to cardiac function, the broad aspects of chemistry, biology and physics had to be known. In addition, electron microscopy has added a new dimension to molecular biology, because the relationship of molecular structure to function is the cornerstone of molecular biology. These developments only occurred during the last 40 years, beginning with the discovery by Avery of the transforming properties of DNA, the discovery of the structure of DNA by Watson and Crick, of cellular protein synthesis, high energy phosphates, molecular role of subcellular elements and organelles, to name just a few.

For this discussion, we have chosen three examples of the relationship of molecular biology with cardiac function, primarily because these fields have a broad impact on cardiac metabolism at the cellular level and on cardiology in general:

I)   Calcium movements in the cell and myocardial failure.

II)   Molecular pathways and cardiac contractility.

III) Molecular basis of vascular reactivity, with special reference to the role of endothelium.

I. Cellular calcium movement and myocardial failure.

The hallmark of myocardial failure is diminished contractility of the heart. As expressed by one of us in the Harvey Lectures in 1954 (1), "One of the basic phenomena of congestive heart failure is inadequate ventricular emptying during systole. It is a condition in which the ratio of residual volume to stroke volume is increased." In 1964 it was proposed by Meerson (2) and later by Gudbjarnason et al (3) that deficient protein synthesis may be responsible for myocardial failure, but later the possibility was mentioned that "inefficient transduction of chemical energy into tension...may be due to abnormality of events that link excitation to contraction." Since then work has been concerned with investigations of the mechanism of heart failure by emphasizing the possible role of cell membranes in calcium transport. Outstanding contribution to the role of membranes in myocardial failure have been made by Dhalla, Katz, Nayler and others (4-8). The work was considerably advanced by the ability to prepare pure preparations of membrane vesicles in vitro (9).

Calcium ions play a pivotal role in contractility of the heart and possibly also in the development of myocardial failure. Nayler (10) has detailed the contributions of Sydney Ringer to the role of calcium in myocardial contractility. It is important to note that Sydney Ringer was both a physician and a scientist. In transfer of calcium from extracelluar spaces to contractile proteins, a group of enzymes play the major role: ATPases, phosphatases, protein kinases, calmodulin, phospholipases, phosphodiesterases and adenylate cyclase.

<u>Sarcolemma</u> is involved in calcium transport by virtue of 1) sodium/potassium ATPase, 2) sodium/calcium exchange, 3) the calcium/magnesium ATPase, and 4) calcium channels (11).

1) <u>Sodium/potassium ATPase</u> hydrolyzes adenosine triphosphate (ATP) at a rate that is increased by sodium or potassium (12). This ATP dependent action pump exchanges sodium which enters the cell. The enzyme is inhibited by digitalis. The primary substrate for the enzyme is ATP and its most characteristic property is the dependence on both Na^+ and K^+. The activity of the enzyme involves the binding of ATP to the enzyme, phosphorylation of the enzyme and breakdown of ATP. Intermediate steps are conformational changes in

5

the enzyme molecule from high Na^+ to high K^+ affinity. Finally there occurs a
K^+ stimulated dephosphorylation. We owe the discovery of the effect of
digitalis on sodium/potassium ATPase to Schatzman, who discovered this phenomenon in red cell membranes (13). 2) $\underline{Na^+/Ca^{++}\text{ exchange in SL}}$: In this
system, the extrusion of Ca^{++} is tightly coupled to the entry of Na^+. The
experimental evidence for Na^+-Ca^{++} exchange has been recognized by the
discoveries of Reuter and Seitz (14), of Blaustein and Hodgkins (15), in 1969.
The process is electrogenic. Stoichiometry of the Na^+-Ca^{++} exchange is 3 to 1
(16). It is important for the understanding of the mechanism of digitalis
action that in sarcolemmal vesicles, calcium influx is promoted by intravesicular Na^+, while Ca^{++} efflux is stimulated by external Na^+ (17). 3)
$\underline{Ca^{++}\text{-}Mg^{++}\text{ activated ATPase}}$: Caroni and Carafoli (18) and Bing and associates
(19) have demonstrated the system in sarcolemma of dog hearts. The function
of this enzyme is to pump calcium out of the muscle cell. The enzyme is
regulated by calmodulin and cAMP-dependent phosphorylase, therefore it
responds to increased influx of Ca^{++} by increased outward pumping, as occurs
with beta-agonists. 4) $\underline{\text{The }Ca^{++}\text{ channel}}$: The Ca^{++} channel is controlled by
voltage-dependent gating, that is its opening and closing is the result of
changes in membrane potential. Possibly, as suggested by Reuter, a voltage
sensor exists in the membrane which may be a protein group and an integral
part of the ion channel (20). Signals which modify channel function are
stimulation by beta-receptors, lipid changes in the sarcolemma such as phosphatidylinositol. Modulation of Ca^{++} channels by neurotransmitters is typical
for the Ca^{++} channel. Consequently beta-blockers can inhibit the cascade of
events (beta-receptors → adenylate cyclase → cAMP-protein kinase → phosphorylation of proteins), which follows binding of beta-agonists to their receptors
and leads to opening of the Ca^{++} channel. Of importance is the finding by
Fleckenstein that movement of Ca^{++} through this channel can be blocked by a
variety of substances (21).

$\underline{\text{Mitochondria}}$ are able to sequester calcium, representing a sink for
intracellular calcium (12, 22). Lehninger et al found that inorganic phosphate accumulates in mitochondria together with calcium (23). Calcium is
released from mitochondria by the Na^+-promoted Ca^{++}-release pathway (22).
Addition of Na^+ to energized heart mitochondria after small amounts of Ca^{++}
are accumulated, induces a rapid efflux of Ca^{++}. Na^+ which has entered the
mitochondria in exchange for Ca^{++}, is returned to the extramitochondrial space
in exchange for H^+, producing a Ca^{++}-H^+ exchange. Although mitochondria act

as intracellular Ca^{++} regulators, they do not exert a beat to beat control over Ca^{++} movements. The ability of mitochondria to store large amounts of Ca^{++} is related to the simultaneous uptake of inorganic phosphate which stores Ca^{++} as hydroxyapatite.

Sarcoplasmic reticulum (SR) accumulates Ca^{++} in the presence of ATP (24). The Ca^{++}-Mg^{++} dependent ATPase moves Ca^{++} in both directions. The rate of Ca^{++} accumulation and storage is increased by phosphorylation of phospholamban (25). The SR membrane is highly asymmetric (26). The ATPase protein has an amphophilous character with polar ends of the enzyme protruding from the outer surface into the aqueous medium while the hydrophobic ends remain within the bilayer. Phosphorylation of the enzymes, hydrolytic cleavage, protein conformational changes, Ca^{++} binding at the membrane receptors are all involved in Ca^{++} transport into and from the sarcoplasmic reticulum. Some of these changes involve sidedness in relation to SR membranes.

Of the contractile proteins, the regulatory protein, Troponin C is particularly important since it allows physical and chemical interaction to develop between the myosin cross bridges of thin filament and active sites of the thick filament (27). Grand et al demonstrated that cAMP-sensitive protein kinase results in phosphorylation of the inhibitor component of troponin (28). Phosphorylation of Troponin-I is mediated by cAMP. Troponin I phosphorylation appears to have a negative correlation with Ca^{++} sensitivity and the maximal velocity of actomyosin ATPase (29).

In heart failure: There is evidence that membrane systems in heart muscle are involved in myocardial failure. Dhalla has stated that irrespective of the stimulus, membranes may change in such a way that there occurs either an intracellular Ca^{++} deficiency or overload (30). This statement is justified on the basis of intracellular Ca^{++} accumulation in certain conditions such as the ischemia followed by reperfusion or ischemia alone (19, 31-33). The difficulty in investigation of the molecular mechanism of myocardial failure lies in a lack of a suitable model. There exists at the present no model which compares with myocardial failure in humans resulting from increased pre or afterload. As early as 1964 efforts have been made to use human autopsy material from failing hearts (34). Peters et al also used myocardial biopsy from patients with congestive cardiomyopathy (35). Implicated in the mechanism of myocardial failure have been changes in receptor regulation (36), deficient cAMP production, deficient Ca^{++} uptake and ATPase activity (37), reduction in Na^{+}-K^{+} ATPase and of Ca^{++} binding (38). Decrease

7

in the rate of Ca^{++} released from SR and deficient calcium binding to SR were
also implicated (39). Isoenzymatic changes in myosin found by Swynghedauw may
also play a role (40).

Therefore the experimental evidence for an involvement of membrane
systems in calcium transport in myocardial failure is not as yet complete.
Other possibilities already mentioned are mitochondrial metabolic changes,
primarily deficient synthesis of energy phosphate and contractile proteins,
particularly regulatory proteins.

There are overlapping features between myocardial ischemia and myocardial
failure. Some of them are deficient synthesis of energy phosphate due to
disturbed respiratory function of mitochondria (41), reduced level of
mitochondrial enzymes with an increased level of lactic dehydrogenase (35).
In addition, membrane functions are disturbed in both conditions. Using SL
vesicles prepared from ischemia and reperfused myocardium, Chemnitius et al
(19) found decreased activity of total adenylate cyclase activity, Ca^{++}-Mg^{++}
dependent ATPase and endogenous phosphorylation, and Bersohn et al (42)
discovered inhibition of Na^{+}-ATPase in purified SL vesicles prepared from
ischemic heart muscle.

For these reasons, although tremendous strides have been made in explor-
ing the molecular biology and its relation to cardiac function, the relevance
of these changes to one of the most common clinical conditions, congestive
heart failure, is as yet not explained. On the other hand, the relationship
of disturbances in molecular biology of membrane system and organelles to
myocardial ischemia is supported by a large number of publications. The
future in this field will undoubtedly see a great many studies to explore the
molecular basis of myocardial failure in models which are more suitable than
those existing at the present time.

II. <u>Molecular Pathways Influencing Myocardial Contractility</u>.

This field is of considerable biochemical and clinical interest, since
recent attempts at therapy of myocardial failure are based on molecular
biological concepts. Much has been learned in recent years through the action
of pharmacological agents which, through stimulation of receptors and subsequent biochemical cascade mechanisms increase the contractility of the myocardium. There exists no common basis of molecular mechanism of positive inotropic action on the myocardium. A variety of possibilities and pathways exist:

8

A) Stimulation of sarcolemmal receptors, resulting in an increase in
adenylate cyclase (beta$_1$ agonists, histamine$_2$ stimulating compounds and
glucagon.

B) Direct stimulation of adenylate cyclase without receptor intermediates: forskolin.

C) Inhibition of phosphodiesterase (selective or unselective): CI 914,
amrinone, milrinone.

D) Increase in myocardial contractility through partial activation of
cAMP (partial agonists): TA-064, prenalterol.

E) Increase in contractility through increased sensitivity of the
myofilaments to Calcium: some phosphodiesterase inhibitors and alpha$_1$ receptor
stimulants.

F) Increase in myocardial contractility through calcium channel activation: BAY k 8644 and alpha$_1$ (postsynaptic receptor stimulation).

G) Increase in mitochondrial respiration with coenzyme Q10:
(ubiquinone).

H) Increase in intracellular calcium through inhibition of sodium/potas-
sium ATPase and the activity of the sodium/calcium exchange: (Digitalis).

I) Increased Ca^{++} availability through activation of the inositol-
triphosphate second messenger system (alpha$_1$ receptor stimulation).

A) Stimulation of sarcolemmal receptors resulting in increase in adenylate cyclase: cAMP activates protein kinases leading to phosphorylation of
proteins and opening of the calcium channel. Phospholamban, protein kinases
are directly involved in this action. Histamine (H$_2$) agonists also increase
cAMP and through it the phosphorylation of proteins responsible for availability of calcium (43-46).

B) Direct stimulation of adenylate cyclase without receptor intermediates: Daly has presented evidence that forskolin, a cardiotonic diterpene,
isolated from roots of a plant, directly activates adenylate cyclase and cAMP.
It appears to be a valuable tool in the exploration of adenylate cyclase
activity in a physiological or biochemical environment (47). Forskolin has
already been used clinically as a positive inotropic agent. For example,
Linderer et al used forskolin on patients with myocardial failure with
improvement in the clinical status (48). The drug is effective when
administered either intravenously or orally. Recent trials in patients with
congestive heart failure have revealed moderate vasodilatory and positive

inotropic effects. The use of this drug is attractive in clinical medicine
since the desensitization which occurs with beta adrenergic agonists may not
occur with forskolin, which bypasses the beta adrenergic receptors acting
directly on the activation of adenylate cyclase.

C) Inhibition of phosphodiesterases (selective or unselective): cAMP
activity is also increased through inhibition of phosphodiesterases. A number
of compounds have been used to achieve this purpose, amongst them CI 914,
amrinone and milrinone (49, 50). CI 914 acts primarily on the cardiac
phosphodiesterase type III, which is a low K_m cAMP specific form of the
phosphodiesterase. The selectivity by which CI 914 inhibits PDE III is
comparable to other cardiotonic agents like amrinone and MDL-17043 (49). The
positive inotropic effects of these compounds are the result of increased Ca^{++}
influx, where the slow inward current increases Ca^{++} release from the
sarcoplasmic reticulum. This is accomplished by phosphorylation of key
proteins in the presence of increased cAMP, which promotes relaxation of the
contractile apparatus (51). Of interest is the peripheral vasodilator effect
of these compounds. For example, we found that in isolated coronary arteries
and aortic strips CI 914 causes relaxation. In the supported perfused rabbit
heart preparation, CI 914 prevents vasoconstriction by histamine of large
coronary arteries (52). The mechanism of this smooth muscle relaxation is not
understood. It has been proposed however that these compounds exert a vasodilatory effect by preventing cAMP dependent Ca^{++} increase or by other
unspecified action (53, 54) or by $beta_2$ receptor stimulation.

D) Increase in myocardial contractility through partial activation of
cAMP (partial agonists): Partial agonists such as prenalterol and and TA-064
are of interest in relating molecular biology to cardiac function. They
present an exception to the rules that increased activation of adenylate
cyclase is essential for increased contractility (55). Nevertheless, they
possess powerful inotropic effect without commensurate activation of cyclic
AMP (56). For this reason they are called partial agonists (57). Why do
these compounds possess a powerful positive inotropic effect? Several mechanisms have been proposed (58): 1) cAMP may not be the second messenger, but
only an intracellular indicator for beta-adrenergic myocardial stimulation.
2) The concentration of cAMP in subcellular compartments may differ. 3)
myocardial beta receptors might be "desensitized" via beta-agonist induced
protein kinases. Beta-agonist induced beta receptor desensitization could
protect myocardial target cells from catecholamine overstimulation. 4) Even

small quantities of cAMP may be sufficient to initiate an increase in the phosphorylation of intracellular target proteins. Thus a small increase in cAMP concentration could result in pronounced cardiac effects. Venter, Ross and Kaplan were able to transform isoproterenol, a powerful beta stimulator and activator of cAMP into a partial beta agonist. Working on cat cardiac muscle, they studied the response of papillary muscle to soluble isoproterenol as compared to isoproterenol immobilized on glass beads. Immobilization of the compound by glass beads maintained the positive inotropic effect, but produced a proportionally lesser degree in activation of cAMP (56).

E) <u>Increase in contractility through increased sensitivity of the myofilaments to calcium</u>: Increased sensitivity of the myofilaments to calcium has been demonstrated by Ruegg, who discovered that nonglycoside, nonadrenergic cardiotonic drugs increased calcium-induced contraction of skinned mammalian fibers (59). With "skinning" the myofilaments become directly accessible to exogenous proteins, drugs and ions. It has been demonstrated that positive inotropic effects of such compounds such as sulmazole and pimobendane exert their pronounced positive inotropic action by increasing the sensitivity of the myofilaments to calcium and, at least in the case of sulmazole, increase calcium affinity to troponin (59, 60).

F) <u>Calcium channel activation</u>: This channel depends upon phosphorylation of proteins either through calmodulin or protein kinases activated by cyclic AMP (11). Inactivation results from Ca^{++} channel blockage (61). Recently it has become apparent that calcium channels can be activated without the interference of cAMP resulting in increased Ca^{++} influx. Examples are dihydropyridine derivatives (Ca^{++} agonists) which act in opposite way to calcium antagonists. Structurally they are related to the calcium blocker nifedipine. Through molecular manipulation the structure can be changed, resulting in calcium entry activation. The agents which are calcium entry activators are devoid of effects on sodium/potassium ATPase and on cellular receptor systems. In addition they do not elevate cAMP in cultured cardiac cells. These compounds appear to act by affecting dihydropyridine sensitive sites rather than allosteric mechanism (62).

G) <u>Myocardial contractility and coenzyme Q_{10}</u>: Coenzyme Q_{10} is a redox coenzyme of the respiratory chain, including the coupled mechanism of electron transfer and oxidative phosphorylation. Q_{10} is the coenzyme of at least five mitochondrial enzymes and there is also apparently a NADH:Q_{10} reductase in the Golgi apparatus. The coenzyme is indispensable in bioenergetics. The concentration of Q_{10} in the human myocardium is high and it has been presumed for years that a myocardial deficiency of Q_{10} might be detrimental to cardiac function (63). Indeed, heart muscle of patients with most severe myocardial failure had lower levels of Q_{10} than those with milder heart failure. Apparently in severe heart failure there exists a myocardial deficiency of Q_{10}.

Q_{10} exists in mitochondria under aerobic conditions in the oxidized quinone form and in the reduced quinol form under anaerobic conditions. Its structure is similar to that of Vitamin K and Vitamin E. It is also similar to plastoquinone, found in chloroplast in plants, another proof that evolution uses the same building stones over billions of years. Cardiac contractility in failing myocardium is influenced by Q_{10} since in severe myocardial disease Q_{10} is deficient. This is also the rational for treatment of patients in severe heart failure (63). Kamikawa et al found that ingestion of Q_{10} by patients with chronic stable angina increased exercise tolerance (64) and Langsjoen found that administration of Q_{10} improved myocardial function and in general resulted in clinical improvement (63). These findings are certainly in line with previous studies which have described deficiencies in oxidative phosphorylation and respiration of mitochondria obtained from failing heart muscle (5).

H) Increase in calcium flux through sarcolemma through inhibition of
sodium/potassium ATPase and the activity of sodium/calcium exchange: Schatzmann discovered that cardiac glycosides inhibit sodium/potassium ATPase in red cell membranes (13). It has been found that the positive inotropic action of digitalis preparations is intimately related to the sodium pump (sodium/potassium ATPase). The action of cardiac glycosides is understood on the basis of the relationship between the action of sodium/potassium ATPase and the Na^+-Ca^{++} exchange. In the latter, calcium influx is promoted by intracellular sodium while calcium efflux is stimulated by external sodium. As sodium concentration increases within the cell due to inhibition of sodium/potassium ATPase, so does intracellular calcium; contractility increases (12). Molecular biology has finally given us a clue to the oldest cardiotonic drug.

I) Increased contractility due to inositol-triphosphate second messenger
system (alpha$_1$ receptor stimulation): Inositol triphosphate (InsP$_3$) is formed from a membrane constituent, phosphatidylinositol 4, 5-biphosphate, one of the lipids located in the inner leaflet of the plasma membrane. It is formed by 2-staged phosphorylation of phosphatidylinositol (65). It is a second

messenger in cellular signal transduction. $InsP_3$ mobilizes calcium from the vesicular pool of the sarcoplasmic reticulum. The rate at which $InsP_3$ is formed after cell stimulation is fast enough for it to be the messenger causing calcium mobilization. Stimulation of alpha-adrenoceptors elevates intracellular calcium, through increased splitting of phosphatidylinositol 4, 5 biphosphate into inositol triphosphate and diacylglycerol. Diacylglycerol appears to activate calcium and phospholipid independent protein kinase C (66, 67).

III. Molecular Basis of Vascular Reactivity, with Special Reference to the Role of the Endothelium.

Many factors are responsible for vascular reactivity. Production of cGMP results in vasodilatation particularly of the coronary arteries (68, 69). Restriction of calcium supply by calcium antagonists causes vascular smooth muscle relaxation (70). Receptors ($alpha_1$, $alpha_2$ and beta) play an important role (71). In recent years the role of the endothelium in promoting vascular relaxation has assumed considerable importance. The presence of a humoral factor in mediating vascular relaxation was first demonstrated by Furchgott and Zawadzki (72). They were able to demonstrate that acetylcholine (ACh) produced marked relaxation of isolated rings of the descending thoracic aorta of the rabbit. They furthermore found that without endothelium, the preparation failed to relax. Endothelium, when stimulated, released the endothelium derived relaxing factor (EDRF) which diffuses to the smooth muscle cell and activates relaxation. Similar findings on the isolated artery preparation have been made by Griffith et al (73) and by Pohl et al (74). Furchgott established the fact that the endothelium receptor on which acetylcholine acts, is of the muscarinic type (72). The nature of EDRF however has remained obscure.

The question remains whether or not the role of the endothelium in relaxing arterial smooth muscle can be demonstrated in coronary arteries perfusing a supported rabbit heart preparation and in coronary arteries of hearts remaining in situ. The role of the endothelium of arteries remaining in contact with the perfused supported heart preparation has been demonstrated in studies with activated platelets injected into coronary arteries denuded of endothelium; this resulted in severe coronary vasoconstriction, while in arteries with intact endothelium, coronary vasoconstriction did not occur (75). Gated photography of the coronary artery after intraatrial injection with Patent Blue dye (color arteriography) was used to determined the internal diameter of the vessels and to calculate large coronary vascular resistance (76). The incidence of vasoconstriction in denuded arteries was significantly higher than that of vessels with intact endothelium. Embolism of aggregated platelets was not responsible for this phenomenon, since filtration of platelet aggregates did not prevent constriction. Equally, injection of non-aggregated platelets was ineffective. Coronary vascular spasm, resulting from injection of activated platelets resulted in prolonged spasm of denuded coronary arteries. It was demonstrated that in the intact preconstricted coronary artery remaining in contact with the beating perfused heart preparation, acetylcholine caused dilatation only when the endothelium was intact, duplicating the results on the isolated artery strip. Acetylcholine decreased both large coronary and total coronary vascular resistance.

Recently, we have been able to demonstrate the protective role of the endothelium of coronary arteries perfusing a rabbit heart in situ (77). Continuous visualization of the coronary arteries containing the dye was accomplished by video recording with a Panasonic video camera (Fig. 1). The light source was a Strobex lamp synchronized with the video camera. The camera was connected to a video cassette recorder and to a color monitor (Fig. 1). The images on the color monitor were digitized and stored in a computer and printed on an Imagewriter. The area of the artery was outlined on the printer and the length, mean diameter, surface area and surface/unit length were obtained (Fig. 1). The computer was programmed to print out the actual vascular diameter by correcting for the ratio of projected to actual diameter.

In order to inactivate the production of EDRF by coronary vascular endothelium, hydroquinone was used. Furchgott and Van de Voorde and Leusen had employed hydroquinone to inactivate EDRF (78, 79). We injected hydroquinone into the left atrium of the heart in situ. This was accomplished during brief cardiac arrest by cooling the heart with ice-cold saline and occlusion of the ascending aorta during injection. Dose response curves were obtained at concentrations of vasopressin of from 0.03 to 1 unit, in the presence and absence of hydroquinone. Scanning electron microscopic pictures of coronary vascular endothelium were obtained with and without injection of hydroquinone. The absence of the effect of EDRF was verified by suspending a strip of coronary arteries exposed to hydroquinone in vivo according to the method of Furchgott and Zawadzki (72). Figure 2 illustrates that in control experiments, coronary arteries obtained from hearts in situ, when suspended in vitro

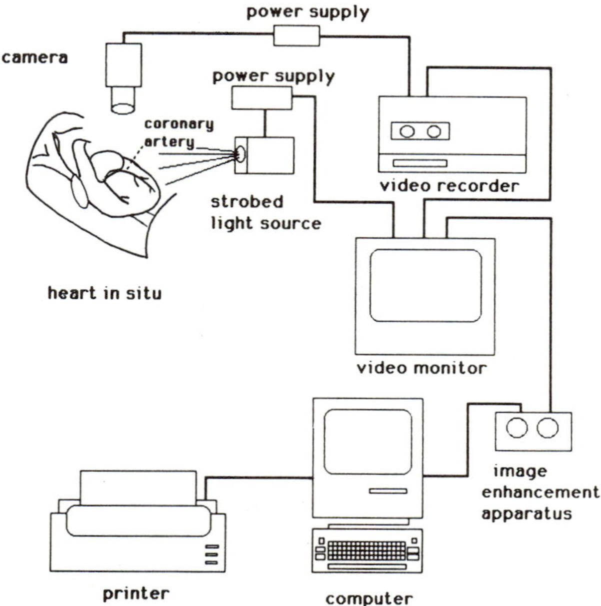

Fig. 1. Diagram describing the system for monitoring and quantitating the internal diameter of the dye injected coronary artery. Shown are the strobex light source, synchronized with the video camera. The images are visualized on a video monitor which can be digitized and stored in a computer and printed on an Imagewriter. The computer is programmed to print out the actual vascular diameter by correcting for the ratio of protected to actual diameter.

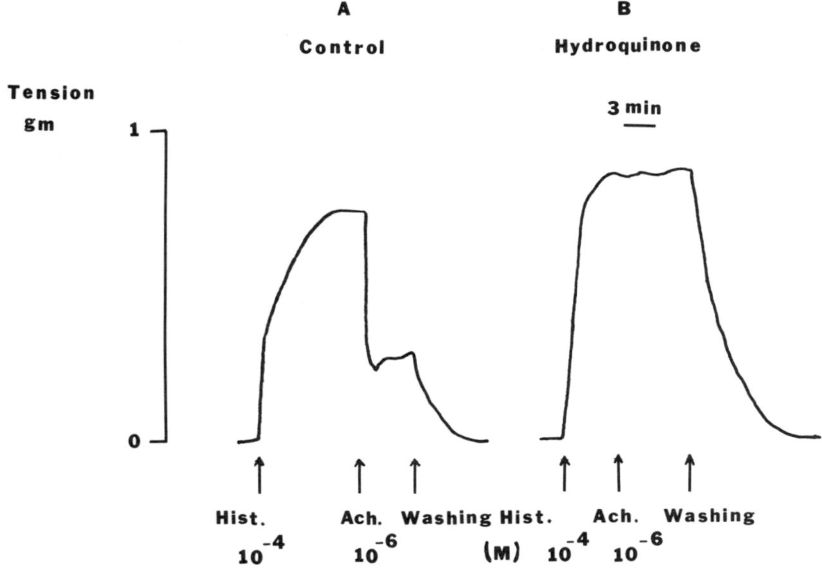

Fig. 2. Illustrates the effect of hydroquinone on the response to acetylcholine of coronary artery strips preconstricted with histamine. The arteries were removed in situ after intraatrial injection of hydroquinone. In the control, acetylcholine produced marked relaxation. In contrast, in the vessel exposed in situ to hydroquinone, acetylcholine resulted in slight constriction. The findings demonstrate that hydroquinone effectively prevented release of EDRF in situ.

relaxed after the addition of acetylcholine. In contrast, arteries exposed in situ to hydroquinone, failed to relax in vitro upon the addition of acetylcholine (Fig. 2). After hydroquinone, vasopressin administered in situ caused a significantly greater decrease in internal diameter as compared to the control (Fig. 3a, 3b, 4a, 4b and 5). These results demonstrate the protective role of the endothelium in the intact beating heart in situ and greatly extend the importance of the original findings by Furchgott and associates (72, 78).

The role of the vascular endothelium as an endocrine organ opens new avenues in the understanding of the molecular basis of vasomotor activity. Bassenge and associates (74) for example have demonstrated that pulsatile

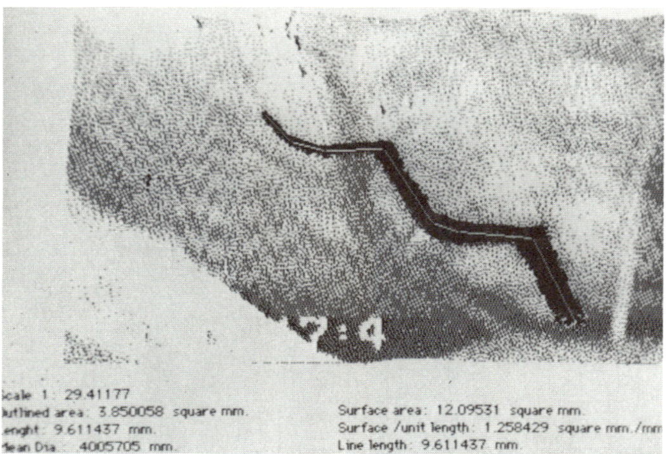

Fig. 3. a) Computerized image of the obtuse marginal coronary artery in situ (control experiment).

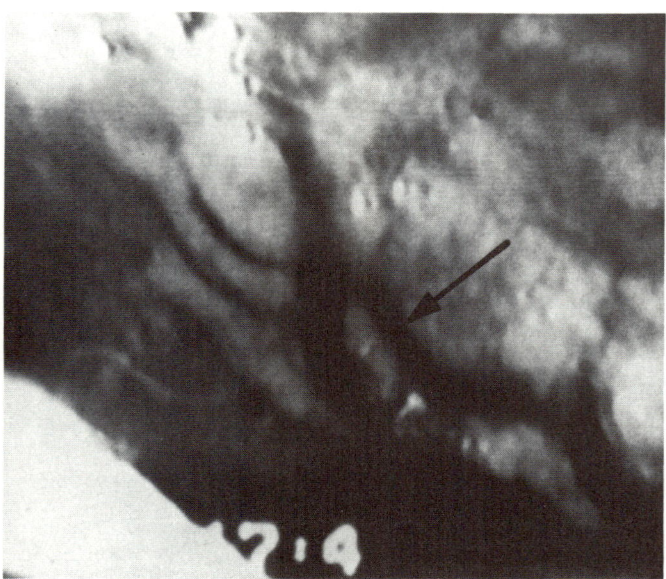

Fig. 3. b) Photographic image of the obtuse marginal artery after injection of patent blue dye into the left atrium of the heart in situ (artery indicated by arrow).

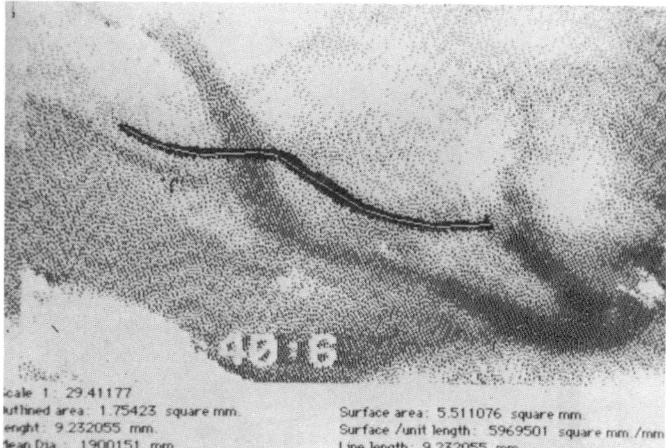

Fig. 4. a) Computerized image of the obtuse marginal coronary artery (see 4b) after injection of hydroquinone followed by 0.1 unit of vasopressin. Marked constriction of the vessel is noticed.

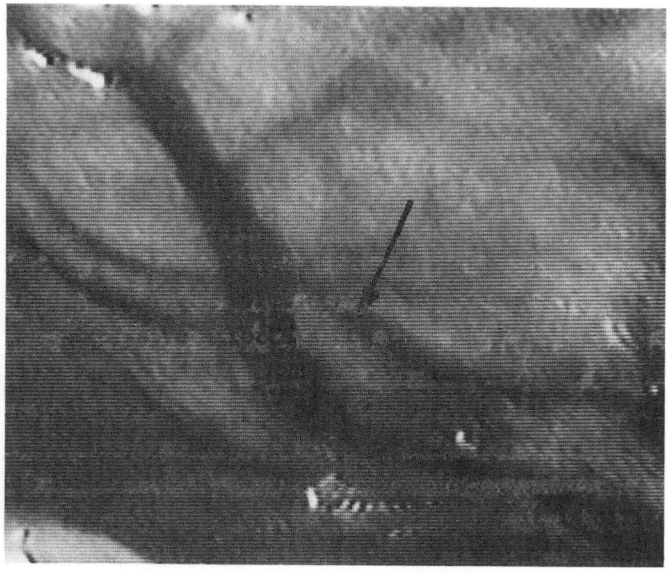

Fig. 4. b) Photographic image of the obtuse marginal coronary artery, as in 4a, after injection of vasopressin (0.1 unit) into the left atrium. The decrease in internal diameter of the vessel is noted (artery indicated by arrow).

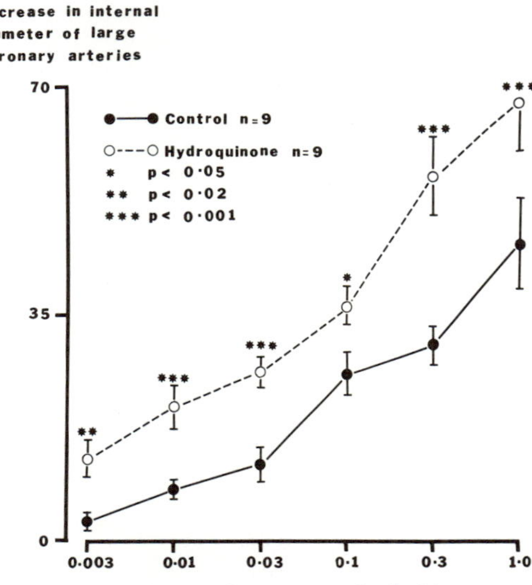

Fig. 5. Concentration response curve (percentage decrease in internal diameter of large coronary arteries with vasopressin). Hydroquinone (2 mg/kg) was injected into the left atrium of the heart in situ. Exposure to hydroquinone resulted in a significantly greater response to vasopressin.

pressure increases the activity of EDRF. Loss of endothelium as occurs in atherosclerosis may predispose the vessel to increased response to vasomotor stimulation, be it neurogenic or humoral. The nature of EDRF is still unknown. It is likely however, that direct contact of endothelium with smooth muscle is not essential for its activity (79, 80).

SUMMARY

Some of the contributions of molecular biology to cardiac functions were discussed. Particular emphasis was placed on the relationship of cellular calcium transport to myocardial failure, on molecular pathways determining cardiac contractility and on molecular mechanisms controlling vascular reactivity. The relationship of events at the molecular level to cardiac function in general was stressed.

ACKNOWLEDGEMENTS

This work was supported by grants from The Council for Tobacco Research, U.S.A., Inc. and The Margaret W. and Herbert Hoover, Jr. Foundation.

REFERENCES

1.   Bing, R.J. In: The Harvey Lectures (Ed. L. Series). Academic Press, New York, 1956, pp. 27-70.
2.   Meerson, F.Z. Circ. Res. 10: 250-258, 1962.
3.   Gudbjarnason, S., Telerman, M. and Bing, R.J. Am. J. Physiol. 206: 294-298, 1968.
4.   Dhalla, N.S., Dzurba, A., Pierce, G.N., Tregaskis, M.G., Panagia, V. and Bea, R.E. In: Myocardial Hypertrophy and Failure (Ed. N.R. Albert). Academic Press, New York, Vol. 7, 1983, pp. 527-534.
5.   Dhalla, N.S., Das, P.K. and Sharma, G.P. J. Mol. Cell. Cardiol. 10: 363-385, 1978.
6.   Katz, A.M. J. Am. Coll. Cardiol. 1: 42-51, 1983.
7.   Nayler, W.G. and Dresel, P.E. J. Mol. Cell. Cardiol. 16: 165-174, 1984.
8.   Nayler, W.G. J. Mol. Cell. Cardiol. 17: 201, 1985.
9.   Jones, L.R., Besch, H.R., Fleming, J.W., McConnaughey, M.M. and Watanabe, A.M. J. Biol. Chem. 254: 530-539, 1979.
10. Nayler, W.G. J. Mol. Cell. Cardiol. 16: 113-116, 1984.
11. Carafoli, E. J. Mol. Cell. Cardiol. 17: 203-212, 1985.
12. Katz, A.M. J. Am. Coll. Cardiol. 5: 16A-22A, 1985.
13. Schatzmann, H.J. Helv. Physiol. Acta. 11: 346-354, 1953.
14. Reuter, H. and Seitz, N. J. Physiol. (London) 195: 451-470, 1968.
15. Blaustein, M.P. and Hodgkins, A.L. J. Physiol. (London) 200: 497-527, 1969.
16. Pitts, B.J.R. J. Biol. Chem. 254: 6232-6235, 1979.
17. Blaustein, M.P. and Nelson, M.T. In: Membrane Transport of Calcium (Ed. E. Carafoli). Academic Press, London and New York, 1982, pp. 217-236.
18. Caroni, P. and Carafoli, E. Nature 283: 765-767, 1980.
19. Chemnitius, J.M., Sasaki, Y., Burger, W. and Bing, R.J. J. Mol. Cell. Cardiol. 17: 1139-1150, 1985.
20. Reuter, H. Nature 301: 569-574, 1983.
21. Fleckenstein, A. Calcium Antagonism in Heart and Smooth Muscle. John Wiley and Sons, New York, 1983.
22. Carafoli, E. In: Membrane Transport of Calcium (Ed. E. Carafoli). Academic Press, London and New York, 1982, pp. 109-139.

23. Lehninger, A.L., Rossi, C.S. and Greenawalt, J.W. Biochem. Biophys. Res. Commun. 10: 444-448, 1983.
24. Hasselbach, W., and Makinose, M. Biochem. Biophys. Res. Commun. 7: 132-136, 1962.
25. Tada, M., Kirschberger, M.A. and Katz, A.M. J. Biol. Chem. 250: 640-647, 1975.
26. De Meis, L. and Inesi, G. In: Membrane Transport of Calcium (Ed. E. Carafoli). Academic Press, London and New York, 1982, pp. 141-186.
27. Katz, A.M. Physiology of the Heart. Raven Press, New York, 1977, p. 109.
28. Grand, R.J., Wilkinson, J.M. and Mole, E.I. Biochem. J. 159: 633-641, 1976.
29. Opie, L.H. Cardiovasc. Res. 16: 483-507, 1982.
30. Dhalla, N.S., Pierce, G.N., Panagia, V., Singal, P.K. and Beamish, R.E. Basic Res. Cardiol. 77: 117-139, 1982.
31. Nayler, W.G., Stone, J., Carson, V. and Chipperfield, D. J. Mol. Cell. Cardiol. 2: 125-143, 1971.
32. Nayler, W.G. and Burian, W. Postgrad. Med. J. 51: 350-356, 1975.
33. Nayler, W.G. J. Mol. Cell. Cardiol. 17: 201, 1985.
34. Bing, R.J., Wu, C. and Gudbjarnason, S. Circ. Res. 14: II64-II69, 1964.
35. Peters, T.J., Wells, G., Oakly, C.M., Brooksby, I.A.B., Jenkins, B.S., Webb-peploe, M.M. and Coltart, D.J. Br. Heart J. 39: 1333-1339, 1977.
36. Heinsimer, J.A. and Lefkowitz, R.J. Hosp. Pract. November: 103-125, 1983.
37. Gertz, E.W., Hess, M.L., Lain, R.F. and Briggs, F.N. Circ. Res. 20: 477-484, 1967.
38. Dhalla, N.S., Sulakhe, D.V., Fedelesova, M. and Yates, J.C. Adv. Cardiol. 13: 282-300, 1974.
39. Sordahl, L.A., McCollum, W.B., Wood, W.G. and Schwartz, A. Am. J. Physiol. 224: 497-502, 1973.
40. Schwartz, K., Lecarpentier, Y., Marth, J.L., Lompre, A.M., Mercadier, J.J. and Swynghedauw, B. J. Mol. Cell. Cardiol. 13: 1071-1075, 1981.
41. Weishaar, R., Sarma, J.S.M., Maruyama, Y., Fischer, R. and Bing, R.J. Cardiology 62: 2-20, 1977.
42. Bersohn, M.M., Philipson, K.D. and Fukushima, J.Y. Am. J. Physiol. 242: C288-C295, 1982.
43. Tsien, W. Adv. Cyclic Nucleotide Res. 8: 363-420, 1977.
44. Klein, J. and Levey, G.S. J. Clin. Invest. 50: 1012-1015, 1971.
45. Baumann, G., Felix, S.B., Riess, G., Loher, U., Ludwig, L. and Bloemer, H. J. Cardiovasc. Pharmacol. 4: 542-553, 1982.
46. Goldstein, R.E., Skelton, C.L., Levey, G.S., Glancy, D.L., Beiser, G.D. and Epstein, S.E. Circulation 44: 638-648, 1971.
47. Daly, J.W.. Adv. Cyclic Nucleotide Protein Phosphoryl. Res. 17: 81-89, 1984.
48. Linderer, T., Biamino, G., Brueggemann, T., Peslin, K. and Schroeder, R. J. Am. Coll. Cardiol. 3: 562, 1984 (Abst.).
49. Weishaar, R.E., Quade, M., Schenden, J.A., Boyd, D.K. and Evans, D.B. Eur. J. Pharmacol. 119: 205-215, 1985.
50. Benotti, J.R., Grossman, W., Braunwald, E., Davolos, D.D. and Alousi, A.A. N. Engl. J. Med. 299: 1373-1377, 1978.
51. Katz, A.M.. J. Am. Coll. Cardiol. 2: 143-149, 1983.
52. Hartmann, A., Saeed, M., Sutsch, G. and Bing, R.J. (submitted).
53. Morgan, J.P., Gwathmey, J., DeFeo, T.T. and Morgan, K.J. Circulation 73(III): 65-76, 1986.
54. Toda, N., Nakajima, M., Nishimura, K. and Miyazaki, M. Cardiovasc. Res. 18: 174-182, 1984.

55. Bing, R.J., Sasaki, Y., Burger, W. and Chemnitius, J.M. Curr. Ther. Res. 36: 1127-1144, 1984.
56. Venter, J.C., Ross, J. and Kaplan, N.O. Proc. Natl. Acad. Sci. USA 72: 824-828, 1975.
57. Hedberg, A. and Mattson, H. J. Pharmacol. Exp. Ther. 219: 798-808, 1981.
58. Chemnitius, J.M. and Bing, R.J. Can. J. Cardiol. 1: 186-190, 1985.
59. Rüegg, J.C. Circulation 73(III): 78-84, 1986.
60. Blinks, J.R. and Endo, M. J. Physiol (London) 353: 63P, 1984.
61. Fleckenstein, A. Ann. Rev. Pharmacol. Toxicol. 17: 149-166, 1977.
62. Rogg, H., Crisciome, L., Truog, A. and Meier, M. J. Cardiovasc. Pharmacol. 7(6): S31-S37.
63. Langsjoen, P.H., Vadhanavikit, S. and Folkers, K. Proc. Natl. Acad. Sci. USA 82: 4240-4244, 1985.
64. Kamikawa, T., Kobayashi, A., Yamashita, T., Hayashi, H. and Yamasaki, N. Am. J. Cardiol. 56: 247-251, 1985.
65. Berridge, M.J. and Irvine, R.F. Nature 312: 315-321, 1984.
66. Fayn, J.N. and Garcia-Sainz, J.A. Life Sci. 26: 1183-1194, 1980.
67. Quist, E. and Sanchez, M. Proc. West. Pharmacol. Soc. 26: 333-335, 1983.
68. Rapoport, R.M., Draznin, M.B. and Murad, F. Proc. Natl. Acad. Sci. USA 79: 6470-6474, 1982.
69. Kukovetz, W.R., Holzmann, S. and Poch, G. Naunyn Schmiedebergs Arch. Pharmacol. 319: 29-33, 1982.
70. Fleckenstein, A. In: Calcium Antagonism in Heart and Smooth Muscle. John Wiley and Sons, New York, 1983.
71. Saeed, M., Holtz, J., Elsner, D. and Bassenge, E. J. Cardiovasc. Pharmacol. 7: 167-173, 1985.
72. Furchgott, R.F. and Zawadski, J.V. Nature 288: 373-376, 1980.
73. Griffith, T.M., Edwards, D.H., Lewis, M.J., Newby, A.C. and Henderson, A.H. Nature 308: 645-647, 1984.
74. Pohl, U., Busse, R., Kuon, E. and Bassenge, E. J. Appl. Cardiol. 1(3): 1986 (in press).
75. Bing, R.J., Burger, W., Chemnitius, J.M., Saeed, M. and Metz, M.Z. Am. J. Cardiol. 55: 1596-1600, 1985.
76. Saeed, M., Schmidli, J., Metz, M. and Bing, R.J. J. Cardiovasc. Pharmacol. 8: 257-261, 1986.
77. Bing, R.J. and Saeed, M. (submitted to Science), 1986.
78. Furchgott, R.F. Ann. Rev. Pharmacol. Toxicol. 24: 175-197, 1984.
79. Van de Voorde, J. and Leusen, I. Eur. J. Pharmacol. 87: 113-120, 1983.
80. Hartmann, A., Saeed, M., Sutsch, G. and Bing, R.J. (In preparation).
81. Ganz, P., Davies, P.F., Leopold, J.A., Gimbrone, Jr., M.A. and Alexander, R.W. Proc. Natl. Acad. Sci. USA 83: 3552-3556, 1986.

B. ELECTRICAL EVENTS AND IONS

2

REGULATION OF CALCIUM SLOW CHANNELS AND POTASSIUM CHANNELS OF CARDIAC MUSCLE
BY CYCLIC NUCLEOTIDES AND METABOLISM

NICHOLAS SPERELAKIS

University of Cincinnati, College of Medicine, Department of Physiology and
Biophysics, Cincinnati, OH 45267

TABLE OF CONTENTS

A. Introduction

Protein phosphorylations are a means whereby the force of contraction of
the heart can be regulated, e.g., by phosphorylation of the contractile proteins, the sarcoplasmic reticulum (SR) membrane, and the sarcolemma. This
article will focus on evidence that cyclic nucleotides regulate the Ca^{2+}
influx into the myocardial cells during each cardiac cycle. This regulation
is presumably mediated by phosphorylation(s) of the Ca^{2+} slow channel protein

and/or of associated regulatory protein(s). Such phosphorylation increases the number of Ca^{2+} slow channels available for voltage activation during the action potential (AP), presumably by increasing the probability of their opening and increasing their mean open time. A greater density of open Ca^{2+} slow channels increases the inward Ca^{2+} slow current (Ca^{2+} influx) during the AP, and so increases the force of contraction. Excessive Ca^{2+} influx can lead to Ca^{2+} overload, arrhythmias, and cell necrosis, if the cells are metabolically incapable of handling the Ca^{2+}.

The force of contraction of the heart is controlled by the Ca^{2+} influx across the cell membrane during the AP. This Ca^{2+} influx occurs through the voltage-dependent and time-dependent gated slow channels of the cell membrane. The Ca^{2+} entering directly elevates $(Ca)_i$ and indirectly elevates $(Ca)_i$ further by releasing Ca^{2+} from the intracellular SR stores (Fabiato and Fabiato, 1979). Although the source of Ca^{2+} for contraction is from two pools, the extracellular fluid and the SR stores, the Ca^{2+} entry across the cell membrane is the major regulatory factor of the force of contraction. Blockade of the slow channels, and hence Ca^{2+} influx, by Ca^{2+}-antagonistic agents (such as nifedipine and Mn^{2+}) depresses or abolishes the contractions without greatly affecting the normal fast AP, i.e., contraction is uncoupled from excitation. The Ca-Na exchanger in the sarcolemma, which normally exchanges 1 Ca_i ion for 3 Na_o ions, reverses in direction during the AP depolarization because of energetic considerations, and might be an important accessory pathway of Ca^{2+} influx during the AP. Relaxation is produced by re-sequestration of the free myoplasmic Ca^{2+} into the SR and pumping of Ca^{2+} out of the cell using Ca-ATPase activity. In addition, the Ca-Na exchange system acts to bail Ca^{2+} out of the cell, using the energy of the Na^+ electrochemical gradient maintained by the (Na,K)-ATPase.

If the net membrane current is inward (e.g., I_{Na} and I_{Ca}), depolarization is produced. If the net current is outward (e.g., I_K), hyperpolarization or repolarization is produced. The important effects of the currents are mediated by the depolarization and repolarization, i.e., by the AP, with the exception of I_{si}, a major part of its effect being mediated by Ca^{2+} ion acting as a second messenger. The Ca^{2+} influx brings about the release of more Ca^{2+} from the SR stores, and besides activating the contractile proteins, activates at least two types of ion channels ($g_{K(Ca)}$ and $g_{Na,K(Ca)}$) and regulates a number of enzymes involved in metabolism and phosphorylations.

There are a number of different ionic currents that contribute to the electrogenesis of the cardiac APs, after-potentials, and pacemaker potentials (diastolic depolarization). Each of these currents passes through a special set of membrane ion channels. These ion channels are proteins floating in the lipid bilayer matrix of the cell membrane, and each channel has a water-filled central pore for ion passage. Some of the ion channels are very selective for only one cation, e.g., for Na^+, Ca^{2+}, or K^+. Other ion channels are nonselective or mixed channels that allow several types of cations to pass through, e.g., Na^+ and K^+. A cation passing through its ion-selective channel probably binds to two or three negatively charged sites on its journey through the channel down its electrochemical (electrical plus concentration) gradient. The flow of ions through these channels is approximately 6×10^6 ions/sec. The voltage-dependent fast Na^+ channels and Ca^{2+} slow channels have an activation (A, m, or d) gate centrally located and an inactivation (I, h, or f) gate at the inner surface of the membrane.

The kinetics of turn-on of the specific conductance may be fast or slow. For example, there is an inward fast Na^+ current $I_{Na(f)}$ carried through fast Na^+ channels that underlie the fast Na^+ conductance $g_{Na(f)}$. There is an inward slow Ca^{2+} current (I_{si}) carried through slow Ca^{2+} channels that underlie the slow Ca^{2+} conductance $g_{Ca(s)}$. The slow channels appear to be kinetically slower than the fast Na^+ channels, that is, they behave as if their gates open, close, and recover more slowly. The apparent slower kinetics is due to the statistical behavior of the population of slow channels, i.e., the gates in any one channel may open and close quickly.

The slow channel gates operate over a less negative (more depolarized) voltage range; that is, their threshold potential and the inactivation voltage range are higher (less negative). These two types of channels for carrying inward (depolarizing) current also are blocked by different drugs: tetrodotoxin (TTX) blocks fast Na^+ channels (by binding to the outer mouth of the channel and acting as a physical plug) but does not affect the slow channels. In contrast, the organic calcium-antagonistic drugs, such as nifedipine and diltiazem, and inorganic ions such as Mn^{2+}, Co^{2+}, La^{3+}, block the slow channels with relatively little or no effect on the fast Na^+ channels. Tetraethylammonium ion (TEA^+) or Ba^{2+} ion selectively block K^+ channels.

Some channels are rectifying, i.e., allow ions to pass through more readily in one direction than in the other. Those K^+-channels that allow K^+ to pass more readily in the outward direction (K^+ efflux), down the resting electrochemical gradient for K^+, underlie *outward-going rectification*. Those K^+ channels that allow K^+ to pass more readily in the inward direction (K^+ influx), against the electrochemical gradient, underlie *inward-going rectification or anomalous rectification*. The kinetics of turn-on of an outward-going K^+ channel is slower than that of the fast Na^+ conductance, and so is often termed the *delayed K^+ rectifier*. Although most of the channel types are turned on (gates opened) by depolarization and turned off (gates closed) by repolarization, there are some types of channels that are turned on (activated) by hyperpolarization (repolarization), i.e., behave in an anomalous manner. One such channel is the channel for the so-called funny current (I_f), also known as the hyperpolarization-activated current (I_H). In addition to the standard voltage-dependent channels, there are several types of Ca^{2+}-operated ion channels. These Ca^{2+}-activated channels, e.g., the Ca^{2+}-activated K^+ conductance ($g_{K(Ca)}$), also exhibit some voltage sensitivity.

B.   Fast Ca^{2+} Channels

Besides the more standard garden-variety slow Ca^{2+} channel, a fast-type of Ca^{2+} channel was found in cardiac muscle, vascular smooth muscle, and neurons (dorsal root ganglion cells) on the basis of kinetics (Chad and Eckert, 1985a; Bean, 1985; Nowycky *et al.*, 1985). The fast Ca^{2+} channels are unaffected by cyclic AMP and phosphorylation, and they are less sensitive or insensitive to Ca antagonistic drugs and Ca agonists (e.g., Bay-K-8644). The fast Ca^{2+} channels have a more negative threshold potential than the slow Ca^{2+} channels, and they conduct a considerably smaller current. They are more sparce than the slow Ca^{2+} channels. The fast Ca^{2+} channels are much more rapidly inactivated than the slow Ca^{2+} channels, having a $t_{1/2}$ of about 10-40 msec. Thus, they are often called transient Ca^{2+} channels or rapidly-inactivating Ca^{2+} channels.

These fast Ca^{2+} channels may be functionally important because Fabiato and Baumgarten (1984) has demonstrated that the most important factor for Ca_i release of Ca^{2+} from the SR is not the steady-state Ca_i, but rather the rate of change of Ca_i, i.e., $d Ca_i/dt$. Thus, the Ca^{2+} influx through the fast Ca^{2+} channels would be more effective in Ca^{2+} release from the SR, whereas Ca^{2+} influx through the slow Ca^{2+} channels may be more involved in loading the SR with more Ca^{2+} for release in the subsequent excitation.

C. Special Properties of the Ca^{2+} Slow Channels

1. Assessment of Ca^{2+} Slow Channel Function

One method of detecting the effect of agents on the Ca^{2+} slow channels is to first block the fast Na^+ channels and excitability by TTX, or to voltage-inactivate them by partially depolarizing the cells (e.g., to -40 mV) in elevated K_o (e.g., 25 mM) (Fig. 1 B,F). Then, addition of agents, such as catecholamines (beta-adrenergic receptor agonists), histamine (H_2 receptor agonist), and methylxanthines (phosphodiesterase inhibitors), which rapidly increase the number of open slow channels during activation by stimulation, causes the appearance of slowly-rising overshooting APs, which resemble the plateau component of the normal fast AP (Shigenobu and Sperelakis, 1972; Schneider and Sperelakis, 1975) (Fig. 1 C,G). The inward current during these slow APs is primarily carried by Ca^{2+} ions. The slow APs are accompanied by contractions that are almost as large as the normal contractions (Schneider and Sperelakis, 1974). The slow APs are blocked by agents that block the Ca^{2+} slow channels and inward slow current (Fig. 1D,H), including Mn^{2+}, La^{3+}, verapamil, nifedipine, and diltiazem (Schneider and Sperelakis, 1974; Shigenobu *et al.*, 1974).

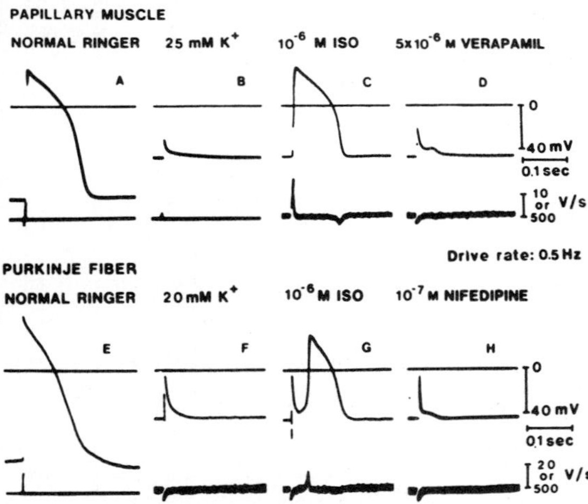

FIG 1 Induction of the slow action potentials (APs) and their block by calcium antagonistic drugs in guinea pig papillary muscle (A-D) and Purkinje fiber (E-H). A,E: Normal fast APs. B,F: Elevation of K_o to 25 mM (B) or 20 mM (F) depolarized to about -45 mV and blocked excitabilty (only shock artifacts remain). C,G: Isoproterenol (10^{-6} M) rapidly induced slow APs. D,H: Verapamil (5 x 10^{-6} M) (D) or nifedipine (10^{-7} M) (H) rapidly depressed and blocked the slow APs. Stimulation rate was 0.5 Hz. Upper straight line in each panel is the zero potential level, and the lower trace is dV/dt, the peak excursion of which gives $\dot{V}_{max}$. The dV/dt calibration bars represent 500 V/s for A and E, and 10 V/s for B-D or 20 V/s for F-H. Modified from Molyvdas and Sperelakis (1983).

Changes in the maximum rate of rise ($\dot{V}_{max}$) of the slow AP may be used as an index of the changes in I_{si}, since $\dot{V}_{max} \propto I_{si}/C_m$. The intensity of I_{si} is a product of the conductance (g_{si}) times the electrochemical driving force. For example, if all of I_{si} is carried by Ca^{2+} ions: $I_{Ca} = g_{Ca}(E_m - E_{Ca})$. Thus, for a constant driving force, I_{si} is directly proportional to g_{si}. The conductance, g_{si}, is proportional to the number of Ca^{2+} slow channels open at any instant in time. Thus, the effect of a drug on depressing $\dot{V}_{max}$ can be translated into an effect on the number of available (unblocked) slow channels, assuming that a channel can either be drug-blocked or unblocked. Although the relationship between $\dot{V}_{max}$ and number of open channels has been reported to be somewhat non-linear, this relationship will be assumed, as an approximation, to be a simple direct linear relationship.

A second method of detecting the effect of agents on the Ca^{2+} slow channels is by use of voltage clamp analysis. Voltage clamp has been done on small cardiac muscle and Purkinje fiber strands (bundles) by various methods. In the past few years, voltage clamp has been done on isolated single adult heart cells using a perfusing electrode technique to measure the macroscopic currents. This preparation and technique has yielded the most reliable and quantitative data for I_{si}. The membrane potential is step-changed from an initial steady-state holding potential (V_h), which is often near the natural resting potential (E_m), to the desired test potential (V_c) and held (clamped) there for a desired time period (e.g., 20-200 msec), and the current (inward and outward) required to hold E_m at V_c measured. The conductance for the ion carrying the current is calculated from $g_i = I_i/(V_c - E_i)$. By clamping to different voltages, the complete relationship between g_i and E_m (V_c) can be obtained. If V_h is about -80 mV, then two inward currents are recorded: an initial fast inward Na^+ current and a second slow inward current carried primarily by Ca^{2+} ions. The two inward currents overlap and are followed by an outward K^+ current, the delayed rectifier K^+ current. If TTX is added to block the fast Na^+ channels, or a V_h of about -50 mV is used to voltage inactivate the fast Na^+ channels, then the fast inward Na^+ current is abolished and the only inward current is I_{si}.

The relatively new technique of patch clamping of small cell membrane areas (e.g., 1-2 μm^2), either left attached to the intact cell (cell-attached patch) or isolated in the tip of the micropipette (isolated patch), has been used to study the Ca^{2+} slow channels and the effects of drugs on these channels (Reuter and Scholz, 1977; Reuter *et al.*, 1982; Reuter, 1983; Reuter *et al.*, 1983; Cavalie *et al.*, 1983; Hess *et al.*, 1984). In the isolated patch method, the patches can be made inside-out or outside-out. Very tight gigohm seals (10-100 GΩ) are formed with the glass tip of the microelectrode to minimize short-circuiting of the patch. The small patch sometimes contains only a single functional ion channel of a given type. It is estimated that there may be only one Ca^{2+} slow channel per 1-10 μm^2 of cell membrane. The density of fast Na^+ channels is about 100 times greater.

The openings and closings of the channels can be examined at different clamp potentials and in the presence of drugs. The probability (p) of the slow channel being open increases at greater depolarizing clamp steps, and decreases at hyperpolarizing clamp voltages. The current that flows through the opened channel is usually about a few picoamperes (pA), and varies with the clamp step and hence the electrochemical driving force. The values for the conductance of the Ca^{2+} slow channel usually range between 5 and 25 pS (pico-Siemens). The Ca^{2+} slow channel typically opens in bursts, and the length of the bursts increases at more depolarized voltages. The relation-ship between the mean current (I) found by time averaging over a time per-iod of, for example, 100 msec is: $I = i_s \cdot N \cdot p$, where i_s is the current through the single channel (for a given driving force), N is the number of channels in the patch (e.g., one), and p is the average probability of the channel being opened during a depolarizing clamp step.

A three-state sequential model, with two closed states (C_1 and C_2) and one open state (O), has been proposed for the Ca^{2+} slow channel (Hess *et al.*, 1984):

$$C_1 \; \underset{k_{-1}}{\overset{k_1}{\rightleftharpoons}} \; C_2 \; \underset{k_{-2}}{\overset{k_2}{\rightleftharpoons}} \; O$$

where k_1 and k_2 are the forward (opening) rate constants, and k_{-1} and k_{-2} are the backward (closing) rate constants. This is the normal operating state of the channels (mode 1 of Hess *et al.*, 1984).

The calcium antagonistic drugs were found to decrease the probability of the channel being opened and to decrease the mean open time (mode 0 of Hess *et al.*, 1984). This can account for the effect of these drugs on decreasing the macroscopic currents (I_{si}) measured from intact cells, and giving rise to a negative inotropic effect in cardiac muscle and vasodilation in vascular smooth muscle. In contrast, the calcium slow channel agonistic drugs, e.g., the dihydropyridine derivative Bay-K-8644, increase the probability of chan-nel opening and the mean open time (mode 2 of Hess *et al.*, 1984). This can account for the effect of this class of drug on increasing the macroscopic currents (I_{si}) measured from intact cells, and giving rise to a positive inotropic effect in cardiac muscle and vasoconstriction in vascular smooth muscle.

2. Blockade of Slow Channels by Calcium Antagonists

The Ca^{2+} influx through the voltage-dependent and time-dependent slow channels of the cell membrane is inhibited by organic compounds like verapamil, nifedipine, diltiazem, and bepridil (Shigenobu *et al.*, 1974; Kohlhardt *et al.*, 1972; Kohlhardt and Fleckenstein, 1977; Vogel *et al.*, 1979; Sperelakis, 1984). Thus, these calcium antagonistic drugs block the slow inward current in myocardial cells, vascular smooth muscle, and skeletal muscle (e.g., Kerr and Sperelakis, 1983). Verapamil, methoxy-verapamil (D600), and nifedipine also block the slow Na^+ channels of young embryonic chick hearts (Shigenobu *et al.*, 1974; Kojima and Sperelakis, 1983). To be a calcium antagonist, a drug must block the slow channel by a direct action on the channel itself, and not indirectly, for example, via metabolic depression or acidosis, and this action must be relatively specific for the slow channels in contrast to the other types of voltage-dependent ion channels. Thus, Ca antagonists act differently, for example, from local anesthetics or metabolic poisons.

The general order of potency of the calcium-antagonistic drugs in blocking the Ca^{2+} slow channels of various heart tissues is nifedipine > diltiazem $\geq$ verapamil > bepridil (Li and Sperelakis, 1983a). Figure 1 illustrates the effect of verapamil and nifedipine on blocking the slow APs in guinea pig papillary muscle and Purkinje fibers driven at a constant rate (Molyvdas and Sperelakis, 1983). The effect of most of the Ca-antagonistic drugs on depression of the slow APs and inward slow Ca^{2+} current (I_{si}) is frequency dependent: the higher the frequency of stimulation, the greater the blocking effect on the slow channels. For example, a dose of drug that completely blocks the slow APs at a drive rate of 1 Hz may exhibit no effect at 0.1 Hz. Nifedipine and other dihydropyridines have a lesser frequency dependence than the other drugs. The drugs might act to slow the recovery process of the slow channel from the inactive state back to the resting state. A slow drive rate or a long quiescent period would allow complete recovery of the drugged slow channel before the next excitation occurred. To exert such an effect on the channel recovery kinetics, the drug may bind to the channel most tightly in the active state or inactive state. Binding of the drug is voltage-dependent, with depolarization favoring binding. Inorganic Ca^{2+} entry blockers, such as Mn^{2+}, Co^{2+}, and La^{3+}, do not exhibit a frequency dependence.

Some analogs of nifedipine (Bay-K-8644 and CGP-28392) possess positive inotropic and vasoconstricting properties (Schramm *et al.*, 1983). These compounds are "Ca-agonists", that activate the Ca^{2+} slow channels. Bay-K-8644 induces slow APs in guinea pig papillary muscles rendered inexcitable by high K^+ and potentiates on-going slow APs (Wahler and Sperelakis, 1984a). It also potentiates on-going Na^+-dependent slow APs present in 3-day-old embryonic chick heart cells (Sada *et al.*, 1985). These findings support the concept that these drugs are slow channel agonists. It has been suggested that such compounds act to stabilize a specific channel conformation state (Triggle and Janis, 1984). Recent results, using voltage clamp and patch clamp analysis, further support the view that slow channels are activated by such drugs (Hess *et al.*, 1984; Thomas *et al.*, 1985; Sanguinetti and Kass, 1984). For example, Hess *et al.*, (1984) reported that Bay-K-8644 increased the probability of the slow channel being in the open configuration and increased the mean open time of the channel, and so increased the peak inward slow current intensity.

A number of other chemicals and drugs also block the myocardial slow channels, including local anesthetics (Josephson and Sperelakis, 1976) and volatile general anesthetics (Lynch *et al.*, 1976). The local anesthetics, lidocaine and procainamide, however, block the slow channels nonspecifically; that is, the dose-response curve for the slow APs is identical to that for the fast APs. However, depressed fast APs (produced in 10 mM $(K)_o$) were about ten times more sensitive to lidocaine. Halothane and enflurane are more selective in inhibiting the slow channels of the heart than the fast Na^+ channels (Lynch *et al.*, 1976). High ouabain concentrations also block the Ca^{2+} slow channels (Josephson & Sperelakis, 1977).

3. Selective Blockade by Acidosis

The myocardial slow channels are selectively blocked by acidosis (Chesnais *et al.*, 1975; Vogel and Sperelakis, 1977). Slow APs induced by isoproterenol, for example, were depressed (decreased rate of rise, amplitude, and duration) as the pH of the perfusing solution was lowered below 7.0 (Vogel and Sperelakis, 1977). The slow AP was 50% inhibited at pH 6.6, and was completely abolished at pH 6.1. The slow APs should be abolished before all the slow channels are blocked because of the requirement of a minimum density of slow channels for regenerative and propagating responses. The contractions were depressed in parallel with the slow APs. Two different buffer systems, HCO_3^--CO_2 and PIPES, gave similar results and were about equally fast. Blockade of the slow channels may occur with acidification of the outer or inner surfaces of the cell membrane. This could change the surface charge of the membrane and/or the conformation of the slow channel proteins.

Acidosis had little or no effect on the normal fast AP, except for the plateau becoming more triangular due to loss of I_{si}. However, the contractions became depressed and abolished as a function of the degree of acidosis. That is, excitation-contraction uncoupling occurred, as expected from a selective blockade of the Ca^{2+} slow channels.

Since the myocardium becomes acidotic during hypoxia and ischemia, it is likely that part of the effect of these metabolic interventions on the slow channels is mediated by the accompanying acidosis, and not solely by a decrease in ATP level. Consistent with this, the effects of hypoxia on the slow AP were almost immediately reversed, but only partially and transiently, by changing the pH of the perfusing solution to 8.0 (Fig. 2). The responses gradually diminished further during the hypoxia even at the alkaline pH (Belardinelli *et al.*, 1979). Consistent with this, slow channel blockade occurs faster during hypoxia at acid pH than at alkaline pH.

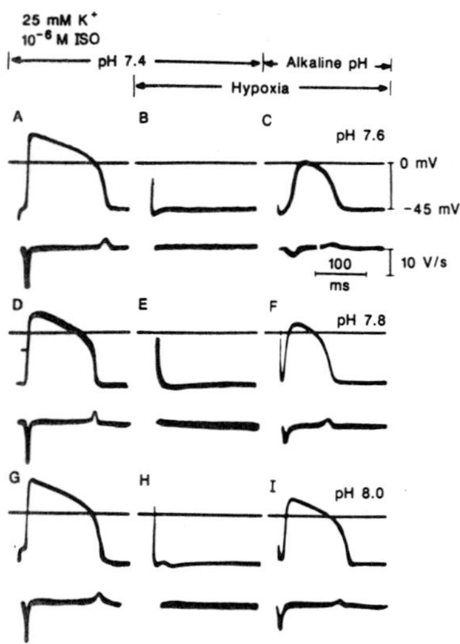

FIG 2 Selective blockade of the slow channels by acid pH. Bicarbonate-CO_2 buffer. A 20-day-old chick embryo heart was perfused with normal Ringer solution and paced at a rate of 0.5/s. **A-C:** Normal fast APs. **A:** Normal fast AP and contractions at pH 7.4. **B:** At pH 6.6, force of contraction was greatly reduced, whereas the APs were almost unaffected. **C:** At pH 6.2, contractions were completely abolished, with almost no effect on the fast APs, i.e., excitation-contraction uncoupling was produced. **D-H:** Blockade of isoproterenol (10^{-6} M)-induced slow AP responses at low pH (25 mM $(K)_o$). **D:** Control slow response and mechanical AP record at pH 7.4. **E-G:** Progressive blockade of slow AP responses and accompanying contractions as pH of perfusing solution was lowered. **H:** At pH 6.1, complete blockade of slow APs and contractions occurred. Upper trace gives dV/dt, from which maximal rate rise of APs was obtained. Modified from Vogel and Sperelakis (1977).

35

4. Metabolic Dependence of the Calcium Slow Channels

Induced slow APs are blocked by hypoxia, ischemia, and metabolic poisons (including cyanide, dinitrophenol, and valinomycin) within 5-15 min, accompanied by a lowering of the cellular ATP level (Schneider and Sperelakis, 1974; Sperelakis, 1980, 1984). An example for a metabolic poison is illustrated in Figure 3. Figure 3 shows that cyanide completely blocked the slow APs and contractions at a time when the fast APs were hardly affected, indicating that the fast Na^+ channels were essentially unaffected. However, the contractions accompanying the normal fast APs were depressed or abolished, indicating that contraction was uncoupled from excitation. Thus, there is a specific dependence of the slow channels on metabolic energy (Irisawa and Kokubun, 1983).

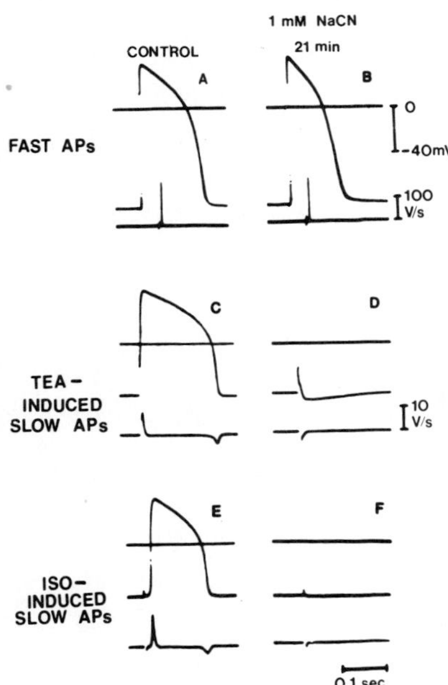

FIG 3 Effect of NaCN on the fast and slow APs of guinea pig papillary muscles. Lower trace gives dV/dt (trace arbitrarily shifted to the right in A-B). A: Control fast AP in 4.7 mM K^+ -Tyrode's solution. B: In the presence of NaCN (1 mM) for 21 min. The AP duration at 50% repolarization (APD_{50}) is substantially shortened, while the amplitude and $\dot{V}_{max}$ of the APs were largely unaffected. C: Slow AP elicited in presence of 10 mM TEA (in 25 mM K^+ -Tyrode's solution). D: 1 mM NaCN abolished these slow APs in 4.3 min. E: Slow AP induced by 10^{-7}M isoproterenol in 25 mM K^+ -Tyrode's solution. F: 1 mM NaCN abolished these slow APs in 4.9 min. From Wahler and Sperelakis (1984b).

Hypoxia and ischemia also blocked the Ca^{2+} slow channels. When the Ca^{2+} -dependent slow APs are blocked by hypoxia, there is a nearly instantaneous partial restoration of the slow APs by changing the pH of the perfusing solution to 7.6, 7.8, or 8.0 (Belardinelli *et al.*, 1979) (Fig. 2). That is, the effect of hypoxia could be counteracted partially, and for a short period, by alkaline pH. Similar results were obtained when the pH of the perfusing solution was varied in advance of the hypoxia; namely, the inhibition produced by hypoxia was less and slower at pH 8.0 than at pH 7.4 or 6.8.

These results suggest that part of the effect of hypoxia was mediated by the accompanying acidosis, which inhibited the Ca^{2+} slow channels.

Global ischemia of Langendorff-perfused hearts also blocked the Ca^{2+} slow channels. The fast APs were greatly shortened in duration after long periods (120 min) of ischemia. However, the contractions were depressed to 10% of control within 5 min. The slow APs were depressed and abolished within 10-20 min of ischemia. In contrast, depressed fast APs (in 10 mM $(K)_o$) were not much affected after 20 min of ischemia. These results suggest that ischemia depresses and blocks the Ca^{2+} slow channels within 5-20 min.

The slow APs blocked by valinomycin or by hypoxia were restored by elevation of the glucose concentration, indicating that the effect of metabolic poisons or hypoxia is indeed mediated by metabolic interference. Slow APs were also potentiated by elevation of the glucose concentration (Wahler and Sperelakis, 1984b; Belardinelli et $al.$, 1979), thus providing further evidence for the metabolic dependence of the myocardial slow channels. Consistent with these results, it was recently demonstrated that intracellular injection of ATP potentiated I_{si} (Taniguchi et $al.$, 1983).

Native slow channels (i.e., those present in cardiac muscle not stimulated by agents such as isoproterenol or histamine) were also blocked by cyanide in a manner and time course similar to that for the isoproterenol-stimulated slow APs (Wahler and Sperelakis, 1984b) (Fig. 3). Thus, no evidence could be obtained by these experiments for a second type of slow channel that might not be metabolically dependent or require phosphorylation.

With prolonged metabolic interference, for example 60-120 min of hypoxia or cyanide, there is a gradual shortening of the plateau duration of the normal fast AP, until only a relatively brief spike-like component remains that is still rapidly rising. Thus, metabolic interference exerts a second, but much slower, effect on the membrane. This effect is probably due to an increase in the kinetics of K^+ conductance (g_K) turn-on, thereby shortening the AP. This effect could be mediated in part by a gradual rise in $(Ca)_i$, which can cause an increase in the Ca-activated g_K ($g_{K(Ca)}$). In addition, it has been found by Noma (1983) that lowering of ATP activates a K^+ channel, which would act to shorten the APD_{50} (see section F). The effect of prolonged metabolic interference on shortening the AP would also help to shut off any residual I_{si}, thereby further reducing the total Ca^{2+} influx per impulse.

5. Extrinsic and Intrinsic Control of Ca^{2+} Influx

The Ca^{2+} influx of the myocardial cell is controlled by extrinsic factors. For example, stimulation of the sympathetic nerves of the heart or circulating catecholamines or other hormones can have a positive inotropic action, whereas stimulation of the parasympathetic neurons has a negative inotropic effect. The mechanism for some of these effects is mediated by changes in the levels of the cyclic nucleotides. This extrinsic control of the Ca^{2+} influx is made possible by the peculiar properties of the slow channels, as, for example, the postulated requirement for phosphorylation.

In addition, there is intrinsic control by the myocardial cell over its Ca^{2+} influx. For example, under conditions of transient regional ischemia, many of the slow channels become unavailable (or silent). This effect may be mediated by lowering the ATP level of the affected cells and by the accompanying acidosis. Thus, the myocardial cell can partially or completely suppress its Ca^{2+} influx under adverse conditions. This causes the affected cells to contract weakly or not at all; since most of the work done by the cell is mechanical, this conserves ATP. Such a mechanism may serve to protect the myocardial cells under adverse conditions, such as transient regional ischemia during coronary vasospasm. If the myocardial cell could not control its Ca^{2+} influx, then the ATP level might drop so low under such conditions that irreversible damage would be done, and the cells would become necrotic. Because of the peculiar properties of the slow channels, they become inactivated, thus uncoupling contraction from excitation and conserving ATP. The cells may then recover fully when the blood flow returns to normal. The effect of prolonged metabolic interference on shortening the fast AP would also help to shut off I_{si} more quickly, thereby reducing the total Ca^{2+} influx per impulse.

D. Regulation of the Ca^{2+} Slow Channels

1. Cyclic AMP Dependence

Cyclic AMP is somehow involved with functioning of the slow channels (Schneider and Sperelakis, 1974; Shigenobu and Sperelakis, 1972; Reuter and Scholz, 1977; Tsien *et al.*, 1972; Watanabe and Besch, 1974; Sperelakis and Schneider, 1976). Histamine and beta-adrenergic agonists, after binding to their specific receptors, lead to rapid stimulation of adenylate cyclase with resultant elevation of cyclic AMP levels. The methylxanthines enter the myocardial cells and inhibit the phosphodiesterase, thus causing an elevation of cyclic AMP. These positive inotropic agents also rapidly induce slow APs, along a parallel time course, presumably by making more slow channels available in the membrane and/or by increasing their mean open time and probability of opening. Dibutyryl cyclic AMP also induces the slow APs after a long lag period of 15-30 min, as expected from slow elevation of intracellular cyclic AMP (Fig. 4).

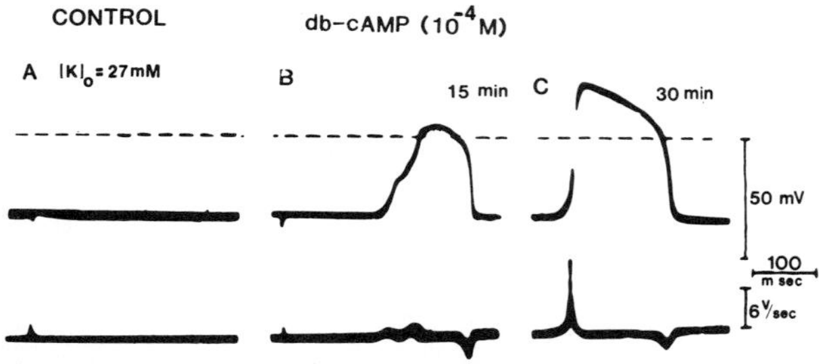

FIG 4 Slow induction of slow APs by perfusing a guinea pig heart with dibutyryl cyclic AMP. **A:** Control condition with heart perfused with 27 mM K^+ - Ringer solution to depolarize the cells to about -35 mV and thereby voltage-inactivate the fast Na^+ channels. **B-C:** Addition of 10^{-4} M db-cAMP produced large slow APs beginning at about 15 min (B), and reaching a peak effect at about 30 min (C). Taken from Schneider and Sperelakis (1975).

Additional evidence for the regulatory role of cyclic AMP has been obtained. Josephson and Sperelakis (1978) showed that a GTP analogue (5'-guanylylimidodiphosphate [GPP(NH)P], 10^{-5} to 10^{-3} M), that directly activates adenylate cyclase, induced the slow APs in cultured reaggregates of chick heart cells within 5-20 min. GPP(NH)P binds to the GTP site on the regulatory component of the adenylate cyclase complex, but cannot be hydrolyzed by the GTPase activity of the enzyme, and so causes an irreversible activation of adenylate cyclase and elevation of cyclic AMP.

Forskolin, another highly potent activator of adenylate cyclase activity, exerts a strong positive inotropic effect in isolated guinea pig atrial muscle (Metzger and Lindner, 1981) and induces and potentiates slow APs (Späh, 1984) (Wahler and Sperelakis, 1986). Prostaglandin $F_{1\alpha}$, which is known to increase cyclic AMP levels in many tissues, induced slow APs in K^+-depolarized cultured chick heart cells within 5 min. These results further support the role of cyclic AMP in regulation of the slow channels of myocardial cells.

Cyclic AMP iontophoretically microinjected into dog Purkinje fibers and guinea pig ventricular muscle cells induced slow APs in the injected cell for a transient period of about 1 min (Vogel and Sperelakis, 1981) (Fig. 5). A second injection of cyclic AMP again induced a slow AP, which again decayed within 1 min. The effect of the injected cyclic AMP occurred immediately, within seconds after the injection was stopped. The amplitude and duration of the induced slow APs were a function of the amount of cyclic AMP injected. Cyclic AMP electrophoretic injections potentiated slow APs induced by theophylline.

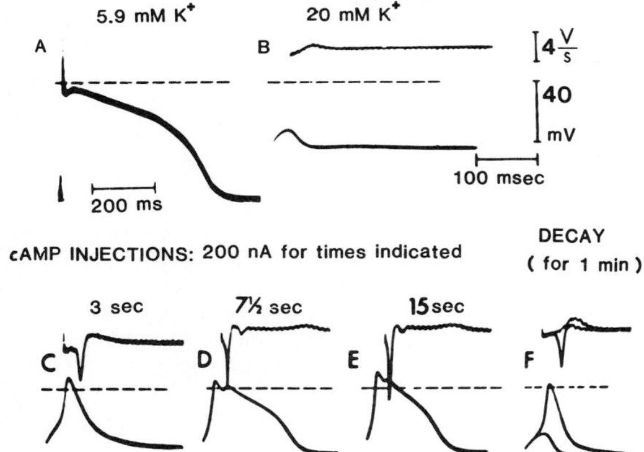

FIG 5 Fast induction of slow APs in a short canine Purkinje fiber by iontophoretic injection of cyclic AMP intracellularly. A: Normal fast AP recorded from a fiber bathed in Krebs-Henseleit solution ($(K)_o$ = 5.9 mM). B: Elevation of $(K)_o$ to 20 mM depolarized the fiber to about -40 mV and abolished excitability. C-F: Induction of slow APs in a single cell by iontophoretic cyclic AMP injections using 200 nA current for 3 s (C), 7.5 s (D), and 15 s (E). The induced responses were allowed to decay completely between injections. F: Decay of induced response. At 1 min after the injection in E, the slow AP had decreased markedly in $+\dot{V}_{max}$ and duration (first sweep) and then disappeared completely (second sweep). Note graded effects of the cyclic AMP injections on the maximal upstroke velocity ($+\dot{V}_{max}$, upper traces). Time calibration in B applies to B-F. Preparation paced at 0.3 Hz. The dV/dt trace was arbitrarily shifted to the right, so as to not be obscured in the AP upstroke. Taken from Vogel and Sperelakis (1981).

Pressure injection of various agents was also done to study the regulation of the Ca^{2+} slow channels by cyclic nucleotides. Pressure injection of cyclic AMP, GPP(NH)P, and cholera toxin into single ventricular myocardial cells of guinea pig papillary muscles rapidly induced and potentiated slow APs (Li and Sperelakis, 1983b). Pressure injection of cyclic AMP induced large slow APs within 10-25 sec after injection was started (Fig. 6). The effect persisted for as long as the pressure was applied, and the slow APs decayed within 25 sec after the injecting pressure was discontinued. Thus, these results confirm the data obtained by iontophoretic injection of cyclic AMP. They also indicate that the upper limit for the life span of one phosphorylated slow channel is 25 sec; the mean life span is likely to be much shorter: a few seconds or even a fraction of a second.

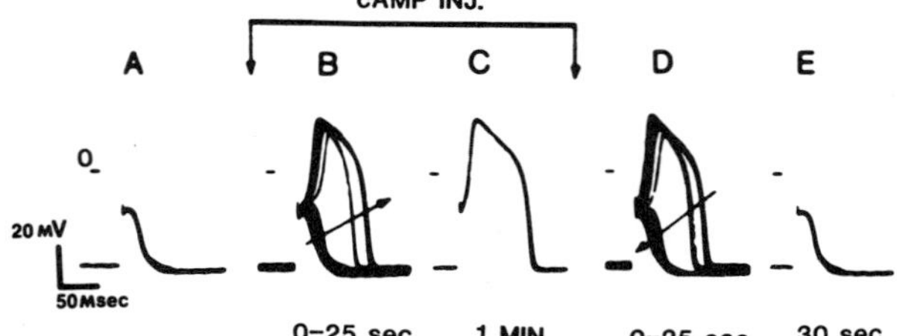

FIG 6 Induction of slow APs in a guinea pig papillary muscle by intracellular pressure injection of cAMP. The muscle was depolarized in 22 mM $(K)_o$ to voltage inactivate fast Na^+ channels. A microelectrode filled with 0.2 M Na^+ -cAMP was used for both pressure injection and intracellular recording. Pressure pulse applied continuously between arrows in B-C. A: Control; small graded response (stimulation rate 30/min). B: Superimposed records showing the gradual build-up of slow APs over a 25-sec period during cAMP injection. C: Presence of stable slow AP during injection for 1 min. D: Gradual decay of slow APs over a period of 25 sec after stopping injection. E: Complete decay of slow APs 30 sec after cessation of cAMP injection. All records were obtained from one cell. Taken from Li and Sperelakis (1983b).

Figure 7 illustrates that intracellular injection of GPP(NH)P (for only 5 sec) produced a very rapid effect; that is, large slow APs were induced within 30-50 sec (Li and Sperelakis, 1983b). This fast effect is in contrast to the relatively slow effect (5-20 min) of GPP(NH)P added to the bathing medium (Josephson and Sperelakis, 1978). The induced slow APs persisted for more than 3 min after the injecting pressure was stopped, indicating the relatively long-acting effect of GPP(NH)P on elevating cyclic AMP.

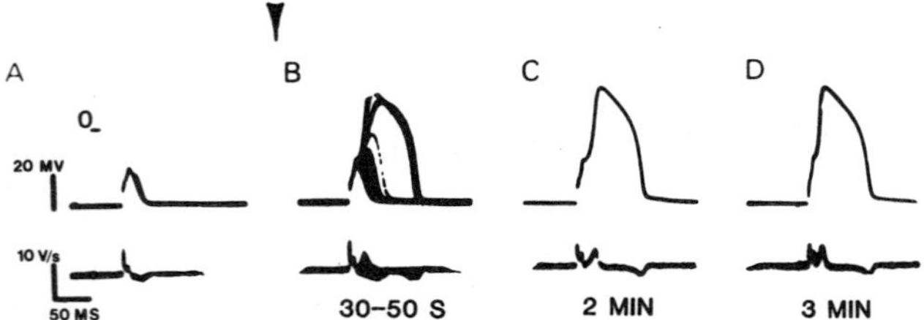

FIG 7 Induction of slow APs by intracellular pressure injection of GPP(NH)P. A: Control; small graded response induced by electrical stimulation (0.5 Hz) in 22 mM K^+-Ringer. B: Induction of slow APs by intracellular injection of GPP(NH)P for 5 sec. A microelectrode filled with 3×10^{-2} M GPP(NH)P in 0.2 M NaCl was used both for injection and membrane potential recording. Superimposed records show the gradual induction and enhancement. C, D: The induced slow APs were stable and persisted for more than 3 min after stopping the injection. Modified from Li and Sperelakis (1983b).

Cholera toxin is known to have an effect on the adenylate cyclase complex similar to that of GPP(NH)P, namely there is an irreversible activation of the regulatory component of the enzyme, due to inhibition of the hydrolysis of the GTP. Injection of cholera toxin rapidly potentiated ongoing slow APs, the effect beginning within 30 sec and reaching maximum within 3 min (Li and Sperelakis, 1983b). The induced slow APs persisted for over 4 min after the injecting pressure was stopped, indicating the relatively long-acting effect of cholera toxin on elevating cyclic AMP.

Cyclic AMP injection by the phosphatidylcholine liposome method confirmed the results obtained by the method of iontophoresis and pressure injection. Cyclic AMP injected simultaneously into the surface cells of cultured heart cell reaggregates by the liposome method also induced slow APs (Bkaily and Sperelakis, 1985).

The results from a number of other laboratories also support a role for cyclic AMP in stimulating the Ca^{2+} slow inward current in myocardial cells. For example, injection of cyclic AMP via a suction pipette enhanced I_{si} in isolated single adult cells (Irisawa and Kokubun, 1983). Similarly, a photochemical activation method for suddenly increasing the intracellular cyclic AMP level enhanced I_{si} in bullfrog atrial cells (Nargeot *et al.*, 1983).

Recent experiments using noise analysis and patch clamp analysis (Cachelin *et al.*, 1983; Trautwein and Hofmann, 1983; Bean *et al.*, 1984) suggest that cyclic AMP increases the number of functional slow channels available in the myocardial sarcolemma and/or the probability of opening of a given channel. The net results would be the same, i.e., an increase in the number of slow channels open at any instant of time. It was demonstrated by Reuter *et al.* (1982) that in patch clamp experiments on single Ca^{2+} slow channels of cultured neonatal rat heart cells, isoproterenol lengthened the mean open time of the channel and decreased the intervals between bursts (clustering of channel open states). The conductance of the single channel was not increased by isoproterenol. Therefore, the increase in the total maximal slow conductance ($\bar{g}_{si}$) produced by isoproterenol could be produced by the observed increase in mean open time of each channel, as well as by an increase in the number of channels participating in the conductance on a stochastic basis.

The cyclic nucleotides also appear to play a role in regulating the Ca^{2+} slow channels of vascular smooth muscle (VSM) cells. However, in VSM cells, cyclic AMP is inhibitory (Ousterhout & Sperelakis, 1986), in contrast to its stimulatory effect in myocardial cells. Furthermore, in VSM, cyclic AMP and cyclic GMP have the same direction of effects, namely inhibitory of I_{Ca} and of contraction, in contrast to cardiac muscle where the two cyclic nucleotides play antagonistic roles.

2. Phosphorylation Hypothesis

Because of the relationship between cyclic AMP and the number of available slow channels, and because of the dependence of the functioning of the slow channels on metabolic energy, it was postulated that a membrane protein must be phosphorylated in order for the slow channel to become available for voltage activation (Shigenobu and Sperelakis, 1972; Tsien *et al.*, 1972; Watanabe and Besch, 1974; Sperelakis and Schneider, 1976; Rinaldi *et al.*, 1982). Elevation of cyclic AMP by a positive inotropic agent activates a cyclic AMP-dependent protein kinase (dimer split into two monomers), which phosphorylates a variety of proteins in the presence of ATP. Several myocardial membrane proteins become phosphorylated under these conditions. A cartoon depiction of the phosphorylation hypothesis is given in Figure 8. The protein that is phosphorylated might be the slow channel protein itself (Fig. 8 A) or a contiguous regulatory type of protein (e.g., phospholamban-like) associated with the myocardial Ca^{2+} slow channel (Fig. 8 B). It was suggested that the function of cardiac slow Ca^{2+} channels in isolated sarcolemmal vesicles is modulated by a cyclic AMP-dependent phosphorylation of a 23,000-mol. wt. sarcolemmal protein ("calciductin") (Rinaldi *et al.*, 1982).

Phosphorylation could make the slow channel available for activation by a conformational change that either allowed the activation gate to be opened upon depolarization or effectively increased the diameter of the water-filled pore (the "selectivity filter" portion) so that Ca^{2+} (and Na^+) could pass through. In this model, the phosphorylated form of the slow channel is the active (operational) form, and the dephosphorylated form is the inactive (inoperative) form. That is, only the phosphorylated form is available to become activated upon depolarization to threshold. Another way to view this is that phosphorylation increases the probability of channel opening with depolarization. The dephosphorylated channels are electrically silent. An equilibrium would probably exist between the phosphorylated and dephosphorylated forms of the slow channels for a given set of conditions, including the level of cyclic AMP. Thus, agents that act to elevate the cyclic AMP level would increase the fraction of the slow channels that are in the phosphorylated form, and hence available for voltage activation. Such agents would increase the force of contraction of the myocardium.

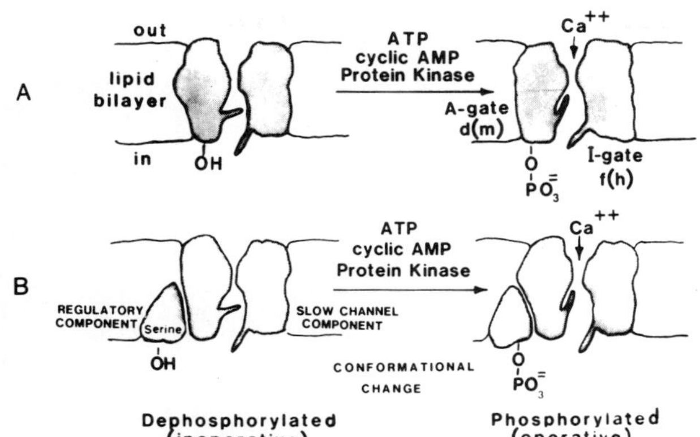

FIG 8 Cartoon model for a slow channel in myocardial cell membrane in two hypothetical forms: dephosphorylated form (left diagrams) and phosphorylated form (right diagrams). The phosphorylation hypothesis assumes that a protein constituent of the slow channel itself (A) or a regulatory protein associated with the slow channel (B) must be phosphorylated in order for the channel to be in a functional state available for voltage activation. Phosphorylation occurs by a cyclic AMP-dependent protein kinase in the presence of ATP. Presumably, a serine or threonine residue in the protein becomes phosphorylated. Phosphorylation may produce a conformation change that effectively allows the channel to function. The dephosphorylated form would be electrically silent. Modified from Sperelakis and Schneider (1976).

As stated above, the mean life span of a phosphorylated channel is likely to be only a few seconds at most. A phosphoprotein phosphatase would hydrolyze and dephosphorylate the slow channel. Thus, agents which affect or regulate the phosphatase would affect the life span of the phosphorylated channel. For example, the phosphatase, calcineurin, was found to increase inactivation of the Ca^{2+} slow channels (Chad and Eckert, 1985b).

There are some positive inotropic agents that induce slow APs but do not elevate cyclic AMP, e.g., angiotensin-II (Freer *et al.*, 1976) and fluoride ion (< 1 mM) (Vogel *et al.*, 1977). Fluoride ion may act by inhibiting the phosphoprotein phosphatase, which dephosphorylates the slow channel protein, thereby resulting in a larger fraction of phosphorylated channels. That is, inhibition of the rate of dephosphorylation should have a similar effect as stimulation of the rate of phosphorylation. Angiotensin may activate a non-cyclic AMP-dependent protein kinase. Thus, the results with angiotensin and fluoride can be fitted within the framework of the phosphorylation hypothesis.

A test of whether the regulatory effect of cyclic AMP is exerted by means of the cyclic AMP-dependent protein kinase and phosphorylation was made by intracellular injection of the catalytic subunit (protein) of the cAMP-dependent protein kinase. Such injections induced and enhanced the slow APs (Bkaily and Sperelakis, 1984) and potentiated I_{si} (Brum *et al.*, 1983). Thus, these results support the phosphorylation hypothesis.

Another direct test of the phosphorylation hypothesis was done by intracellular injection (by the liposome method) of an inhibitor (protein) of the cAMP-dependent protein kinase into cultured chick heart cells (Bkaily and Sperelakis, 1984). It was found that the inhibitor depressed and abolished the slow APs (Fig. 9). Although some depolarization also occurred concomitantly, it was shown, by application of repolarizing current pulses, that the slow channels were blocked even at the larger take-off potentials. The effect of the inhibitor was rapidly reversed by injection of the catalytic subunit of the cAMP-dependent protein kinase (Fig. 9 F). Injection of heat-denatured inhibitor was without effect. Thus, these results further support the phosphorylation hypothesis.

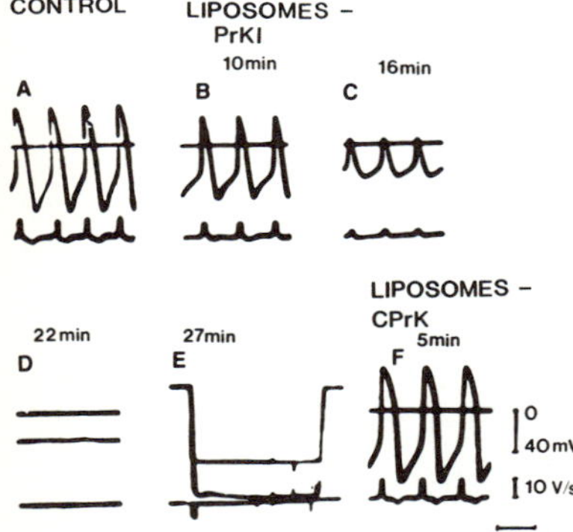

FIG 9 cAMP-dependent protein kinase inhibitor (PrKI) blocked spontaneous slow APs in cultured chick heart cells (reaggregates), and injection of catalytic subunit of PrK reversed these inhibitory effects. Liposome method used for injection. **A:** Control slow APs. After superfusion with solution containing liposomes filled with PrKI, AP amplitude and $+\dot{V}_{max}$ were decreased (B, 10 min; C, 16 min). **D:** At 22 min, the APs were blocked accompanied by depolarization. **E:** Electrical stimulation during hyperpolarizing current pulses could not elicit APs. **F:** Injection of catalytic subunit of protein kinase (CPrK) restored slow APs within 5 min. All records from the same impalement. Taken from Bkaily and Sperelakis (1984).

Consistent with the phosphorylation hypothesis, it has been found that the Ca^{2+} slow channel "dies" within 90 sec in isolated membrane inside-out patches (Reuter, 1983). That is, the Ca^{2+} slow channel activity is permanently lost. This is consistent with the washing away of regulatory components of the slow channels or of the enzymes necessary to phosphorylate the channel.

Even perfusion of excitable cells (Helix neurons in this example) is accompanied by a progressive loss of the Ca^{2+} slow current, and this loss is slowed or partially reversed by any means that enhances cAMP-dependent phosphorylation (Chad and Eckert, 1985a). In addition, however, they found that leupeptin, an inhibitor of Ca-dependent proteases, retards the kinase-irreversible Ca^{2+}-dependent loss of Ca^{2+} slow current. They concluded that an endogenous Ca-dependent protease may account for the irreversible loss of Ca^{2+} slow channel activity in perfused neurons.

In summary, the Ca^{2+} slow channels of the heart are regulated by cyclic AMP in a stimulatory fashion. Elevation of cyclic AMP produces a very rapid increase in number of slow channels available for voltage activation during excitation. The probability of a slow channel opening at a given voltage is increased and the mean open time of a given channel is increased. The mechanism whereby cyclic AMP stimulates the slow channels is by means of the cyclic AMP-dependent protein kinase and phosphorylation of one or more proteins. Presumably a protein that is phosphorylated is the slow channel protein itself or an associated regulatory-type (stimulatory) of protein. Phosphorylation may produce a conformational change that allows the channel gates to operate (open and close) or increases the diameter of the water-filled central pore sufficiently to allow Ca^{2+} ion to pass through. Therefore, any agent that increases the cyclic AMP level of the myocardial cell will tend to potentiate I_{si}, Ca^{2+} influx, and contraction. Such agents include beta-adrenergic agonists (such as norepinephrine and isoproterenol), H_2-histaminic receptor agonists (such as histamine), and cyclic AMP-specific phosphodiesterase inhibitors (such as the methylxanthines caffeine and theophylline, amrinone, and milrinone).

Cyclic AMP has been found to also regulate other types of ion channels. For example, the serotonin-sensitive K^+ channel of Aplysia sensory neurons are closed by cyclic AMP (Siegelbaum *et al.*, 1982). In cell-attached patches, serotonin produced long closures of the K^+ channels, whose gating was weakly dependent on voltage and independent of $(Ca)_i$ (Camardo *et al.*, 1983). In isolated membrane patches, the catalytic subunit of cAMP-PK produced closures of these K^+ channels, simulating serotonin (Shuster *et al.*, 1985). It was concluded that cAMP-PK acts on the internal surface of the cell membrane to phosphorylate the K^+ channel protein or an associated membrane-bound regulatory protein.

46

3. Cyclic GMP Antagonism of Cyclic AMP

Superfusion of isolated guinea pig papillary muscles with 8-Br-cGMP (10^{-5} -10^{-3} M) abolished the Ca^{2+}-dependent slow APs and accompanying contractions within 7-20 min (Wahler and Sperelakis, 1985b). A similar inhibition by cGMP was shown for the slow APs of canine Purkinje fibers (Mehegan *et al.*, 1985). Intracellular injection of cyclic GMP into cells of guinea pig papillary muscle, by the pressure injection method, transiently depressed or abolished slow APs much more quickly (e.g., 1-2 min) (Wahler and Sperelakis, 1985b) (Fig. 10). Injection of cyclic GMP into cultured chick heart cells by the liposome method also depressed and abolished the slow APs (Bkaily and Sperelakis, 1985).

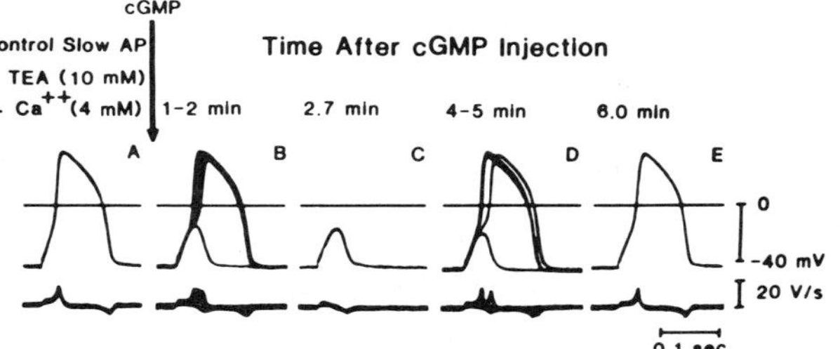

FIG 10 Transient abolition of slow APs by intracellular cGMP injection. A microelectrode filled with 50 mM Na^+-cGMP (in 0.2 M KC1) was used for both pressure injection and potential recording. **A:** Control slow AP induced by 10 mM TEA plus 4.0 mM $(Ca)_o$ (fast Na^+ channels inactivated by 25 mM K^+). **B-C:** 1-2 min following the onset of the cGMP pulse (10 sec duration), the slow APs were depressed and finally abolished. **D-E:** At 4-6 min, the slow APs recovered spontaneously to control levels. All records from the same cell. Taken from Wahler and Sperelakis (1985b).

Nitroprusside, which elevates cyclic GMP levels by stimulation of the guanylate cyclase, also depressed or abolished the slow APs of cultured chick heart cells within 35 min (Bkaily and Sperelakis, unpublished observations). Prostaglandin $F_{2\alpha}$, which is known to increase cyclic GMP levels in many tissues, abolished the naturally-occurring slow APs of cultured chick heart cells within 10 min. (Bkaily and Sperelakis, unpublished observations). The results with nitroprusside and $PGF_{2\alpha}$ further support those with cyclic GMP injection and superfusion, and indicate that cyclic GMP is involved in regulation of the myocardial slow channels, playing a role opposite to that of cyclic AMP.

Therefore, cyclic GMP regulates the functioning of the myocardial Ca^{2+} slow channels in a manner that is antagonistic to that of cyclic AMP. The effect of cyclic GMP may be mediated through phosphorylation of a protein that regulates the functioning of the slow channel. It is possible that the slow channel protein, or an associated regulatory protein, has a second site that can be phosphorylated and which, when phosphorylated, inhibits the slow channel. Another possibility is that there is a second type of regulatory protein that is inhibitory when phosphorylated (Fig. 11). Another mechanism proposed for frog ventricular muscle, in which db-cAMP potentiates the twitch and 8-Br-cGMP depresses it, is based on the fact that cGMP depressed the cAMP level (i.e., there was a reciprocal relationship between cGMP and cAMP), namely that cGMP may be part of a feedback mechanism to regulate cAMP level (Singh and Flitney, 1981).

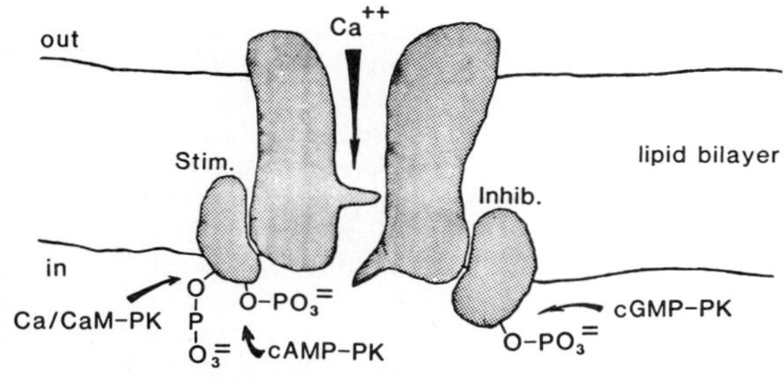

FIG 11 One possible model for modulation of slow channel function by cAMP-, cGMP-, and calmodulin-dependent phosphorylation. A cAMP-dependent protein kinase (PK) and Ca/calmodulin-dependent PK may phosphorylate two sites on a regulatory protein (stim.) which stimulates slow channel activity. Phosphorylation of an inhibitory regulatory protein (Inhib.) by cGMP-dependent PK may result in inhibition of slow channel activity.

4. Acetylcholine and Adenosine

The parsympathetic neurotransmitter acetylcholine (ACh) is well known to increase g_K, and thereby can hyperpolarize SA nodal cells (therefore depressing automaticity) and shorten the duration of the AP in atrial myocardial cells. This would also tend to suppress slow APs in atrial cells by increasing the overlapping outward K^+ current, and so diminishing the net inward (slow) current.

ACh exerts a negative inotropic effect on the ventricular myocardium that has been stimulated by beta-adrenergic agonists. That is, in ventricular myocardial cells, activation of the muscarinic receptor by ACh reverses the stimulation of the adenylate cyclase complex produced by beta-adrenergic agonists. Activation of the beta-adrenergic receptor activates the regulatory (stimulatory) component (N_s protein) of the adenylate cyclase complex, whereas activation of the muscarinic receptor activates an inhibitory regulatory component (N_i protein) of the enzyme (Fig. 12).

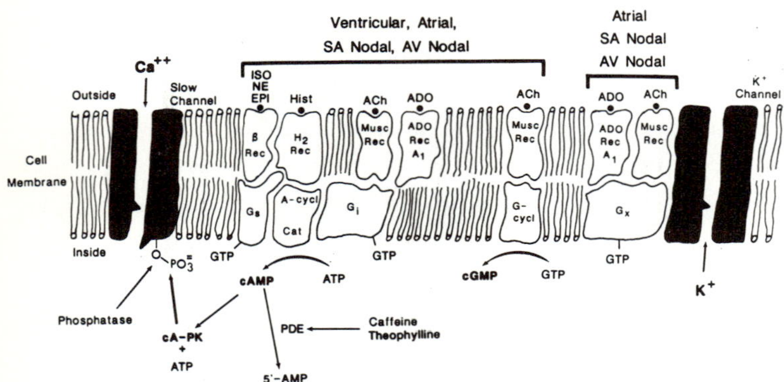

FIG 12 Diagrammatic summary of the relationship between receptors and the slow channels in myocardial cell membrane.

Included are the mechanism of action of some positive inotropic agents, such as beta-adrenergic agonists, histaminic H_2 agonists, and methylxanthines (phosphodiesterase inhibitors). The beta agonists and H_2 agonists act on the regulatory component (guanine nucleotide binding protein) of the adenylate cyclase complex to stimulate cyclic AMP production. The voltage-dependent myocardial slow Ca^{2+} channels are dependent on cyclic AMP and on metabolism, presumably because a protein constituent (or regulatory component) of the slow channel must be phosphorylated in order for it to be in a form that is available for voltage activation. Cyclic AMP stimulates the Ca^{2+} slow channels via phosphorylation by a cyclic AMP-dependent protein kinase (cA-PK). Other types of phosphorylation, by calmodulin-dependent, phospholipid-dependent, or cGMP-dependent protein kinases, may also regulate slow channel function. Also depicted are the mechanisms for the negative inotropic effects of acetylcholine (ACh) and adenosine (ADO) in various cardiac tissues, e.g., ventricular, atrial, SA nodal, and AV nodal. ACh and ADO activate, respectively, muscarinic receptors and ADO receptors (A_1) which inhibits the catalytic subunit of adenylate cyclase via the G_i (N_i) coupling protein. This action antagonizes or reverses the stimulatory effects of activation of the beta-adrenergic receptor or histaminic H_2 receptor on the adenylate cyclase exerted via the G_s (N_s) coupling protein, thereby returning the cyclic AMP level back towards the basal level. As illustrated, muscarinic receptor activation also stimulates the guanylate cyclase, and thereby elevates the cyclic GMP level. Cyclic GMP inhibits the Ca^{2+} slow channels. In all cardiac tissues except ventricular, ADO and ACh act, via their respective receptors, to activate a special K^+ channel via a G_x (G_O or N_O) type of coupling protein, as depicted at the right side of the diagram. This effect increases a K^+ conductance ($g_{K(ACh)}$ and $g_{K(ADO)}$), and therefore gives rise to ADO-induced and ACh-induced K^+ current.

Activation of the muscarinic receptor by ACh exerts an inhibitory effect on adenylate cyclase and cyclic AMP level, via the N_i (inhibitory) coupling protein, to reverse the stimulation of adenylate cyclase produced by means of the N_s coupling protein due to, for example, activation of the beta-adrenoceptor or H_2 receptor. That is, the muscarinic receptor antagonizes or opposes the stimulation of adenylate cyclase produced by other receptors such as the beta-adrenoceptor or H_2 receptor. Thus, ACh depresses Ca^{2+} influx and contraction not only by elevation of cyclic GMP, but also by reversing cyclic AMP elevation produced by beta-adrenergic agonists and H_2 agonists.

Josephson and Sperelakis (1982), in voltage-clamp experiments on cultured chick ventricular cells stimulated by isoproterenol, demonstrated that ACh depresses the inward slow current, I_{si}. It is possible that the depression of the ISO-potentiated I_{si} is also mediated by a lowering of the cyclic AMP level which was elevated by activation of the beta-adrenergic receptor. It is not known whether part of this effect of ACh is also mediated through elevation of the intracellular cyclic GMP level, which would act to antagonize the effects of cyclic AMP (see Section D-3 above). ACh did not increase the outward K^+ current (I_K) in these ventricular cells. This indicates that the ACh-activated K^+ channel is absent from ventricular cells (see Fig. 12).

Wahler and Sperelakis (1986) found that, in guinea pig papillary muscles, ACh not only depressed the slow APs induced by isoproterenol, but also the slow APs that were induced by forskolin. If forskolin's action resulted from a direct stimulation of the catalytic subunit of the adenylate cyclase complex, then activation of the muscarinic receptor may somehow reverse this stimulation. Alternatively, the action of ACh on inhibiting the forskolin response could have been mediated by an increase in g_K or by stimulation of guanylate cyclase and consequent elevation of cyclic GMP.

Adenosine (ADO) has effects on the heart that are virtually identical to those of ACh. For example, in isolated rabbit SA node, both ADO and ACh depress automaticity and hyperpolarize (West and Belardinelli, 1985). In atrial cells, both ADO and ACh markedly shorten the action potential and produce a small hyperpolarization and depression of automaticity (Belardinelli and Isenberg, 1983). In contrast, in ventricular muscle of birds (Shigenobu and Sperelakis, 1975) and mammals (Schneider *et al*, 1976), ACh and ADO do not shorten the APD_{50} and do not hyperpolarize. For example, Belardinelli and Isenberg (1983) showed that ADO did not shorten the APD in isolated ventricular myocytes from both bovine and guinea pig hearts. However, if the APD_{50} is first prolonged by addition of isoproterenol (ISO), then adenosine is effective in counteracting the effects of ISO, including the effects on the plateau overshoot (Belardinelli & Isenberg, 1983).

50

In the case of the slow AP in mammalian (guinea pig) ventricular muscle, induced by ISO (10^{-7} M) in 27 mM K^+-Ringer, ADO, in concentrations as high as 10^{-4} M, had little or no effect (Schneider *et al.*, 1976). This was confirmed in voltage clamp measurements of I_{si} (I_{Ca}) in isolated guinea pig ventricular myocytes (in 25 mM $(K)_o$ to suppress the fast I_{Na}) by Isenberg and Belardinelli (1984). The stimulation of I_{Ca} by ISO (10^{-8} M) was not counteracted by ADO (2 x 10^{-4} M). However, if these experiments were repeated in normal low $(K)_o$ (5.4 mM), ADO (2 x 10^{-4} M) was able to counteract the stimulatory effect of ISO (10^{-8} M) (Isenberg & Belardinelli, 1984) (Fig. 13). Hence, for some unknown reason, in high $(K)_o$, ADO cannot antagonize the potentiating effect of ISO on I_{Ca}.

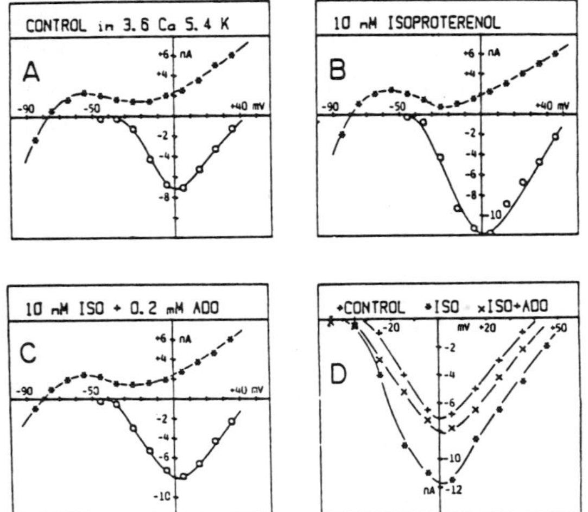

FIG 13 Ability of ADO to antagonize the stimulatory effect of ISO on I_{Ca} in isolated guinea pig ventricular myocytes in normal $(K)_o$ (5.4 mM). **A:** Control I/V curves for I_{Ca} (unfilled cirlces) and for the delayed outward I_K (asterisks). **B:** Increased I_{Ca} after addition of 10^{-8} M ISO. **C:** Addition of 2 x 10^{-4} M ADO in continued presence of the ISO reduced the peak I_{Ca} to nearly the control level. **D:** The I/V curves for I_{Ca} are superimposed: control (+), ISO (*), and ADO + ISO (x). Taken from Isenberg & Belardinelli (1984) with permission.

The Ca^{2+}-dependent slow APs of atrial muscle of guinea pig are blocked by ADO (Schrader *et al.*, 1975). The effects of ADO on the dose/response curves for ISO stimulation of the Ca^{2+}-dependent slow APs in rat cardiac muscle were studied (Knabb *et al.*, 1983). In atrial muscle, ADO (10^{-6} M) produced a pronounced shift to the right in the dose/response curve. In contrast, in ventricular muscle, the shift in the dose/response curve was much less prominent. These results on rat ventricular muscle are essentially in agreement with those of Schneider *et al.* (1976) on guinea pig ventricular muscle. As might be expected, theophylline (5 x 10^{-5} M) shifted the dose/response curves to the left in both atrial and ventricular muscles. A micro-

adenosine deaminase also shifted the dose/response curves to the left, suggesting that endogenously-produced ADO had a depressant effect on the ISO response under normal conditions. It has been found that endogenous ADO increases significantly during systole compared to diastole (Thompson *et al.*, 1980).

Consistent with the ability of ADO to counteract the stimulatory effect of ISO on I_{Ca} in ventricular muscle, it was shown that ADO (10^{-5} M) reversed the elevation of cyclic AMP produced by ISO (3×10^{-8} and 10^{-7} M) to nearly the control (basal) level in embryonic chick (12-day-old) ventricular muscle (Belardinelli *et al.*, 1982). Further support for the view that the anti-adrenergic effect of ADO in ventricular muscle is due to inhibition of adenylate cyclase was provided by West *et al.* (1986). They showed that the positive inotropic, increased I_{Ca}, and increased APD responses to forskolin (150 nM) were antagonized by ADO (50-200 µM), whereas the similar responses to dibutyryl cAMP were not antagonized.

Consistent with the ability of ADO to antagonize the stimulatory effect of ISO on I_{Ca} in ventricular muscle, Belardinelli and Isenberg (1983) found that ADO (20 µM) counteracted the potentiating effect of ISO (1 mM) on the delayed after-depolarization (DAD) in isolated bovine ventricular myocytes. Other agents that decrease I_{Ca}, such as the calcium antagonist drugs, have a similar effect.

The mechanism whereby ADO and ACh shorten the normal AP and hyperpolarize in atrial muscle, in addition to inhibition of I_{Ca}, is an increase in K^+ conductance (g_K). For example, Belardinelli and Isenberg (1983) measured the steady-state outward I_K using voltage clamp of isolated guinea pig atrial myocytes. They found that ADO (2 µM) increased outward I_K in spontaneously firing myocytes, as well as in quiescent myocytes, and that ACh (1 µM) had a similar effect. That is, there was similarity between the ADO-induced current and ACh-induced current. The increased outward K^+ current would, of course, tend to shorten the APD and hyperpolarize (more towards E_K).

The effects of ADO and ACh in various cardiac tissues are summarized diagrammatically in Figure 12. As depicted, the ventricular cell does not possess the ADO-or ACh-activated K^+ conductance channel, whereas the atrial and nodal cells do. This would explain why the normal AP is not shortened in ventricular muscle, whereas it is shortened in atrial muscle and nodal cells and hyperpolarization is produced. As depicted, all cardiac tissues possess ADO and ACh receptors, which when hooked to the G_i (N_i) coupling protein,

52

antagonizes the stimulatory effects of the beta-adrenergic and histaminic H_2 receptors exerted on the catalytic subunit of adenylate cyclase via the G_s (N_s) coupling protein. This would explain the lowering of the cyclic AMP level by ADO or ACh that was elevated by ISO and the reversal of the increase in I_{Ca} produced by ISO. Stimulation of the guanylate cyclase by muscarinic receptor activation, with consequent elevation of cyclic GMP, would also act to depress I_{Ca} (see Section D-3 above).

ADO inhibits the Ca^{2+}-dependent APs and contractions of VSM cells from small dog coronary arteries, whereas ADO has little or no effect on the VSM of large coronary arteries (Harder *et al.*, 1979).

5. Calmodulin and Protein Kinase C

Inhibitors of calmodulin, namely trifluoperazine (TFP) and calmidazolium, were found to inhibit the slow APs of cultured chick heart cells (Bkaily *et al.*, 1984; Bkaily and Sperelakis, 1986). The inhibition of the slow APs produced by calmidazolium, injected intracellularly by the liposome method, is illustrated in Figure 14. Also illustrated is the finding that subsequent injection of calmodulin could reverse the inhibition produced by calmidazolium.

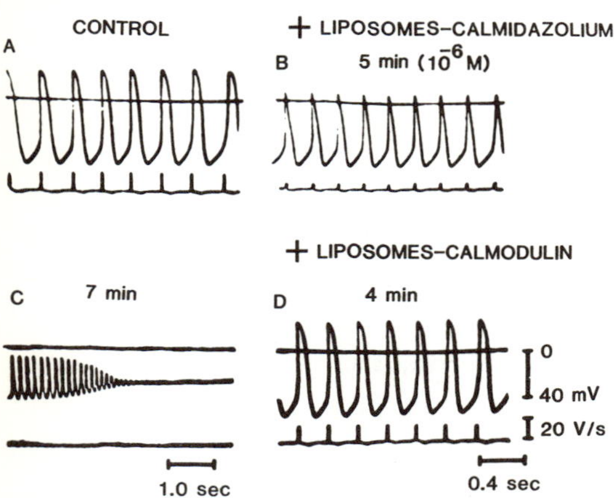

FIG 14 The calmodulin inhibitor, calmidazolium, blocks spontaneous slow APs occurring naturally in cultured chick heart cells (reaggregates), and injection of calmodulin reverses the inhibitory effects. **A:** Control slow APs. **B:** 5 min after superfusion with Tyrode solution containing liposomes filled with 10^{-6}M calmidazolium, $+\dot{V}_{max}$ decreased without any change in the resting potential. **C:** At 7 min, there was further decrease in $+\dot{V}_{max}$ accompanied by depolarization, and finally all spontaneous activity stopped. Hyperpolarizing pulses could not induce any APs (not shown). **D:** Injection of calmodulin restored slow APs within 4 min. All records were from the same impalement. Taken from Bkaily and Sperelakis, 1986).

In the presence of calmidazolium and the inhibitor of cAMP-dependent protein kinase, calmodulin injection had no effect, whereas subsequent injection of the catalytic subunit of cAMP-dependent protein kinase restored the slow APs (Bkaily and Sperelakis, 1986). When the catalytic subunit was injected first, the slow APs recovered only partially; full recovery of the slow APs required subsequent injection of calmodulin.

Therefore, it appears that calmodulin also plays a potentiating role in the regulation of the myocardial Ca^{2+} slow channels. This effect may be mediated by the Ca^{2+}-calmodulin protein kinase, and phosphorylation of a protein that affects the functioning of the slow channel (Fig. 11). It is possible that a regulatory protein associated with the slow channel, when phosphorylated, acts to make that slow channel become available for voltage activation. That is, a protein associated with the slow channel may be phosphorylated by the Ca^{2+}-calmodulin dependent protein kinase, which may, in some manner, potentiate the effects of cAMP-dependent phosphorylation of the slow channel. Thus, it appears that maximal activation of the slow channels requires two separate phosphorylation steps. These may be on the same protein (Fig. 11) or on two separate proteins (i.e., two stimulatory regulatory components).

High concentrations of the α-adrenergic agonist, phenylephrine, has been shown to cause a positive inotropic effect and to increase APD and to increase I_{Ca} in bovine cardiac muscle (Bruckner and Scholz, 1984). There is still controversy with respect to the effect of activation of the α-adrenoceptors of myocardial cells on the level of cyclic AMP, some investigators reporting increases and others finding no changes. However, the α-adrenoceptor stimulates the phosphatidyl inositol (PI) cycle and breakdown and generation of inositol trisphosphate (IP_3) and diacyl glycerol (DG) (Brown, 1985). IP_3 has been implicated as a second messenger to act on the SR to release Ca^{2+} stored in this compartment. DG and Ca^{2+} activate protein kinase C, which phosphorylates a number of proteins. It is not known at present whether protein kinase C is involved in regulation of the myocardial Ca^{2+} slow channels.

6. Possible Action of Some Drugs on Phosphorylation/Dephosphorylation Cycle

Some agents that affect the force of contraction of the heart may do so without changing the levels of the cyclic nucleotides. For example, fluoride ion is a potent positive inotropic agent and potentiates the Ca^{2+}-dependent slow APs and Ca^{2+} influx (I_{si}), but yet does not elevate cyclic AMP, as stated above. Fluoride is known to permeate the cell membrane

readily and to be a potent inhibitor of a number of enzymes, including phosphoprotein phosphatases. Therefore, fluoride may act by inhibiting the phosphatase which dephosphorylates the slow channel protein (or associated regulatory protein). This would prolong the life span of the phosphorylated
channel, and so would increase the number of slow channels in the phosphorylated state at any instant in time. Thus, potentiation of I_{si} and contraction can be produced by inhibition of the rate of dephosphorylation, as well
as by stimulation of the rate of phosphorylation.

Consistent with the hypothesis of a phosphorylation/dephosphorylation
cycle for the Ca^{2+} slow channels, it was reported that the phosphoprotein
phosphatase, calcineurin, increases the rate of inactivation of I_{si} in snail
neurons, and it was suggested that phosphorylation may regulate the rate of
inactivation (Chad and Eckert, 1985b).

It is also possible that some negative inotropic drugs may depress the
rate of phosphorylation. It would be difficult to distinguish electrophysio-
logically between a drug that depressed the rate of phosphorylation of the
Ca^{2+} slow channel (e.g., by inhibiting the cAMP-PK) and one that blocked the
slow channel directly (e.g., by acting as a physical plug). For example, if
a Ca antagonistic drug, such as verapamil, were to inhibit cAMP-dependent
phosphorylation of the slow channel, it would, in effect, "block" the channel
by an indirect means; even the frequency dependency of a drug could be
accounted for by such an action.

E. Effect of Cyclic GMP on K^+ Channels

In cell-attached patch clamp experiments, single-channel currents from
inwardly-rectifying K^+ channels were observed in single ventricular cells
isolated from 16-17-day-old embryonic chick hearts and cultured for 2-10 days
(Wahler and Sperelakis, 1986). The patch pipettes were filled with 150 mM
KCl to reduce the K^+ equilibrium potential, E_K, across the patch membrane to
about 0 mV. At an applied pipette potential of 0 mV, the membrane potential
across the patch membrane would be equal to the resting potential of the
cell, about -70 mV. Thus, the electrochemical gradient for K^+ ion ($E_m - E_K$)
would be -70 mV, and would drive K^+ current inward through the K^+ channels.
Under this steady-state voltage, the inward K^+ currents were about 1.0 pA,
and the single-channel conductance was about 8 pS (Fig. 15 A, C). There was
a second conductance state of this K^+ channel of about 26 pS. The channel
was identified as being a K^+ channel by the measured reversal potential of 0

mV (applied pipette potential of -70 mV; $V = -V_{pip}$; $E_C = V_{pip} - E_m = (-70 - (-70)) = -70 + 70 = 0$ mV). The channel was identified as inwardly rectifying by plotting I/V curves, and showing that the conductance increased at more negative membrane potentials and decreased at more positive membrane potentials. The channel openings ranged between a few ms to 280 ms, with the average channel open-time being 41 ms; there was an approximate exponential distribution of open-times, with the greatest frequency of occurrence being short openings.

Addition of 8-Br-cGMP (10^{-4} or 10^{-3} M) to the medium superfusing the cell inhibited or blocked channel activity within 3-10 min (Fig. 15B). However, this inhibitory effect was only transient; the channels spontaneously recovered activity in the continued presence of the cyclic GMP analog. As can be seen in Figure 15D, in a record taken after 15 min in the presence of 8-Br-cGMP, the channel openings now included openings that were much longer than in the control condition (Fig. 15C). Under this condition of "long-term" exposure to the cyclic GMP analog, the frequency distribution of channel open-times showed two components, one averaging 33 ms (which is close to the control value of 41 ms) and a second component averaging 740 ms. Such long openings were rarely observed in the absence of 8-Br-cGMP. As a control, superfusion with the non-cyclic analog, 8-Br-GMP, had no effect.

Hence, it appears that cyclic GMP plays a regulatory role on the K^+ channels as well as on the Ca^{2+} slow channels. Cyclic GMP inhibits the Ca^{2+} slow channels (section D-3), whereas the inward-rectifying K^+ channels are initially inhibited but subsequently recovered or even stimulated. The great prolongation of the mean open-time produced by cyclic GMP is somewhat similar to the prolongation of open-time of the Ca^{2+} slow channels produced by Ca agonists such as Bay-K-8644 (see section C-1). Since the inwardly-rectifying K^+ channel ocnductance is heavily involved in determining the P_{Na}/P_K ratio or g_{Na}/g_K ratio in a resting membrane, and hence the resting potential (E_{diff} value), the initial inhibitory phase of cyclic GMP action could affect the excitability of the myocardial cell because of the decreased g_K (depolarization, increased R_m, AP prolongation). If the later recovery phase actually includes stimulation, this would increase g_K and depress excitability (hyperpolarization, decreased R_m, AP shortening).

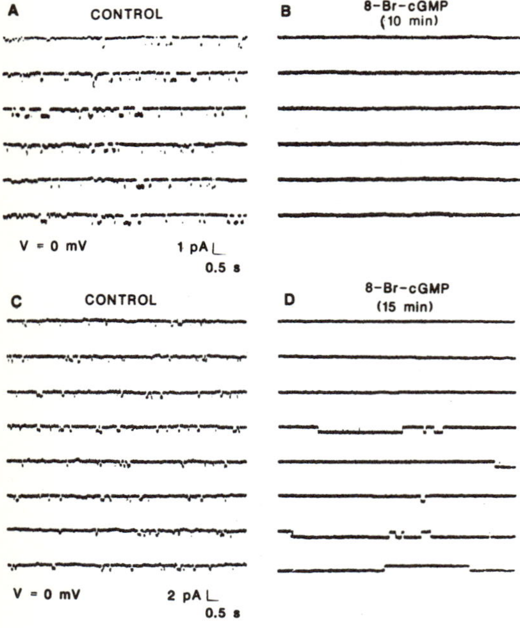

FIG 15 Biphasic effects of cyclic GMP on the single-channel currents of an inwardly-rectifying, K^+ channel recorded from two single cultured embryonic (16-17-day-old) chick heart cells (A-B, and C-D) by the cell-attached patch clamp technique. **A-B:** Experiment illustrating the initial inhibitory effects of cyclic GMP. **A:** Control channel openings illustrated in six consecutive oscilloscope sweeps. **B:** Superfusion of the cell with the lipid-soluble cyclic GMP analog, 8-Br-cGMP (10^{-3} M), abolished the channel openings within 3-10 min; records illustrated taken at 10 min. **C-D:** Experiment illustrating the later stimulatory effects of cyclic GMP. **C:** Control records. **D:** Superfusion with 8-Br-cGMP (10^{-4} M) produced initial inhibition followed by stimulation. Records illustrated taken after 15 min exposure to 8-Br-cGMP. The crucital inhibitory phase persisted up through the upper three sweeps, and was followed by the stimulatory phase depicted in the lower five sweeps. In each panel, all sweeps are consecutive. Calibrations (current, time) for A-B given in panel A, and those for C-D are given in panel C. In these two experiments, the pipette potential was 0 mV, and the pipette was contained 150 mM KCl to bring E_K across the patch membrane to about 0 mV. (Wahler and Sperelakis, 1986.)

F. ATP-Regulated K^+ Channels

Single inwardly-rectifying K^+ channel currents have been shown to be dependent on ATP levels in cardiac cells (Noma, 1983; Trube and Hescheler, 1984; Noma and Shibasaki, 1985). At normal ATP levels, the inwardly-rectifying K^+ channels have a slope conductance of approximately 25 pS (145 mM KCl in pipette (Trube and Hescheler, 1984)). In the presence of metabolic inhibitors (cell-attached patch) or in the absence of ATP in the solution bathing the cytoplasmic side (inside-out patch), this type of single-channel current disappears, and a new type appears. The new current is also an inwardly-rectifying K^+ current, but the slope conductance is approximately 80 pS. That is, the 80 pS channel appeared only after inhibition of cellular metabolism by DNP to lower the ATP level. Thus, the type and conductance of K^+ channel current depends on the ATP level in the heart. ATP stimulates the normal low-conductance (25 pS) inwardly-rectifying K^+ channel, and inhibits the high conductance (80 pS) inwardly-rectifying K^+ channel. It was suggested (Noma, 1983) that this ATP-sensitive K^+ channel underlies the increased outward K^+ current which occurs in conditions of hypoxia or metabolic poisons, and that the ATP-inhibited K^+ channel may serve as a link between cellular energy metabolism and regulation of membrane excitability. ATP depletion produces shortening of the APD_{50}, and this results in a negative inotropic effect, thus sparing ATP. Hence, when ATP is lowered by hypoxia and ischemia, activation of the ATP-inhibited K^+ channel prevents further depletion of ATP, and thus would help to protect the ischemic cells from irreversible damage (see section C-5).

When the cell was dialzed with a solution containing only 0.5 mM ATP, the Ca^{2+} slow current was decreased to less than 10% of the control value; the delayed rectifier outward time-dependent K^+ current was also depressed (Noma and Shibasaki, 1985). However, there was an increase in the time-independent inwardly-rectifying outward K^+ current, as described above.

In isolated single ventricular cells from adult guinea pig heart, two-microelectrode voltage clamp studies showed that the marked shortening of the APD_{50} produced by 0.1 mM DNP was accompanied by a pronounced increase of the time-independent outward-rectifying activated K^+ current (Isenberg *et al.*, 1983). In addition, DNP caused a smaller and slower increase in an inward-rectifying K^+ current; this latter current caused hyperpolarization but did not contribute to shortening of the APD_{50}.

G.   Summary and Conclusions

The voltage- and time-dependent slow channels in the myocardial cell membrane are the major pathway by which Ca^{2+} ions enter the cell during excitation for initiation and regulation of the force of contraction of cardiac muscle. These slow channels appear to behave kinetically, on a population basis, as if their gates open, close, and recover more slowly than those of the fast Na^+ channels. In addition, the slow channel gates operate over a less negative (more depolarized) voltage range. Tetrodotoxin does not block the slow channels, whereas the calcium antagonistic drugs, Mn^{2+}, Co^{2+}, and La^{3+} ions do.

The slow channels have some special properties, including functional dependence on metabolic energy, selective blockade by acidosis, and regulation by the intracellular cyclic nucleotide levels. Because of these special properties of the slow channels, Ca^{2+} influx into the myocardial cell can be controlled by extrinsic factors (such as autonomic nerve stimulation or circulating hormones) and by intrinsic factors (such as cellular pH or ATP level). During transient regional ischemia, the selective blockade of the slow channels, which results in depression of the contraction and work of the afflicted cells, might protect the cells against irreversible damage by helping to conserve their ATP content. Reperfusion arrhythmias may be caused by the breakdown of this protective mechanism, in that, upon reperfusion, the Ca^{2+} slow channels may recover before the cells are capable of handling the greater Ca^{2+} influx. The Ca^{2+} slow channels may recover their function before the ATP level is sufficiently recovered to allow bail-out of the intracellular Ca^{2+}. In addition, the generation of free radicals upon reperfusion may injure the Ca-ATPase and other enzymes involved in Ca^{2+} metabolism. The net effect of this would be to cause Ca^{2+} overload of the cells and SR, with subsequent delayed after-depolarizations (DADs) leading to triggered automaticity and arrhythmias.

Following blockade of the fast Na^+ channels in myocardial cells with TTX or by voltage-inactivating them in 25 mM $(K)_o$, catecholamines, angiotensin-II, histamine, and methylxanthines rapidly allow the production of slowly-rising Ca^{2+}-dependent APs by increasing the number of Ca^{2+} slow channels available for voltage activation and/or their mean open time. Concomitantly, these compounds rapidly elevate intracellular cyclic AMP levels, suggesting that cyclic AMP is somehow related to the functioning of the slow channels. Exogenous cyclic AMP produces the same effect, but much more slowly.

Exposure of intact myocardial cells to agents which directly stimulate the adenylate cyclase (e.g., GPP(NH)P and cholera toxin), also induces slow APs within 10-20 min. Intracellular injection of cyclic AMP, GPP(NH)P, and cholera toxin rapidly (within seconds) induce or potentiate ongoing slow APs in the injected cell. Thus, the time delay between exposure to the agent and an observed effect is greatly reduced by intracellular application of the agent. These results clearly indicate the key role played by cyclic AMP in regulation of the Ca^{2+} slow channels, and hence in controlling Ca^{2+} influx and force of contraction.

The Ca^{2+} slow channels are very sensitive to blockade by metabolic poisons, hypoxia, and ischemia. The slow AP is blocked at a time when the rate of rise and duration of the normal fast AP is essentially unaffected. However, the contraction accompanying the fast AP is depressed or abolished; that is, contraction is uncoupled from excitation, as expected from selective slow channel blockade. The ATP level is greatly reduced by the metabolic poisons, for example, by valinomycin and DNP, at the same time that the slow channels are blocked. Therefore, the slow channels are metabolically dependent, presumably on ATP, whereas the fast Na^+ channels are not. Part of the effect of ischemia in blocking the slow channels appears to be mediated by the concomitant acidosis, since the slow channels are selectively sensitive to blockade by acid pH; in contrast, the fast APs are not much affected, but excitation-contraction uncoupling occurs.

The dependence of the myocardial slow channels on the cyclic AMP level and on metabolism suggests that phosphorylation of a membrane protein constituent of the slow channel, or of an associated regulatory protein, by a cyclic AMP-dependent protein kinase and ATP, may make the channel available for voltage activation during excitation; that is, the dephosphorylated channel would be electrically silent. A direct test of the phosphorylation hypothesis, namely injection of an inhibitor of the cAMP-protein kinase, supported the view that the cyclic AMP regulation of the slow channels is mediated by phosphorylation of some protein (stimulatory-type).

The parasympathetic neurotransmitter ACh depresses the inward slow current (I_{si}) stimulated by beta-adrenergic agonists or forskolin. ADO has effects on cardiac tissues that are similar to those of ACh, but ADO and ACh each act on their own receptors. In atrial and nodal cells, ADO hyperpolarizes and shortens the APD by activating a receptor-operated K^+ conductance channel. This ADO-activated K^+ current is not present in ventricular cells of mammals and birds. In ventricular muscle, ADO antagonizes the effects of beta-adrenoceptor agonists, by reversing the stimulation of adenylate cyclase by the beta agonists. Thus, the augmentation of I_{Ca} by beta agonists is reversed by ADO.

The myocardial Ca^{2+} slow channels are also regulated by cyclic GMP, in a manner that is opposite to that of cyclic AMP. The effect of cyclic GMP is presumably mediated by means of phosphorylation of a protein, as for example, a regulatory protein (inhibitory-type) associated with the slow channel.

Calmodulin also may play a role in regulation of the myocardial slow Ca^{2+} channels, possibly mediated by the Ca^{2+}-calmodulin-protein kinase and phosphorylation of some regulatory-type of protein.

Thus, it appears that the Ca^{2+} slow channel is a complex structure, perhaps consisting of several proteins, including perhaps two associated regulatory proteins, one stimulatory and one inhibitory, both of which may require phosphorylation in order to express their regulatory function. Some cardioactive drugs, including perhaps some of the calcium antagonistic drugs, could conceivably affect the phosphorylation-dephosphorylation steps. Although it is not known how long a given site on the slow channel complex remains phosphorylated, the transient effect of the intracellular injection of cyclic AMP sets an upper limit of about 30 sec; the mean life span is more likely to be of the order of 1 sec or less.

Not only are the myocardial Ca^{2+} slow channels regulated by cyclic nucleotides, but some K^+ channels are also affected by these second messenger compounds. For example, it was found that cyclic GMP has a dual effect on an inwardly-rectifying K^+ channel: initially there is inhibition of the channel followed by recovery. In the later recovery phase, the mean open-time of the channels is greatly increased.

The Ca^{2+} slow channels located in cultured vascular smooth muscle cells from the rat aorta are also modulated by cyclic nucleotides, but in this tissue both cyclic AMP and cyclic GMP act in the same direction to block the Ca^{2+} slow channels and inhibits Ca^{2+} influx (Ousterhout and Sperelakis, 1986). This action of the cyclic nucleotides can account, at least in part, for their inhibition of contraction and vasodilating properties.

Acknowledgments

The research data from the author's laboratory reviewed in this article were supported primarily by NIH grant HL-31942. The author wishes to acknowledge his major former and present research colleagues and collaborators relevant to this article: Drs. K. Shigenobu, J.A. Schneider, S.M. Vogel, I. Josephson, T. Li, G. Bkaily, and G.M. Wahler.

REFERENCES

Bean BP (1985). Two kinds of calcium channels in canine atrial cells. J Gen Physiol 86:1-30.

Bean BP, Nowysky MC, Tsien RW (1984). β-adrenergic modulation of calcium channels in frog ventricular heart cells. Nature 307:371-375.

Belardinelli L, Isenberg G (1983). Actions of adenosine and isoproterenol on isolated mammalian ventricular myocytes. Circ Res 53:287-297.

Belardinelli L, Vogel SM, Sperelakis N, Rubio R, Berne RM (1979). Restoration of inward slow current in hypoxic heart muscle by alkaline pH. J Mol Cell Cardiol 11:877-892.

Belardinelli L, Vogel S, Linden J, Berne RM (1982). Antiadrenergic action of adenosine on ventricular myocardium in embryonic chick hearts. J Mol Cell Cardiol 14:291-294.

Bkaily G, Sperelakis N (1984). Injection of protein kinase inhibitor into cultured heart cells blocks calcium slow channels. Am. J. Physiol. 246 (Heart Circ. Physiol. 15):H630-H634.

Bkaily G, Sperelakis N (1985). Injection of cyclic GMP into heart cells blocks the slow action potentials. Am J Physiol (Heart Circ Physiol) 248:H745-H749.

Bkaily G, Sperelakis N (1986). Calmodulin is required for a full activation of the calcium slow channels in heart cells. J Cyclic Nucleotide & Prot Phosph Res 11:25-34.

Bkaily G, Sperelakis N, and Eldefrawi M (1984). Effects of the calmodulin inhibitor, trifluoperazine, on membrane potentials and slow action potentials of cultured heart cells. Europ J Pharmacol 105:23-31.

Brown JH (1985). α_1-adrenergic and muscarinic cholinergic stimulation of phosphoinositide hydrolysis in adult rat cardiomyocytes. Circ Res 57:532-537.

Bruckner R, Scholz H (1984). Effects of α-adrenoceptor stimulation with phenylephrine in the presence of propranolol on force of contraction, slow inward current and cyclic AMP content in the bovine heart. Br J Pharmacol 82:223-232.

Brum G, Flockerzi V, Hofmann F, Osterreider W, Trautwein W (1983). Injection of catalytic subunit of cAMP-dependent protein kinase into isolated cardiac myocytes. Pflugers Arch 398:147-154.

Cachelin AB, dePeyer JE, Kokubun S, Reuter H (1983). Ca^{2+} channel modulation by 8-bromocyclic AMP in cultured heart cells. Nature 304:462-464.

Camardo JS, Shuster MJ, Siegelebaum SA, Kandel ER (1983). Modulation of a specific potassium channel in sensory neurons of Aplysia by serotonin and cAMP-dependent protein phosphorylation. Cold Spring Harbor Symp Quant Biol 48:213-220.

Cavalie A, Ochi R, Pelzer D, Trautwein W (1983). Elementary currents through Ca^{2+} channels in guinea pig myocytes. Pflugers Archiv 398:284-297.

Chad J, Eckert R (1985a). Leupeptin, an inhibitor of Ca-dependent proteases, retards the kinase-irreversible, Ca-dependent loss of calcium current in perfused snail neurons. Biophys J 47:266a (abst).

Chad J, and Eckert R (1985b). Calcineurin, a calcium-dependent phosphatase, enhances Ca-mediated inactivation of Ca current in perfused snail neurons. Biophys J 47:266a (abst).

Chesnais JM, Coraboeuf E, Sauvain MP, Vassas JM (1975). Sensitivity to H, Li, and Mg ions of the slow inward sodium current in frog atrial fibers. J Mol Cell Cardiol 7:627-642.

Fabiato A, Fabiato F (1979). Calcium and cardiac excitation-contraction coupling. Ann Rev Physiol 41:473-484.

Fabiato, A, Baumgarten, C (1984) Methods for detecting calcium release from the sarcoplasmic reticulum of skinned cardiac cells and the relationships between calculated transsarcolemmal calcium movements and calcium release. In: <u>Physiology and Pathophysiology of the Heart</u>, edited by N. Sperelakis, Martinus Nijhoff, pp. 215-254.

Freer RJ, Pappano AJ, Peach MJ, Bing KT, McLean MJ, Vogel SM, Sperelakis N (1976). Mechanism of the positive inotropic effect of angiotensin II on isolated cardiac muscle. Circ Res 39:178-183.

Harder D, Belardinelli L, Sperelakis N, Rubio R, Berne RM (1979). Differential effects of adenosine and nitroglycerin on the action potentials of large and small coronary arteries. Circ Res 44:176-182.

Hess P, Lansman JB, Tsien RW (1984). Different modes of Ca channel gating behavior favoured by dihydropyridine Ca agonists and antagonists. Nature 311:538-544.

Irisawa H, Kokubun S (1983). Modulation by intracellular ATP and cyclic AMP of the slow inward current in isolated single ventricular cells of the guinea pig. J Physiol 338:321-327.

Isenberg G, Belardinelli L (1984). Ionic basis for the antagonism between adenosine and isoproterenol on isolated mammalian ventricular myocytes. Circ Res 55:309-325.

Isenberg, G, Vereecke J, vanderHeyden G, Carmeliet E (1983). The shortening of the action potential by DNP in guinea-pig ventricular myocytes is mediated by an increase of a time-independent K conductance. Pflugers Arch 397:251-259.

Josephson I, Sperelakis N (1976). Local anesthetic blockade of Ca^{2+} -mediated action potentials in cardiac muscle. Eur J Pharmacol 40:201-208.

Josephson I, Sperelakis N (1977). Ouabain blockade of inward slow current in cardiac muscle. J Mol Cell Cardiol 9:409-418.

Josephson I, Sperelakis N (1978). 5'-Guanylimidodiphosphate stimulation of slow Ca^{2+} current in myocardial cells. J Mol Cell Cardiol 10:1157-1166.

Josephson I, and Sperelakis N (1982). On the ionic mechanism underlying adrenergic-cholinergic antagonism in ventricular muscle. Eur J Pharmacol 40:201-208.

Kerr LM, Sperelakis N (1983). Ca^{2+}-dependent slow action potentials in normal and dystrophic mouse skeletal muscle. Am J Physiol 245:C415-C422.

Knabb MT, Rubio R, Berne RM (1983). Potentiation of slow action potential with theophylline or "micro" adenosine deaminase. Am J Physiol 244:H454-H457.

Kohlhardt M, Bauer B, Krause H, Fleckenstein A (1972). Differentiation of the transmembrane Na and Ca channels in mammalian cardiac fibres by the use of specific inhibitors. Pflügers Arch 335:309-322.

Kohlhardt M, Fleckenstein A (1977). Inhibition of the slow inward current by nifedipine in mammalian ventricular myocardium. Naunyn-Schmied Arch Pharmacol 298:267-272.

Kojima M, Sperelakis N (1983). Calcium antagonistic drugs differ in blockade of slow Na^+ slow channels in young embryonic chick hearts. Eur J Pharmacol 94:9-18.

Li T, Sperelakis N (1983a). Calcium antagonist blockade of slow action potentials in cultured chick heart cells. Can J Physiol Pharmacol 61:957-966.

Li T, Sperelakis N (1983b). Stimulation of slow action potentials in guinea pig papillary muscle cells by intracellular injection of cAMP, Gpp(NH)p, and cholera toxin. Circ Res 52:111-117.

Lynch C, Vogel S, Sperelakis N (1976). Halothane depression of myocardial slow action potentials. Anesthesiology 55:360-368.

Mehegan JP, Muir WW, Unverferth DV, Fertel RH, McGiurk SM (1985). Electrophysiological effects of cyclic GMP on canine cardiac Purkinje fibers. J Cardiovasc Pharmacol 7:30-35.

Metzger H, Lindner E (1981). The positive inotropic-acting forskolin, a potent adenylate cyclase activator. Arzneim-Forsch/Drug Res 31:1248-1250.

Molyvdas PA, Sperelakis N (1983). Comparison of the effects of several calcium-antagonistic drugs (slow-channel blockers) on the electrical and mechanical activities of guinea pig papillary muscle. J Cardiovasc Pharmacol 5:162-169.

Nargeot J, Nerbonne JM, Engels J, Lester HA (1983). Time course of the increase in the myocardial slow inward current after a photochemically generated concentration jump of intracellular cAMP. Proc Natl Acad Sci (USA) 80:2395-2399.

Noma A (1983). ATP-regulated K^+ channels in cardiac muscle. Nature 305:147-148.

Noma A, Shibasaki T (1985). Membrane current through adenosine-triphosphate-regulated potassium channels in guinea-pig ventricular cells. J Physiol 363:463-480.

Nowycky MC, Fox AP, and Tsien RW (1985). Three types of neuronal calcium channel with different calcium agonist sensitivity. Nature 316:440-443.

Ousterhout JM, Sperelakis N (1986). Depression of Ca^{2+}-dependent action potentials by cyclic nucleotides in cultured aortic smooth muscle cells. (Submitted).

Reuter H (1983). Calcium channel modulation by neurotransmitters, enzymes and drugs. Nature 301:569-574.

Reuter H, Cachlin AB, DePeyer JE, Kokubun S (1983). Modulation of calcium channels in cultured cardiac cells by isoproterenol and 8-bromo-cAMP, Cold Spring Harbor Symposium on Quant Biol 48:193-200.

Reuter H, Scholz H (1977). The regulation of the calcium conductance of cardiac muscle by adrenaline. J Physiol (London) 264:49-62.

Reuter H, Stevens CF, Tsien RW, Yellen G (1982). Properties of single calcium channels in cardiac cell culture. Nature (London) 297:501-504.

Rinaldi ML, Capony J-P, Demaille JG (1982). The cyclic AMP-dependent modulation of cardiac sarcolemmal slow calcium channels. J Mol Cell Cardiol 14:279-289.

Sada H, Sada S, Sperelais N (1985). Actions of the slow channel activator, Bay-K-8644, on the electrical activity of 3-day-old embryonic chick hearts. Clin & Exper Pharm & Physiol 12:57-61.

Sanguinetti MC, Kass RS (1984). Dihydropyridine derivatives: Voltage-dependent modulation of calcium channel current. Biophys J 45:394a.

Schneider JA, Shigenobu K, Sperelakis N (1976). Valinomycin inhibition of the inward slow current of cardiac muscle. In Roy PE, Dhalla NS (eds): series "Recent Advances in Studies on Cardiac Structure and Metabolism", Vol. 9, University Park Press, Baltimore, pp. 33-52.

Schneider JA, Sperelakis N (1974). The demonstration of energy dependence of the isoproterenol-induced transcellular Ca^{2+} current in isolated perfused guinea pig hearts -- an explanation for mechaical failure in ischemic myocardium. J Surg Res 16:389-403.

Schneider JA, and Sperelakis N (1975). Slow Ca^{2+} and Na^+ responses induced by isoproterenol and methylxanthines in isolated perfused guinea pig hearts exposed to elevated K^+. J Mol Cell Cardiol 7:249-273.

Schrader J, Rubio R, Berne RM (1975). Inhibition of slow action potentials of guinea pig arterial muscle by adenosine: A possible effect on Ca^{2+} influx. J Mol Cell Cardiol 7:427-433.

Schramm M, Thomas G, Towart R, Franckowiak G (1983). Activation of calcium channels by novel 1,4-dihydropyridines. Arzneim Forsch/Drug Res 33:1268-1272.

Singh J, Flitney FW (1981). Inotropic responses of the frog ventricle to dibutyryl cyclic AMP and 8-bromo cyclic GMP and related changes in endogenous cyclic nucleotide levels. Biochem Pharmacol 30:1475-1481.

Shigenobu K Schneider, JA, Sperelakis N (1974). Verapamil blockade of slow Na$^+$ and Ca^{2+} responses in myocardial cells. J Pharmacol Exp Ther 190:280-288.

Shigenobu K, Sperelakis N (1972). Ca^{2+} current channels induced by catecholamines in chick embryonic hearts whose fast Na$^+$ channels are blocked by tetrodotoxin or elevated K$^+$. Circ Res 31:932-952.

Shigenobu K, Sperelakis N (1975). PRolongation of the action potential plateau of embryonic chick hearts organ cultured in the presence of cyclic AMP. Jap J Pharmacol 25:481-484.

Shuster MJ, Camardo JS, Siegelbaum SA, and Kandel ER (1985). Cyclic AMP-dependent protein kinase closes the serotonin-sensitive K$^+$ channels of Aplysia sensory neurones in cell-free membrane patches. Nature 313:392-395.

Siegelbaum SA, Camardo JS, Kandel ER (1982). Serotonin and cyclic AMP close single K$^+$ channels in Aplysia sensory neurones. Nature 299:413-417.

Späh F (1984). Forskolin, a new positive inotropic agent, and its influence on myocardial electrogenic cation movements. J Cardiovasc Pharmacol 6:99-106.

Sperelakis N (1980). Changes in membrane electrical properties during development of the heart. In Zipes DP, Bailey JC, Elharrar V (eds): "The Slow Inward Current and Cardiac Arryhthmias," Boston: Martinus Nihhoff, pp 221-262.

Sperelakis N (1984). Cyclic AMP and phosphorylation in regulation of Ca^{2+} influx into myocardial cells, and blockade by calcium-antagonistic drugs. Am Heart J 107:347-357.

Sperelakis N, Schneider JA (1976). A metabolic control mechanism for calcium ion influx that may protect the ventricular myocardial cell. Am J Cardiol 37:1079-1085.

Taniguchi J, Noma A, Irisawa H (1983). Modification of the cardiac action potential by intracellular injection of adenosine triphosphate and related substances in guinea pig single ventricular cells. Circ Res 53:131-139.

Thompson CI, Rubio R, Berne RM (1980). Changes in adenosine and glycogen phosphorylase activity during the cardiac cycle. Am J Physiol 238:H389-H398.

Thomas G, Chung M, Cohen CJ (1985). A dihydropyridine (Bay k 8644) that enhances calcium currents in guinea pig and calf myocardial cells. Circ Res 56:87-96.

Trautwein W, Hofmann F (1983). Activation of calcium current by injection of cAMP and catalytic subunit of cAMP-dependent protein kinase. Proc Internat Union Physiol Sci 15:75-83.

Triggle DJ, Janis RA (1984). Calcium channel antagonists: Pharmacologic and radioligand binding approaches to mechanisms of action. In: Sperelakis N (ed): "Calcium Antagonists, Mechanisms of Action on Cardiac Muscle and Vascular Smooth Muscle", Boston: Martinus Nijhoff, pp. 11-20.

Trube G, Hescheler J (1984). Inward-rectifying channels in isolated patches of the heart cell membrane: ATP-dependence and comparison with cell-attached patches. Pflugers Arch 401:178-184.

Tsien RW, Giles W, Greengard P (1972). Cyclic AMP mediates the effects of adrenaline on cardiac Purkinje fibers. Nature (London) New Biol 240:181-183.

Vogel S, Crampton R, Sperelakis N (1979). Blockade of myocardial slow channels by bepridil (CERM-1978). J Pharmacol Exp Ther 210:378-385.

Vogel S, Sperelakis N (1977). Blockade of myocardial slow inward current at low pH. Am J Physiol 233:99-103.

Vogel S, Sperelakis N (1981). Induction of slow action potentials by micro-iontophoresis of cyclic AMP into heart cells. J Mol Cell Cardiol 13:51-64.

Vogel S, Sperelakis N, Josephson I, Brooker G (1977). Fluoride stimulation of slow Ca^{2+} current in cardiac muscle. J Mol Cell Cardiol 9:461-475.

Wahler GM, Sperelakis N (1984a). The new Ca^{2+} agonist (Bay K 8644) potentiates and induces slow action potentials. Am J Physiol (Heart and Circ Physiol) 247:H337-H340.

Wahler GM, Sperelakis N (1984b). Similar metabolic dependence of stimulated and unstimulated myocardial slow channels. Canad J Physiol Pharmacol 62:569-574.

Wahler GM, and Sperelakis N (1985). Intracellular injection of cyclic GMP depresses cardiac slow action potentials. J Cyclic Nucleotide Prot Phosphorylation Res 10:83-95.

Wahler GM, Sperelakis N (1986). Cholinergic attenuation of the electrophysiological effects of forskolin. J Cyclic Nucleo & Prot Phosphory Res 11:1-10.

Watanabe AM, Besch HR Jr (1974). Cyclic adenosine monophosphate modulation of slow calcium influx channels in guinea pig hearts. Circ Res 35:316-324.

West GA, Belardinelli L (1985). Correlation of sinus slowing and hyperpolarization caused by adenosine in sinus node. Pflugers Arch 403:75-81.

West GA, Isenberg G, Belardinelli L (1986). Antagonism of forskolin effects by adenosine in isolated hearts and ventricular myocytes. Am J Physiol 250:H769-H777.

3

POTASSIUM CHANNELS IDENTIFIED WITH SINGLE CHANNEL RECORDINGS AND THEIR ROLE IN CARDIAC EXCITATION

Akinori Noma and Hiroko Matsuda

Dept. of Physiology, Faculty of Medicine Kyushu University, Fukuoka, 812 JAPAN

INTRODUCTION

Since the introduction of the voltage clamp technique in cardiac muscles (1), the potassium current has been extensively studied and various components of K current have been dissected (2-4). Organic blockers of K currents, such as tetraethylammonium (TEA) and 4-aminopyridine, or the ionic blockers such as Ba^{2+} and Cs^+, were never selective to a given component of the potassium current, even though the sensitivity of each component was different. Therefore, separation into current components was made only on the basis of different kinetics. The time-independent current could not be separated into components until the invention of the patch clamp tecnique (5).

In the single channel current recording, the individual K channel is definitely characterized with the single channel conductance, life time of the open- and closed-state channel and sensitivity to various neuro-transmitters. If single channels are recorded from the isolated-patches, or the whole-cell current recordings are made under the intracellular dialysis, their sensitivity to different chemicals are also tested. Until now 6 different classes of K channels have been identified in the mammalian cardiac muscle. In this study recent patch clamp studies of the cardiac K channels will be reviewed and the role of each K channel in the cardiac excitation will be discussed. The comparison of the channels may also be facilitated since different mechanisms are proposed for the inward-going rectification (6), which is one of the almost common characteristics of the cardiac K channels.

Table 1.

	Inward-going rectification	Mechanism	Single channel conductance	Kinetics	Function	Correspondence
Inward rectifier K channel	+	rapid closure & Mg block	40–50 pS	activation (hyper) inactivation (depo)	Resting G_K	I_{K1}
Delayed rectifier K channel	+	rectification	10 pS	activation (depo)	Repolarization & pacemaker	I_K
Muscarinic recept. operated K Channel	+	Mg block	60 pS	activation (hyper)	Vagal regulation	$I_{K.ACh}$
ATP-regulated K channel	+	Na, Mg block	85 pS	weak voltage dependence	Sensor of ATP_i	$I_{b.g.}$
Ca-activated K channel	+	open channel noise on strong depo.	200 pS	activation & inactivation (depo)	rapid repolarization sensor of Ca_i	Transient outward current
Na-activated K channel	+	Mg block	200 pS	—	sensor of Na_i	$I_{b.g.}$

RESULTS AND DISCUSSION

General characteristics of the cardiac K channels

Table 1 summarizes the characteristics of the K channels so far identified in the cardiac cells. Usually a high potassium ion (K^+) solution (150 mM) is used for the pipette solution facing to the external surface of the membrane in order to increase the single K channel current. The single channel conductace increases proportional to the 0.3-0.5th power of the external K concentrations (K_o), varying with different types of the K channels. In the table, conductances at 140-150 mM K^+ are described. Under such a condition, the equilibrium potential for K^+ is nearly zero mV across the patch membrane under the suction pipette. With the pipette potential of 0 mV, therefore, K^+ carries an inward current driven by the resting membrane potential. If the driving force for K^+ is changed by varying the pipette potential, the amplitude of the inward K current varies almost in an ohmic manner. However, when the driving force for K^+ is reversed, the amplitude of the outward-going current of most of the K channels is smaller than that of the inward-going current driven by the same magnitude of the potential difference. In certain types of the K channel the outward-going signal has not been clearly identified under the cell-attached conditions, because of its small size or rapid closure of the channel on depolarization. These characteristics are called inward or anomarous rectification (7).

Inward rectifier K channel

The inward rectifier K channel was first analysed when the patch clamp technique was introduced in the cardiac muscle (8-11). This channel is a cardiac representative of the class of K channel which has been described in other tissues under a category of the inward rectifier K channel (12-16). The channel conductance has been examined in the inward direction, since it was difficult to identify the outward current through this channel. The slope conductance is roughly proportional to the square root of K_o, which was varied over the range of 20-150 mM.

Transient outward current through the inward rectifier K channel was recorded in the whole cell recording under the condition of internal perfusion with Cs-rich internal solution (17). Recently, the outward current was also recorded with K-rich internal solution and also single channel recording of the outward current was succeeded in a modified inside-out patch recording configuration (18). At 15°C, the outward current was deactivated with an average time constant of less than 10 ms at around the potassium equilibrium potential (E_K). The time constant exponentially decreased for potentials more positive to E_K. The instantaneous current-voltage relation for the whole cell current and the single channel current-voltage (i-V) relation were almost linear. It was also found that the outward single channel currents were blocked by an application of Mg^{2+} into the bath facing to the inner surface of the membrane. Thus, the rectification of the current can be explained by a rapid closure of the channel on depolarization and by Mg^{2+} block of the outward current.

The whole cell current carried by the inward rectifier K channel most probably corresponds to the I_{K1} defined by Noble (19) in Purkinje fibers. I_{K1} has also been described in ventricular cells (20-21) and in atrial cells (22). The density of distribution of the inward rectifier K channel is quite high and the open probability of the inward rectifier K channel is near its maximum at around the resting membrane potential (9, 11). Thus, the resting K conductance of the ventricular and atrial cells is mostly generated by this channel. It should be noted that the channel is scarcely found in the nodal pacemaker tissues (23).

Most of other K channels also show inward-going retification and were often called inward rectifier. For example, the muscarinic receptor-operated K channel is sometimes called as inward rectifier. However, the nature of the muscarinic receptor-operated K channel is completely different from that of the inward rectifier K channel (24). In order to avoid confusion in designation, the term inward rectifier should be used for the K channel discussed above.

<u>Delayed rectifier K channel.</u>

The pacemaker tissue of the S-A node or those having a potency of generating the spontaneous action potential, such as the A-V node cell, atrial cells or the Purkinje fibers, show the outward current, which activates during depolarization and decays slowly on repolarization (outward current tail) to the potential range of the pacemaker potential (see for review, 25, 26). Depending on different kinetics, the current was separated into various components, such as I_{K2}, I_x and I_K in different tissues. Except the current defined as I_{K2}, these outward currents have been considered to be carried by K channels. The estimation of the limiting conductance at various potentials (or the fully-activated current-voltage relation), consistently suggested inward-going rectification of the channel.

Single channel currents of the delayed rectifier K current (I_K) were recently recorded from the isolated nodal cells (27). The reversal potentials, estimated by extrapolating the i-V relations at different K^+ concentrations, well agreed with E_K and indicated that the channel is a selective K channel. It has a rather small unit conductance of about 10 pS at 150 mM K_o. The single channel conductance was approximately proportional to the square root of K_o and was voltage-independent over the negative potential range. The correspondence of this channel to the delayed rectifier K current was demonstrated by calculating the ensemble average of the single channel current records. After a conditioning depolarization to activate the channel, the hyperpolarization induced inward-going single channel current at the initial part of the voltage jump. The open probability of the channel decreased exponentially after the onset of the repolarization. The time constant for deactivation well agreed with that of the whole cell recordings of I_K.

The outward unitary current through the channel has not been identified. The mechanism of rectification is not yet clarified.

The single kinetic parameter has been assumed for simplicity to describe the time-dependent changes in I_K, although the tail current showed at least two exponential components (28-30). In the single channel analysis the kinetics of the channel was more complicated than expected from the single gating kinetics (Shibasaki, personal communication). The activation of the delayed rectifier K channel during depolarization may play a role in terminating the action potential. Following deactivation may underlie the slow diastolic depolarization (31). In the pacemaker tissue the background K conductance is relatively small, because of the negligible population of the inward rectifier K channel. Thus,

the K conductance of the nodal cell is dominated by the delayed
rectifier K channel and the amplitude of the slow diastolic
depolarization is large enough to generate the significant pacemaker potential. When the background K conductance is increased by
acetylcholine (ACh) stimulation of the muscarinic receptor (see
below), the contribution of the delayed rectifier becomes relatively small and the pacemaker potential is depressed.

Muscarinic receptor-operated K channel.

The negative chronotropic control of the heart rate by the vagal
nerve is mediated by ACh, which increases the membrane K conductance through interaction with the muscarinic receptor in the
pacemaker tissue (32, 33). The conventional voltage clamp
experiments on the ACh-induced K current disclosed that the current
has a peculiar voltage-dependent kinetics, which is different from
those of the delayed rectifier K current or the inward rectifier
(34). Therefore, a discrete class of K channels was suggested to
underlie the muscarinic response.

The single channel recording indicated, in fact, that the
muscarinic receptor-operated K channel has larger single channel
conductance than the inward rectifier K channel (24). The average
life time of the open-channel current is quite short, less than
1/30 of the inward rectifier K channel. The kinetics of the
channel is mostly determined by the concentration of ACh, but the
voltage-dependent kinetics is also present. The open-probability
decreases on depolarization and increases on hyperpolarization.
Even in the absence of agonists, the channel can open at a very low
open probability (35).

Because of the presence of certain delay before the initiation
of the muscarinic response, it has long been suggested that an
unknown intracellular second messenger is involved. However,
experiments injecting possible second messengers into the single
cell preparation failed to identify the second messenger (36).
Furthermore, the single K channel responded to ACh applied in the
patch pipette, but did not respond to ACh applied in the bath (35).
Recent findings strongly suggested that a type of GTP-binding
protein couples the muscarinic receptor with the K channel. This
view was proved by the following findings (37-40). (1) In the

absence of GTP in the internal solution, the K current was not activated by the agonists. (2) The pertussis toxin, which is a selective blocker of the inhibitory GTP-binding protein, blocked the muscarinic response. (3) In the presence of GTPγS, the agonist activated the K current irreversibly. The characteristic delay of the muscarinic ACh response may be explained by the delayed interactions between the receptor, GTP-binding protein and the channel on the plane of the surface membrane (35).

The outward current is usually difficult to record with the cell-attached patch recording. Thus, inward-going rectification was suggested. Recently, effects of intracellular Mg^{2+} was examined in the inside-out patch recording (Horie and Irisawa, personal communication). They found that in the absence of intra-cellular Mg^{2+}, the channel conductance was almost ohmic.

ATP-regulated K channel.

A class of K channels is activated when the intracellular ATP concentration is decreased below a certain level ($<$2 mM, in heart cells), and these channels were found not only in the cardiac muscle (41-47), but also in the skeletal muscle (48, 49) and in the pancreatic b-cells (50, 51). The existence of the ATP-regulated K channel has been demonstrated in the adult ventricular, atrial and nodal cells and also in the cultured neonatal cells at a relatively high density.

The conductance of the ATP-regulated K channel is large, about 80 pS at 150 mM K_O. The dependence of the channel conductance on K_O is relatively shallow than expected from the constant field theory. The i-V relation also shows an apparent inward-going rectification. The slope conductance is almost constant over the potential range negative to E_K, but the unit amplitude becomes smaller than expected from the linear relationship as the potential is shifted toward positive potentials. The depression of the outward current was partially explained by a voltage-dependent block of the channel by the intracellular Na^+ (47). Recently, Mg^{2+} ions were also found to block the channel only from the intra-cellular side and the blockage became stronger with depolarization (52). In the absence of both Na^+ and Mg^{2+}, the i-V relationship is almost linear. The Mg^{2+} effect was consistent with a simple model for the open channel blocker, in which Mg^2 can enter the inner mouth of the channel, but cannot pass through the channel pore. Thereby, Mg^{2+} interfers the passage of the outward-going K^+. It was concluded that under anoxic conditions, the channel is activated and the membrane K conductance is increased. However, excess loss of intracellular K^+ during the plateau of the cardiac action potential is inhibited by the voltage-dependent block of the channel by the intracellular Na^+ and Mg^{2+}.

The channel knetics is mainly determined by the intracellular ATP concentration. The voltage-dependent kinetics is practically not significant. In this sense, it may be said that the channel generates a time-independent background K current. The channel is closed not only by ATP but also by GTP and UTP. ADP at relatively high concentrations also blocks the channel, but AMP or adenosin fails to affect the channel at physiological concentrations. The non-hydrolysable ATP analogue, AMPPNP, also closes the channel. The relationship between the ATP concentration and the channel open probability was consistent with 3-4:1 binding and a half-maximum concentration of 0.5 mM. In the skeletal muscle, 1:1 binding and a dissociation constant of 0.13 mM were obtained (49). It is likely that the channel itself has a receptor site facing toward the intracellular media or that an independent ATP-receptor molecule is directly coupled to the K channel and regulate the open probability of the channel. It might be viewed that the channel plays a role as a chemical sensor in transducing the intracellular ATP concentration into a electrical signal and regulating the cardiac excitability.

<u>Ca-activated K channel.</u>

A class of K channels is activated when the intracellular Ca^2 concentration is raised in various cells, i.e. cultured muscle cells (53, 54), ganglion cells (55), chromaffin cells (56) and smooth muscle cells (see also for more extensive references, 57). Such a Ca-activated K channel has been assumed also in the cardiac muscle to be involved in the transient outward current (58-60) and also in the alteration of the cardiac excitation during Ca injection (61, 62). However, trials to see the Ca-activated K channel in the inside-out patch, which was exposed to a Ca-containing solution, failed to disclose such a channel in the ventricular and atrial cells. Recently large conductance Ca-activated K channel was found in cow cardiac Purknje fibers when the internal Ca concentration was raised from 0.01 μM to 1 μM (63). The single channel conductance depended on the external K concentration; 200 pS at 140 mM K_o, 140 pS at 70 mM K_o and 120 pS at 10.8 mM K_o. The i-V relation was almost linear in the voltage range between +10 and 110 mV. With stronger depolarization the open channel noise was found accompanied with an apparent decrease in the unit amplitude.

The ensemble average of the single channel current showed rapid activation of the channel (tau = 5-20 ms) and following inactivation (tau = 30-100 ms). The channel may be responsible for the transient outward current in the cow Purkinje fiber.

Na-activated K channel.

A class of K channel was found in the ventricular cell, which was activated by the intracellular Na^+ of $>$20 mM, but not by the intracellular Ca^{2+} (64). An increase of the K conductance was confirmed in the whole cell current recording when the cell was dialysed using the high Na^+ pipette solution. The single channel conductance of about 200 pS is the largest within the cardiac K channels. The slope conductance decreased at potentials more positive to the E_K, indicating an inward-going rectification of the single channel current. Opening of the channel was usually accompanied by repetitive brief closures and the open channel current appeared as a burst of openings. It seems that the burst at least in the outward current is caused by a flickery block by the intracellular Mg^{2+} and Na^+ (Horie and Irisawa, personal communication).

The kinetics is almost voltage-independent, but depends on Na_i. The relationship between Na_i and the open probability could be explained by 3:1 binding and the half maximum concentration of 66 mM of Na_i.

The contribution of this channel under physiological conditions is not totally clear, because its sensitivity is rather low compared to the normal Na_i of less than 10 mM. The density of distribution seems to be relatively low, according to the infrequent apperance of the channel in the single channel recording.

Conclusion.

The number of types of cardiac K channels revealed by the single channel recording is almost equal or even larger than the number of current components defined in the conventional voltage clamp experiments, such as I_{K1}, I_{K2}, I_{X1}, I_{X2}, I_K, etc. However, we can now define individual channel not only in terms of different kinetics, but also by the single channel conductance, and by the sensitivity to physiological substances, which are present inside and outside the cell. It became evident that each type of K channel has its own unique functions in the genesis of cardiac excitation or in reflecting the change in the intracellular media to the membrane excitability.

The inward-going rectification of the K channels except that of the delayed rectifier K channel seems to be due to blockade of the channel pore by the intracellular Mg^{2+} and/or Na^+. The blockade becomes stronger with depolarization. Thus, the mechanism may be very useful in providing the low K conductance during plateau of the action potential and also to inhibit an excess loss of intracellular K.

Acknowledgement; This work was supported by a Grant-in-Aid for Special Project Research from the Japanese Ministry of Education, Science and Culture.

1. Deck, K.A. and Trautwein, W. Pflugers Arch. 280:63-80, 1964.
2. Noble, D. and Tsien, R.W. J. Physiol. (Lond) 195:185-214, 1968.
3. Noble, D. and Tsien, R.W. J. Physiol. (Lond) 200:205-231, 1969a.
4. Noble, D. and Tsien, R.W. J. Physiol. (Lond) 200:233-254, 1969b.
5. Hamill, O.P., Marty, A., Neher, E., Sakmann, B. and Sigworth, F.J. Pflugers Arch. 391:85-100, 1981.
6. Hille, B. In: Ionic Channels of Excitable Membranes, Sinauer Associates Inc., Sunderland, Massachusetts, 1984.
7. Adrian, R.H. Prog. Biohys. Mol. Biol. 19:340-369, 1969.

8. Trube, G., Sakmann, B. and Trautwein, W. Pflugers Arch. 391:R7, 1982.
9. Kameyama, M., Kiyosue, T. and Soejima, M. Jpn. J. Physiol. 33:1039-1056, 1983.
10. Sakmann, B. and Trube, G. J. Physiol. (Lond) 347:641-657, 1984a.
11. Sakmann, B. and Trube, G. J. Physiol. (Lond) 347;659-683, 1984b.
12. Adrian, R.H., Chandler, W.K. and Hodgkin, A.L. J. Physiol. (Lond) 208:645-668, 1970.
13. Hagiwara, S., Miyazaki, S. and Rosenthal, N.P. J. Gen. Physiol. 67:621-638, 1976.
14. Fukushima, Y. Nature 294:368-371, 1981.
15. Fukushima, Y. J. Physiol. (Lond) 331:311-331, 1982.
16. Ohmori, H., Yoshida, S. and Hagiwara, S. Proc. Natl. Acad. Sci. U.S.A. 78:4960-4964, 1981.
17. Matsuda, H. and Noma, A. J. Physiol. (Lond) 357:553-573, 1984.
18. Matsuda, H., Saigusa, A. and Irisawa, H. Proc. Int. Uni. Physiol. Sci. 16:P266.04, 1986.
19. Noble, D. J. Physiol.(Lond). 160:317-352, 1962.
20. Beeler, G.W.Jr. and Reuter, H. J. Physiol. (Lond) 207: 165-190, 1970.
21. McDonald, T.F. and Trautwein, W. J. Physiol. (Lond) 274:217-246, 1978.
22. Rougier, O., Vassort, G. and Stampfli, R. Pflugers Arch. 301:91-108, 1968.
23. Noma, A., Nakayama, T., Kurachi, Y. and Irisawa, H. Jpn. J. Physiol. 34:245-254, 1984.
24. Sakmann, B., Noma, A. and Trautwein, W. Nature 303:250-253, 1983.
25. Carmeliet, E. and Vereecke, J. In: Handbook of Physiology, Sec. 2, The Cardiovascular System, Vol. 1, The Heart, Am. Physiol. Soc., Bethesda, Maryland, 1979, pp. 269-297.
26. Irisawa, H. Physiol. Rev. 58:461-498, 1978.
27. Shibasaki, T. and Irisawa, H. Proc. Int. Uni. Physiol. Sci. 16:P266.07, 1986.
28. Noma, A. and Irisawa, H. Pflugers Arch. 366:251-25, 1976.
29. DiFrancesco, D., Noma, A and Trautwein, W. Pflugers Arch. 381:271-279, 1979.
30. Yanagihara, K. and Irisawa, H. Pflugers Arch. 388:255-260, 1980.
31. Yanagihara, K., Noma, A. and Irisawa, H. Jpn. J. Physiol. 30:841-857, 1980.
32. Harris, E.J. and Hutter, O.F. J. Physiol. (Lond) 133:58P, 1956.
33. Trautwein, W. and Dudel, J. Pflugers Arch. 266:324-334, 1958.
34. Noma, A. and Trautwein, W. Pflugers Arch. 381:263-269, 1978.
35. Soejima, M. and Noma, A. Pflugers Arch. 400:424-431, 1984.

36. Trautwein, W., Taniguchi, J. and Noma, A.   Pflugers Arch. 392:307-314, 1982.
37. Pfaffinger, P.J., Martin, J.M., Hunter, D.D., Nathanson, N.M. and Hille, B.   Nature 317:536-538, 1985.
38. Breitwieser, G.E. and Szabo, G. Nature 317:538-540, 1985.
39. Sorota, S., Tsuji, Y., Tajima, T. and Pappano, A.J.   Circ. Res. 57:748-758, 1985.
40. Endoh, M., Maruyama, M. and Iijima, T.   Am. J. Physiol. 249:H309-320, 1985.
41. Trube, G. and Hescheler, J.   Naunyn-Schmiedebergs Arch. of Pharmacology 322:R64, 1983.
42. Trube, G. and Hescheler, J.   Pflugers Arch. 401:178-184, 1984.
43. Noma, A.   Nature 305:147-148, 1983.
44. Kakei, M. and Noma, A.   J. Physiol. (Lond) 352:265-284, 1984.
45. Kakei, M., Noma, A. and Shibasaki, T.   J. Physiol. (Lond) 363:441-462, 1985.
46. Noma, A. and Shibasaki, T.   J. Physiol.(Lond) 363:463-480, 1985.
47. Noma, A.   Biomed. Res. 7(Suppl):95-98, 1986.
48. Spruce, A.E., Standen, N.B. and Stanfield, P.R.   Nature 316:736-738, 1985.
49. Spruce, A.E., Standen, N.B. and Stanfield, P.R.   J. Physiol. (Lond) in press.
50. Cook, D.L. and Hales, C.N.   Nature 311:271-273, 1984.
51. Ashcroft, F.M., Ashcroft, S.J.H. and Harrison, D.E.   J. Physiol. (Lond) 369:101P, 1985.
52. Horie, M., Noma, A. and Irisawa, H.   Proc. Int. Uni. Physiol. Sci. 16:P266.05, 1986.
53. Pallotta, B.S., Magleby, K.L. and Barrett, J.N.   Nature 293:471-474, 1981.
54. Barrett, J.N., Magleby, K.L. and Pallotta, B.S.   J. Physiol. (Lond) 331:211-230, 1982.
55. Lux, H.D., Neher, E. and Marty, A.   Pflugers Arch. 389:293-295, 1981.
56. Marty, A.   Nature 291:497-500, 1981.
57. Inoue, R., Kitamura, K. and Kuriyama, H.   Pflugers Arch. 405:173-179, 1985.
58. Deck, K.A., Kern, R. and Trautwein, W.   Pflugers Arch. 280:50-62, 1964.
59. Kenyon, J.L. and Gibbons, W.R.   J. Gen. Physiol. 73:139-157, 1979.
60. Siegelbaum, S.A. and Tsien, R.W. J. Physiol. (Lond) 299:485-506, 1980.
61. Isenberg, G.   Pflugers Arch. 371:71-76, 1977a.
62. Isenberg, G.   Pflugers Arch. 371:77-84, 1977b.
63. Callewaert, G., Vereecke, J. and Carmeliet, E.   Pflugers Arch. 406:424-426, 1986.
64. Kameyama, M., Kakei, M., Sato, R., Shibasaki, T., Matsuda, H. and Irisawa, H.   Nature 309:354-356, 1984.

4

Na AND Ca CHANNELS IN THE HEART

ARTHUR M. BROWN, DIANA L. KUNZE and ANTONIO E. LACERDA

Department of Physiology and Molecular Biophysics, Baylor College of Medicine, One Baylor Plaza, Houston, Texas 77030

INTRODUCTION

Thanks to the development of the gigaseal patch-clamp method (34) cardiac membrane electrophysiology has entered the molecular phase thus allowing single- Na- and Ca-channel proteins to be studied in the living state. The application of this approach has been particularly fortuitous because the development of viable isolated adult cell preparations (48,49,78,79,93) so important for adequate voltage clamping involved enzymatic dispersion which also prepared the cell membranes in such a way as to allow gigaseals to be made. Although the single-channel method has the highest resolution of any electrophysiological method presently available, data analysis is tedious and the method itself suffers from bandwidth limitation. Therefore, application of the voltage-clamp method to single cells (11) has been very important and provides a necessary reference for interpreting the single-channel results.

CALCIUM CURRENTS

Ca-current measurements in single cardiac myocytes have confirmed many of the previous results obtained in multicellular preparations, however there are important quantitative differences. In single myocytes, Ca-current density seems to be larger than expected from measurements on multicellular preparations and the activation and inactivation kinetics are faster (50), but see Hume and Giles (46), Mitchell et al. (69), and Noble (74). Part of this discrepancy may be due to the series resistance in multicellular preparations, but other possibilities, such as nonuniformities and time-varying changes of electrochemical potentials in the clefts (62,90), may also be of importance. Another interesting property of Ca current originally discovered in intact preparations was its relatively negative reversal potential (E_{rev}) which does not agree with the much more positive Ca equilibrium potential (E_{Ca}). In internally dialyzed cells it was shown that the negative shift of E_{rev} resulted from a small permeability to K ions (58,60) as previously suggested for intact preparations (83). More recently, outward current, presumably carried by K ions through single Ca channels, has been reported in channels that have been treated with large doses of BAY K8644, a dihydropyridine (DHP) Ca-channel agonist that at these concentrations markedly prolongs the single-channel lifetime (36).

As a rule, Ca channels are much more selective for divalent versus monovalent cations (60,66,83) and Sr and Ba have been found to carry inward current as well as Ca ions (33,81). It has been known for some time that Ca channels acquire the ability to pass monovalent cations such a Na, Li, N_2H_5, and NH_3OH under conditions in which divalent cations are completely removed and Ca-chelating substances such as EDTA or EGTA are added. This was first described in amphibian heart (18,85) and has since been found in other excitable cells (2,55,38). The result has been explained using a rate-theory model of ion permeation in which two ions can occupy the channel at one time. When they are both Ca ions, the repulsive force between the two lowers the apparent affinity at one of the sites, thereby increasing the effective mobility. When the other ion is a monovalent ion, the divalent ion binds with a high affinity, thereby reducing the likelihood that the monovalent cation will pass on through the channel (38).

Ca current is also dependent on intracellular Ca concentration (52,65), but see Noble (74). When Ca is injected into the ventricular cell, the duration of the action potential rapidly shortens, transient depolarization is elicited, and, finally, the action potential disappears. However, when EGTA is injected, prolongation of the action-potential duration is observed (67). Ca current is abolished within 5 min when the concentration of Ca within the patch pipette increases from 10^{-9} to 10^{-7} M, without changing inactivation kinetics during a step pulse (28,47). It is probable that the process is too slow to be detected during the usual test pulse durations that are employed.

Recently single-channel cardiac Ca currents have been recorded (9,17,37,84). These studies have shown that at the single-channel level the behavior is stochastic, but at the population level the behavior is deterministic, in this case voltage-dependent. At a given potential the amplitude is constant. Single-channel slope conductance with 90 to 96 mM Ba in the pipette ranges from 15 to 25 picosiemens, whereas with 50 mM Ca or Ba it is 9 to 10 picosiemens. The I-V relationship is approximately ohmic over a rather narrow potential range, but seems to agree with earlier results obtained from tail-current analysis over a far wider range of potentials (83). The relationship between open-state probability, p, and voltage also seems to be similar, although, again, for technical reasons referred to earlier, the comparison was made over a fairly narrow range. All the evidence suggests only two conducting states: open and closed. As we shall discuss subsequently, the interpretation of the data favors a single open state and multiple closed states. There is also compelling evidence for an inactivated state that is accessed from the open state (Ca-current-dependent inactivation) by the single channel (64).

The basic properties of voltage-dependent single Ca channels appear to be very similar in various tissues (8). More recently, however, a second clearly-defined Ca channel has been described in dorsal root ganglion (DRG) cells (16,76) and may be present in other cells as well. As a result Bean (6) has reported this possibility in dog atrial cells, and similar properties have been observed in GH_3 cells, an anterior pituitary tumor cloned cell line (68). The newly identified channel has a lower threshold (ca. -60 mV), with rapid, voltage-dependent inactivation. It has a slow tail current and possibly a greater relative permeability to Ca ion than to Ba ion. There are also pharmacological differences between the two sets of channels. In what follows, we the more customary high-threshold channels will be dealt with because thus far there have been no descriptions of the single-channel behavior of the low-threshold channels in cardiac muscle.

The most complete single-channel studies on cardiac Ca channels are those of Cavalié et al. (17). These investigators have shown that the activation kinetics can be realized by a minimum three-state model. They have shown, as have others, that the open time distribution is described by a single exponential function consistent with a single open state.

The closed times are described by at least two exponentials, as will be discussed later. Additionally, a comparison of Ba and Ca conductions was made. The Ba permeability was higher, but the differences in the various state occupancies were subtle and probably cannot entirely account for the obvious kinetic differences present in the whole-cell currents, i.e., the very much slower inactivation of Ba currents. An interesting feature of these studies was the fact that prolonged recordings showed clearly the occurrence of clustering in addition to the well-known bursting. The clustering can be regarded, in a way, as bursting of bursts. The implication is that the inactivation process is clearly related to this process. If this interpretation is correct, it means that one of the inactivated states is not absorbing. Moreover, there were no changes in amplitude or open times, indicating that inactivation resides entirely in the kinetics with which the various states of the Ca channel are traversed.

Unlike Na channels, Ca channels are modulated by hormones and neurotransmitters (82,98,99). In agreement with earlier results from syncytial preparations (53), β-adrenoceptor agonists increase Ca current in single mammalian myocytes without changing kinetics (50,102), although in frog cells the activation and inactivation kinetics were slowed (7). At the single-channel level, the effect appears to be due to a reduction in nulls and a reduction of the dwell time in an early closed state C_1 (15).

It is still controversial as to whether or not β-agonists make an additional contribution by changes in the number of functional channels (N_F). Bean et al. (54) reported that β-adrenergic stimulation increased N_F per cell. On the other hand, Brum et al. (13) concluded that on β-adrenergic stimulation, N_F remained unchanged. Studies recently appearing in the literature have modified the single-Ca-channel activity. Among them, DHP compounds are the most interesting. For example, BAY K8644 and CGP 28,392, both similar in structure to the DHP Ca-channel antagonist nifedipine, increase cardiac contractility and divalent cation influx (87,88,96).

There is evidence that the function of Ca current is closely related to the metabolic state of the intracellular milieu. Possibly one of the most striking findings is that Ca-channel activity disappears quite rapidly after excising a membrane patch. This does not occur with Na and most K channels, although a slow decline can occur for these channels as

well. In other experiments, injections of the various adenine
nucleotides other than ATP (i.e., ADP, AMP, and CP) all enhanced the
action-potential amplitude and prolonged its duration (94). The
prolongation of the action potential may suggest a concomitant increase
in Ca current. Application of CN-Tyrode or DNP solution invariably
caused a shortening of the action potential, whereas a reduction in Ca
current was not so obvious, and an increase in the outward current was
responsible for the shortening of the action-potential duration (51,94).

Ca channels can be blocked by various organic compounds. The
mechanisms of action of some of these Ca-channel blockers have been
analyzed recently in multicellular (97) and single-cell cardiac
preparations (59). Verapamil and its derivatives (D600) block Ca
channels predominantly from the inside surface of the membrane (35) by
entering the channel preferentially when it is open. This also applies
to diltiazem (59). The blocking potencies of these charged tertiary
amines depend on membrane potential (voltage dependence) and on the rate
of stimulation (use dependence). This is in contrast to the effects of
the DHPs (nifedipine, nitrendipine, nisoldipine), which are uncharged at
physiological pH and do not show voltage and use dependence (53,59).
However, important discrepancies exist if one compares the blocking
effects of DHP on I_{Ca} with radioligand binding (32) of this class of
compounds to putative Ca channels in homogenates or crudely purified
particular fractions of cardiac sarcolemma. The K_d value estimated from
the blocking potency of Ca current by nitrendipine is two to three orders
of magnitude higher than the K_d values obtained in radioligand-binding
studies (59). However, the discrepancy appears to have been resolved by
Sanguinetti and Kass (86) and Bean (5) who showed that K_d was much
smaller when cardiac membrane was held at depolarized potentials at which
most channels are inactivated (10). Another discrepancy is that in the
electrophysiological experiments Ca ions compete with nitrendipine at its
binding site, an opposite effect has been reported for radioligand
binding (63). Ca and other divalent cations in the micromolar-to-
millimolar range even facilitate ^{3}H-nitrendipine and ^{3}H-nimodipine
binding.

Also suggested by receptor binding studies is that nitrendipine and
DHP bind to a common receptor site that differs from, but is

allosterically linked to, the site or sites at which other Ca antagonists such as diltiazem and verapamil bind (26). Thus, as Ca-channel labels, they seemed to be useful toward eventual biochemical isolation, purification, and reconstitution of Ca channels.

We have studied the Ca agonist and Ca antagonist effects on whole-cell and single-channel Ca currents of single heart cell. Bay K8644 and CGP 28,392 increased whole-cell Ca current in a dose-dependent manner, and ED_{50} values were similar to those reported for contractility in rabbit aorta and guinea pig heart. The measured ED_{50} was also consistent with the apparent dissociation constant (K_d) of a high-affinity binding site present in cardiac sarcolemmal vesicles. We proposed that the molecular basis for these results in an increase in the probability that a single Ca channel, having opened and closed, will subsequently reopen during membrane depolarization. At high concentrations of BAY K8644 and in the presence of 96 mM Ba, different effects are observed, primarily a marked prolongation of open time (9).

SODIUM CURRENTS

Progress has also been rapid in this area for similar reasons. Furthermore, experience with the structural features of syncytial preparations has allowed better delineation of the limits of these preparations and therefore facilitated comparison with the more rigorously controlled situations in single-cell and single-channel experiments. Experiments in rabbit Purkinje fibers with wide intercellular clefts (21,22), in tightly coupled cell aggregates (27,72), and in isolated single mammalian ventricular cells (12,57,61) have provided useful comparative information. One finding of importance that has emerged is the pronounced nonlinear relation between g_{Na} and V_{max} of the action potential, as suggested earlier from calculations of g_{Na} and V_{max} in nerve (20,100).

A voltage clamp with two suction pipettes allowed Brown et al. (11,12) to analyze Na current quantitatively in rat ventricular cells. The Na current produced by single depolarizing steps from a holding potential of -80 mV had a threshold between -70 and -60 mV and a peak at -30 to -20 mV. The peak current was on the order of 70 to 140 nA. Current densities at peak currents in 145 mM Na were 0.5 to 1.0 mA/cm^2, based on an average cell surface area of 15,000 μM^2 (77). Maximum Na conductance (g_{Na}) was calculated to be 25 mS/cm^2 in a 145 mM Na solution. In cultured spherical cells prepared from one-day-old neonatal rats, the peak amplitude was less than 300 pA which was more than likely due to the small size of the cell (14), but see Yatani and Brown (101). The work of Brown and associates also showed that the kinetics of cardiac Na currents could be described by two inactivation processes; one fast, the other slower. The ratio of the fast τ and the activation τ was similar to that described for mammalian nerve, and the voltage dependences were similar also. The slower process could be associated with Na-current involvement in the plateau of the action potential, because this cannot be attributed to a window current, which would not be present at such potentials (4). This component is striking in single-channel recordings of Na channels (56) and is a clue that allowed certain kinetic models to be excluded.

Direct single-channel recordings by means of the patch-clamp method have shown similarities of certain features of Na-channel behavior in various excitable cells. Ensemble averages of hundreds of single-channel records yield mean currents, I, identical with the macroscopic Na currents obtained from whole-cell recordings. The Na-channel density per unit surface area ranges from about 1 to 2 channels μM^{-2} in cultured cardiac cells (14) to about 16 μM^{-2} in neuroblastoma cells (80).

Single-Na-channel slope conductance at 16 to 18°C is about 15 picosiemens in cultured cardiac cells from neonatal rat hearts (14), a value similar to that obtained in cultured muscle cells (45,89), neuroblastoma cells (80), and chromaffin cells (28). The I-V relation flattens at hyperpolarized potentials, probably because of Ca effects on single-channel conductance (103). Gating of the channels (i.e., their opening, closing, and inactivation properties as functions of voltage) also shares features with other cell types. Channel open times increase with depolarization and inactivation of the channels during depolarization and, in the steady state, after conditioning clamp steps results from a reduced opening probability, not a decrease in single-channel current. However, the occurrence of the slower inactivation process was also responsible for certain differences. Therefore, in neuroblastoma cells, a channel, having opened, was more likely to have passed to an absorbing inactivated state than to a state from which it could reopen (1). This, in addition to a rather wide dispersion of latencies to first opening or waiting times, led to the proposal that the kinetic scheme for Na channels differed grossly from that proposed by Hodgkin and Huxley (41). In the early model, activation was assumed to occur quickly and inactivation slowly, and state models of the chemical-kinetics variety (29) assumed this to be the case. In the new model, the opposite is the case. Activation occurs slowly and is widely dispersed in time, and inactivation is fast. The results in cardiac cells, however, are not consistent with this idea (56) and may indicate fundamental differences.

Single-channel observations provided evidence that there may be more than one set of Na channels in neural cells (71), and suggestions along these lines have derived from single-channel studies in heart cell as well (14,56). It has been reported that in heart cells the Na channels functioning during the window current are more sensitive to tetrodotoxin (TTX) than the Na currents that flow during the upstroke (23), and it has been noted in single-channel studies that a differential TTX sensitivity occurs for channels having shorter waiting times (95). It also has been reported that in nerve cells there is a set of threshold channels that deactivate very slowly (30), but this has not been observed in ventricular cells (56).

Another set of questions regarding Na channels is their pharmacology (31). It is well known that the doses of TTX necessary for blockage of cardiac Na channels are about 100 times those required in nerve (12,19). Conversely, the required doses of local anesthetics are much less in heart. Two theories have been proposed for local anesthetics actions: the modulated-receptor hypothesis (25,39,40,42-44,92) and the guarded-gate hypothesis (91).

CONCLUSION

Technological advances resulting from the use of isolated single cells, internal dialysis combined with voltage clamp, and patch-clamp methods are revolutionizing cardiac electrophysiology. Other techniques not covered here, but certain to have equally profound effects, include reconstitution and channel isolation. Coronado and Latorre (24) have incorporated K and Cl channels prepared from bovine cardiac sarcolemmal membranes into lipid bilayers. The K channels seem to have many of the properties observed in intact preparations. The similar incorporations of functioning Na and Ca channels into lipid bilayers seem feasible (70,73).

The Na channel has been cloned and its primary structure is known (75). It is likely that the same techniques will be applied to the Ca channel and, of course, other membrane channels. This will open the way for site-specific mutagenesis, in which case the problem of the details of channel function at the structural level can be dealt with directly.

REFERENCES

1. Aldrich, R.W., Corey, D.P., and Stevens, C.F. Nature. 306:436-441, 1983.

2. Almers, W., and McLeskey, E.W. J. Physiol. 353:585-608, 1984.

3. Armstrong, C. J. Gen. Physiol. 50:491-503, 1966.

4. Attwell, D., Cohen, I., Eisner, D., Ohba, M., and Ojeda, C. Pfluegers Arch. 379:137-142, 1979.

5. Bean, B.P. Proc. Natl. Acad. Sci. USA 81:6388-6392, 1984.

6. Bean, B.P. Biophys. J. 47:497a, 1985.

7. Bean, B.P., Nowycky, M.C., and Tsien, R.W. Nature. 307:371-375, 1984.

8. Brown, A.M., Camerer, H., Kunze, D.L., and Lux, H.D. Nature. 299:156-158, 1982.

9. Brown, A.M., Kunze, D.L., and Yatani, A. Nature. 311:570-572, 1984.

10. Brown, A.M., Kunze, D.L., and Yatani, A. J. Physiol. (Lond.). 347:59P, 1984.

11. Brown, A.M., Lee, K.S., and Powell, T. J. Physiol. (Lond.). 318:455-477, 1981.

12. Brown, A.M., Lee, K.S. and Powell, T. J. Physiol. (Lond.). 318:479-500, 1981.

13. Brum, G., Osterrieder, W., and Trautwein, W. Pfluegers Arch. 401:111-118, 1984.

14. Cachelin, A.B., de Peyer, J.E., Kokubun, S., and Reuter, H. J. Physiol. (Lond.). 340:389-401, 1983.

15. Cachelin, A.B., de Peyer, J.E., Kokubun, S., and Reuter, H. Nature. 304:462-464, 1983.

16. Carbone, E., and Lux, H.D. Nature. 310:501-502, 1984.

17. Cavalié, A., Ochi, R., Pelzer, D. and Trautwein, W. Pfluegers Arch. 398:284-297, 1983.

18. Chesnais, J.M., Coraboeuf, E., Sauviat, M.P., and Vassas, J.M. J. Mol. Cell. Cardiol. 7:627-642, 1975.

19. Cohen, C.J., Bean, B.P., Colatsky, T.J., and Tsien, R.W. J. Gen. Physiol. 78:383-411, 1981.

20. Cohen, I., Attwell, D., and Stricharz, G. Proc. R. Soc. Lond. B214:85-98, 1981.

21. Colatsky, T.J. J. Physiol. (Lond.). 305:215-234, 1980.

22. Colatsky, T.J., and Tsien, R.W. J. Physiol. (Lond.). 290:227-252, 1979.

23. Coraboeuf, E., Deroubaix, E., and Coulombe, A. Am. J. Physiol. 237:H561-567, 1979.

24. Coronado, R., and Latorre, R. Nature. 298:849-852, 1982.

25. Courtney, K.R. J. Pharmacol. Exp. Ther. 195:225-236, 1975.

26. Depover, A., Matlib, M.A., Lee, S.W., Dube, G.P., Grupp, I.L., Grupp, G., and Schwartz, A. Biochem. Biophys. Res. Commun. 108:110-117, 1982.

27. Ebihara, L., Shigeto, N., Lieberman, M., and Johnson, E.A. J. Gen. Physiol. 75:437-456, 1980.

28. Fenwick, E.M., Marty, A., and Neher, E. J. Physiol. (Lond.). 331:599-635, 1982.

29. Fitzhugh, R. J. Cell. Comp. Physiol. (Suppl.). 66:111-117, 1965.

30. Gilly, W.F., and Armstrong, C.M. Nature. 309:448-450, 1984.

31. Grant, A.O., Starner, C.F., and Strauss, H.C. Circ. Res. 55:427-439, 1984.

32. Grossman, H., Ferry, D.R., Lübbecke, F., Mewes, R., and Hofmann, F. Trends Pharmacol. Sci. 3:431-437, 1982.

33. Hagiwara, S., and Byerly, L. Annu. Rev. Neurosci. 4:69-125, 1981.

34. Hamill, O.P., Marty, A., Neher, E. Sakmann, B., and Sigworth, F.J. Pfluegers Arch. 391:85-100, 1981.

35. Hescheler, J., Pelzer, D., Trube, G., and Trautwein, W. Pfluegers Arch. 392:287-291, 1982.

36. Hess, P., Lansman, J.B., and Tsien, R.W. J. Physiol. (Lond.). 359:9P, 1984.

37. Hess, P., Lansman, B., and Tsien, R.W. Nature. 311:538-544, 1984.

38. Hess, P., and Tsien, R.W. Nature. 311:453-456, 1984.

39. Hille, B. J. Gen. Physiol. 69:475-496, 1977.

40. Hille, B. J. Gen. Physiol. 69:497-515, 1977.

41. Hodgkin, A.L., and Huxley, A.F. J. Physiol. (Lond.). 117:500-544, 1952.

42. Hondeghem, L.M., and Katzung, B.G. Biochem. Biophys. Acta. 472:373-398, 1977.

43. Hondeghem, L.M., and Katzung, B.G. Circulation. 61:1217-1224, 1980.

44. Hondeghem, L.M., and Katzung, B.G. Annu. Rev. Pharmacol. Toxicol. 24:387-423, 1984.

45. Horn, R., Patlak, J., and Stevens, C.F. Nature. 291:426-427, 1981.

46. Hume, J.R., and Giles, W. J. Gen. Physiol. 81:153-194, 1983.

47. Insawa, H., and Kokubun, S. J. Physiol. (Lond.). 338:321-337, 1983.

48. Isenberg, G., and Klöckner, U. Nature. 284:358-360, 1980.

49. Isenberg, G., and Klöckner, U. Pfluegers Arch. 395:6-18, 1982.

50. Isenberg, G., and Klöckner, U. Pfluegers Arch. 395:30-41, 1982.

51. Isenberg, G., Vereecke, J., Van der Heyden, G., and Carmeliet, E. Pfluegers Arch. 397:251-259, 1983.

52. Josephson, I.R., Sanchez-Chapula, J., and Brown, A.M. Circ. Res. 54:144-156, 1984.

53. Kass, R.S. J. Pharmacol. Exp. Ther. 223:445-456, 1982.

54. Kostyuk, P.G., and Krishtal, O.A. J. Physiol. (Lond.). 270:545-568, 1977.

55. Kostyuk, P.G., Mironov, S.L., and Shuba, Y.M. J. Membr. Biol. 76:83-93, 1983.

56. Kunze, D.L., Lacerda, A.E., Wilson, D.L., and Brown, A.M. J. Gen. Physiol. 86:691-719, 1985.

57. Lee, K.S., Akaike, N., and Brown, A.M. J. Neuroscience Methods. 2:51-78, 1980.

58. Lee, K.S., and Tsien, R.W. Nature. 297:498-501, 1982.

59. Lee, K.S., and Tsien, R.W. Nature. 302:790-794, 1983.

60. Lee, K.S., and Tsien, R.W. J. Physiol. (Lond.). 354:253-272, 1984.

61. Lee, K.S., Weeks, T.A., Kao, R.L., Akaike, N., and Brown, A.M. Nature. 278:269-271, 1979.

62. Levis, R.A., Mathias, R.T., and Eisenberg, R.S. Biophys. J. 44:225-248, 1983.

63. Luchowski, E.M., Yousif, F., Triggle, D.J., Maurer, S.C., Sarmiento, J.G., and Janis, R.A. J. Pharmacol. Exp. Ther. 230:607-613, 1984.

64. Lux, H.D., and Brown, A.M. Science. 225:432-434, 1984.

65. Marban, E., and Tsien, R.W. Biophys. J. 33:143a, 1981.

66. Matsuda, H., and Noma, H. J. Physiol. (Lond.). 357:553-573, 1984.

67. Matsuda, H., Noma, A., Kurach, Y., and Irisawa, H. Circ. Res. 51:142-151, 1982.

68. Matteson, D.R., and Armstrong, C.M. J. Gen. Physiol. 83:371-394, 1984.

69. Mitchell, M.R., Powell, T., Terrar, D.A., and Twist, T. Proc. R. Soc. Lond. B219:447-469, 1983.

70. Moczydrowiski, E.G. Biophys. J. 47:190a, 1985.

71. Nagy, K., Kiss, T., and Hoff, D. Pfluegers Arch. 399:302-308, 1983.

72. Nathan, R.D., and DeHaan, R.L. J. Gen. Physiol. 73:175-198, 1979.

73. Nelson, M.T., French, R.J., and Krueger, B.K. Nature. 308:77-80, 1984.

74. Noble, D. J. Physiol. (Lond.). 353:1-50, 1984.

75. Noda, M., Shimizu, S., Tanabe, T., Takai, T., Kayano, T., Ikeda, T., Takahashi, H., Nakayma, H., Kanaoka, Y., Minamino, N., Kangawa, K., Matsuo, H., Raftery, M.A., Hirose, T., Inayama, S., Hayashida, H., Miyata, T., and Numa, S. Nature. 312:121-127, 1984.

76. Nowycky, M.C., Fox, A.P., and Tsien, R.W. Biophys. J. 45:36a, 1984.

77. Page, E., and McAllister, L.P. J. Ultrastruct. Res. 43:388-411, 1973.

78. Powell, T., Terrar, D.A., and Twist, V.W. J. Physiol. (Lond.). 302:131-153, 1980.

79. Powell, T., and Twist, V.W. Biochem. Biophys. Res. Commun. 72:327-333, 1976.

80. Quandt, F.N., and Narahashi, T. Proc. Natl. Acad. Sci. USA. 79:6732-6736, 1982.

81. Reuter, H. Prog. Biophys. 26:1-43, 1973.

82. Reuter, H. Annu. Rev. Physiol. 41:413-424, 1979.

83. Reuter, H., and Scholz, H. J. Physiol. (Lond.). 264:17-47, 1977.

84. Reuter, H., Stevens, C.F., Tsien, R.W., and Yellen, G. Nature. 297:501-504, 1982.

85. Rougier, O., Vassort, G., Garnier, D., Gargoul, Y.M., and Coraboeuf, E. Pfluegers Arch. 308:91-110, 1969.

86. Sanguinetti, M.C., and Kass, R.S. Circ. Res. 55:336-348, 1984.

87. Schramm, M., Thomas, G., Towart, R., and Franckowiak, G. Nature. 303:535-537, 1983.

88. Schramm, M., Thomas, G., Towart, R., and Franckowiak, G. Arzneim. Forsch. 33:1268-1272.

89. Sigworth, F.J., and Neher, E. Nature. 287:447-449, 1980.

90. Spray, D.C., Harris, A.L., and Bennet, M.V.L. Science. 204:432-434, 1979.

91. Starmer, C.F., Grant, A.O., and Strauss, H.C. Biophys. J. 46:15-27, 1984.

92. Strichartz, G.R. J. Gen. Physiol. 62:37-57, 1973.

93. Taniguchi, J., Kokubun, S., Noma, A., and Irisawa, H. Jpn. J. Physiol. 31:547-558, 1981.

94. Taniguchi, J., Noma, A., and Irisawa, H. Circ. Res. 53:131-139, 1983.

95. Ten Eick, R., Yeh, J., and Matsuki, N. Biophys. J. 45:70-73, 1984.

96. Thomas, G., Gross, R., and Schramm, M. J. Cardiovasc. Pharmacol. 6:1170-1176, 1984.

97. Trautwein, W., Pelzer, D., and McDonald, T.F. Circ. Res. (Suppl. I). $\underline{52}$:60-68, 1983.

98. Tsien, R.W. Adv. Cyclic Nucleotide Res. $\underline{8}$:363-420, 1977.

99. Tsien, R.W., and Siegelbaum, S. <u>In</u>: The Physiological Basis for Disorders of Biomembranes (Eds. T. Andreioli, J. F. Hoffman, and D. D. Fanestil), Plenum, New York, 1978, pp. 517-538.

100. Walton, M., and Fozzard, H.A. Biophys. J. $\underline{25}$:407-420, 1979.

101. Yatani, A., and Brown, A.M. Circ. Res. $\underline{57}$:868-875, 1985.

102. Yatani, A., Imoto, Y., and Goto, M. Jpn. J. Physiol. $\underline{34}$:337-349, 1984.

103. Yeh, J. <u>In</u>: Proteins in the Nervous System: Structure and Function (Eds. B. Haber, J. R. Perez-Polo, and J. D. Coulter), Alan R. Liss, New York, 1982, pp. 17-99.

5

SODIUM PATHWAYS IN AND OUT OF THE CARDIAC CELLS : RELATIONSHIP
TO INOTROPY

M. LAZDUNSKI, J. BARHANIN, M. FOSSET, C. FRELIN, D. PAURON, U.
QUAST*, J.F. RENAUD, G. ROMEY, P. VIGNE

Centre de Biochimie du CNRS, Parc Valrose, 06034 Nice Cedex, France

*Sandoz, Pharmaceutical Division, Preclinical Research, CH-4002 Basle,
Switzerland

The main systems involved in the regulation of the internal Na^+ level in the
cardiac cells are presented in Fig. 1. They include **(i)** the (Na^+,K^+)ATPase that is
the major efflux system for Na^+ (1), **(ii)** the Na^+/H^+ exchange system that is the
major influx system (2, 3), **(iii)** the $Na^+/K^+/Cl^-$ co-transport, **(iv)** the Na^+/Ca^2
exchange system. This latter system works in both directions (Na^+ influx coupled to
Ca^{2+} efflux or vice-versa) but only the mode corresponding to Ca^{2+} influx coupled
to Na^+ influx will be considered here in relation with inotropy.

The (Na^+,K^+)APase and its pharmacology in relation with inotropy

Our work has been carried out using chick cardiac cells in culture. These cells
have a high and a low affinity digitalis receptor but only one of them, the low
affinity receptor, is associated with the inotropic effects of the drug (1).
There are 1.4×10^6 low affinity sites (Na^+ pumps) for ouabain per cardiac cell.

Binding of $[^3H]$ouabain to the low affinity site corresponded closely to
ouabain inhibition of ^{86}Rb influx, to ouabain-induced accumulation of intracellular
Na^+ and to ouabain-induced increase in rate of Ca^{2+} entry. This Ca^{2+} entry, that
was not inhibited by Ca^{2+} channel blockers but was suppressed in the presence of
Li^+, was due to the Na^+/Ca^{2+} exchanger (1).

Dose-response curves for the ouabain induced inotropic effect were closely
correlated to ouabain concentration dependences of Na^+ accumulation and Ca^{2+}
entry (1). Therefore, the sequence of events leading to digitalis induced inotropy
is : ouabain inhibition of Na^+ efflux through the (Na^+,K^+)ATPase $\longrightarrow$ increase
of internal Na^+ concentration $\longrightarrow$ triggering of the activity of the Na^+/Ca^{2+}
exchanger $\longrightarrow$ more Ca^{2+} entry and more contraction (1).

It turns out that inotropic effects were observed as long as about 50% of the
total pumps are still active. A larger inhibition of the (Na^+,K^+)ATPase lead to
arythmia and cardiotoxic effects (1). The reason for these cardiotoxic effets is not

totally understood. It may be due to depolarization following inhibition of the Na^+ pump. It may also be due to the increase of Ca^{2+}_i which may activate non-specific, Ca^{2+}-dependent ionic channels (4). Activation of these channels would also lead to depolarization.

The Na+/H+ exchange system and diuretics of the amiloride family

The activity of the exchange system can be measured by a variety of techniques including **(i)** $^{22}Na^+$ influx techniques, **(ii)** H^+ efflux, **(iii)** changes of internal pH (2, 3, 5-9). The system is electroneutral and can work in both directions. However under normal conditions Na^+ entry is coupled to H^+ efflux (Fig. 1).

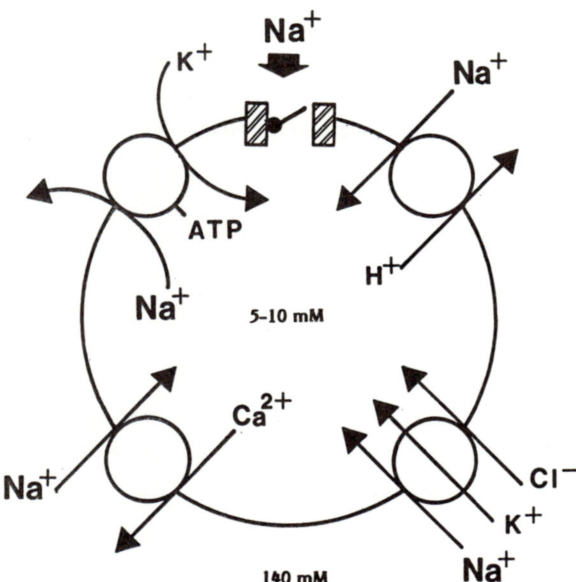

Fig. 1. The different Na^+ transport systems that regulate the internal sodium concentration in cardiac cells.

This system is the major entry pathway for Na^+ (2). It is responsible for nearly 50% of the Na^+ entry under steady-state conditions.

The Na^+/H^+ exchanger is inhibited by amiloride and a number of its derivatives. N-5 substituted derivatives are very potent (2, 10). One particularly active molecule is ethyl-isopropyl amiloride (EIPA) (11) (Fig. 2).

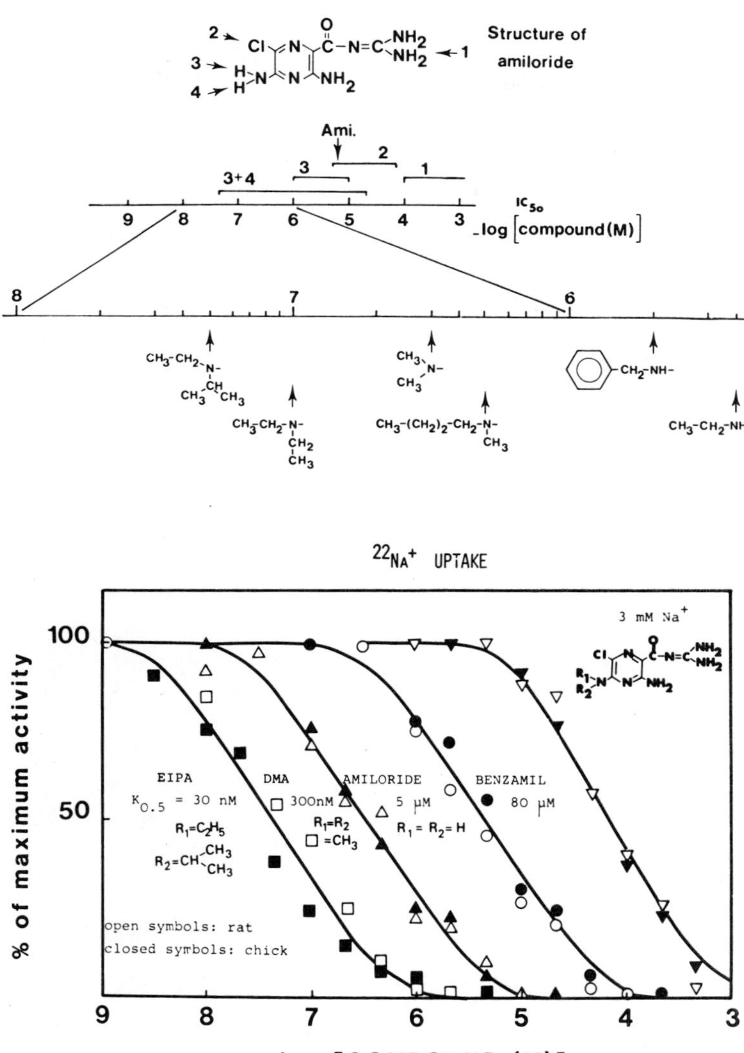

Fig. 2. Structure-function relationships in the amiloride series for blockade of the Na+/H+ exchange system. Higher part : results of different types of substitutions on the IC50 value for inhibition of the exchanger. Lower part : pharmacology of amiloride derivatives in rat and chick cardiac cells using 22Na+ flux experiments.

The inotropic effect of digitalis is due, as we have seen before, to Na^+_i accumulation which triggers Ca^{2+} entry through the Na^+/Ca^{2+} exchanger. Na^+_i accumulation is produced by inhibiting Na^+ efflux through partial blockade of the (Na^+,K^+)ATPase. However, one will of course expect that Na^+_i accumulation will not occur if, while inhibiting the major efflux system (the (Na^+,K^+)ATPase), one also inhibits the major influx system (the Na^+/H^+ exchanger). Amiloride has indeed been shown to decrease the cardiotonic and cardiotoxic effects of ouabain (2, 3).

Another interesting aspect of the Na^+/H^+ exchanger is its involvement in internal pH control and probably its close linkage with Na^+_i and Ca^{2+}_i accumulation following reperfusion after ischemia (3).

External and internal pH dependences of the cardiac Na^+/H^+ exchange system are presented in Fig. 3. It is clear that in conditions of ischemia, when both external and internal pH's are acidic, near pH 6, the Na^+/H^+ exchange system has very little activity because of the low value of the external pH. After reperfusion, the external pH becomes alkaline while, at least in the initial period following reperfusion, the internal pH remains acidic. pHo and pHi dependences of the activity of the Na^+/H^+ exchanger (Fig. 3) indicate that these conditions ensure a high activity of the Na^+/H^+ exchanger which rapidly evacuates the excess of internal H^+ at the expense of massive Na^+ entry. Na^+ entering the cardiac cell following reperfusion cannot be rejected outside the cardiac cell using the (Na^+,K^+)ATPase **(i)** because the ATP level has decreased during ischemia, **(ii)** because the activity of the transport enzyme itself has been decreased during the ischemic period and the acidosis (3). Then, the only pathway available to Na^+ to leave the cardiac cell is the Na^+/Ca^{2+} exchange system. Na^+_i accumulation following reperfusion is then due to the activation of the Na^+/H^+ exchange. Ca^{2+}_i accumulation, that is directly linked to reperfusion-induced toxicity and cell death, is probably secondary to Na^+_i accumulation and occuring through the Na^+/Ca^{2+} exchanger (3).

The $Na^+/K^+/Cl^-$ co-transport and diuretics of the furosemide family

The cardiac cells, as most other cells, has a membrane integrated $Na^+/K^+/Cl^-$ co-transport (12, 13). This co-transport is inhibited by a series of drugs including furosemide or bumetanide (Fig. 4). The most potent molecule is benzmetanide ($K_{0.5} = 0.3\,\mu M$).

The $Na^+/K^+/Cl^-$ co-transporter is, together with the (Na^+,K^+)ATPase, the main entry system for K^+ (Fig. 4, inset A). It represents 50% of $^{86}Rb^+$ transport ($^{86}Rb^+$ being used as a K^+ substitute). Ouabain plus bumetanide inhibit more than 85% of $^{86}Rb^+$ entry.

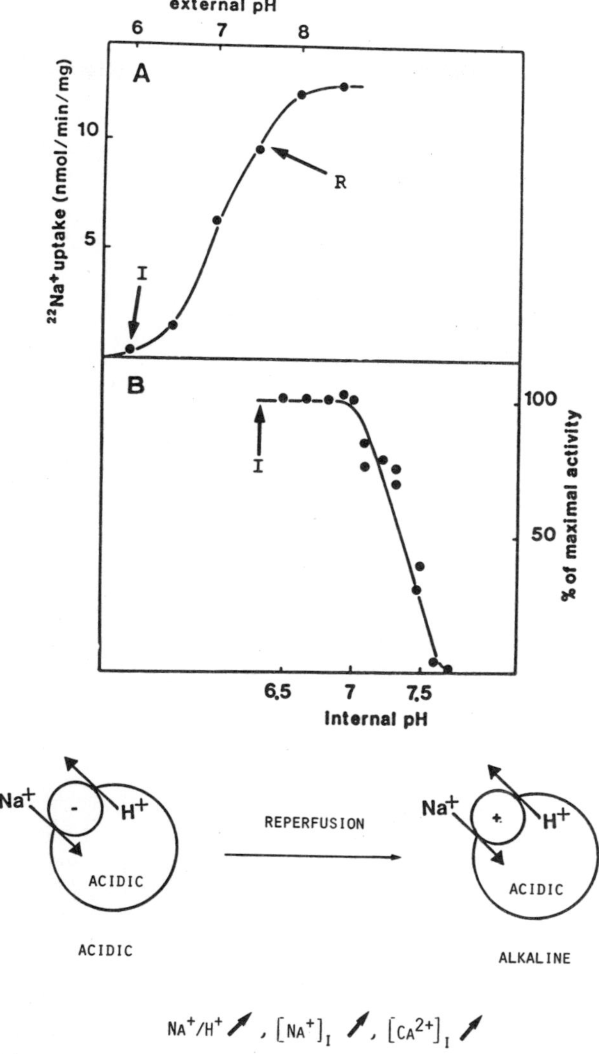

$$NA^+/H^+ \nearrow \;,\; [NA^+]_I \nearrow \;,\; [CA^{2+}]_I \nearrow$$

Fig. 3. External and internal pH dependences of the activity of the Na$^+$/H$^+$ exchanger (higher part) and their consequences in reperfusion following ischemia (lower part). I. External and internal pH values during ischemia. R. External pH value during the first moments of reperfusion. Lower part : signs - and + mean that the Na$^+$/H$^+$ exchanger is inactive (-) at acidic pH (internal and external) during ischemia whereas it is very active (+) following reperfusion, when the external pH is alkaline and the internal pH acidic.

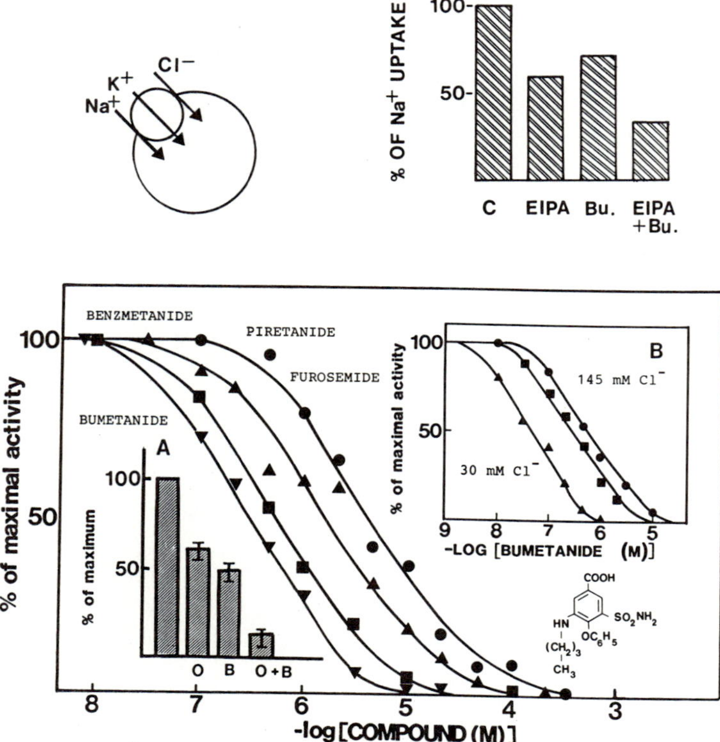

Fig. 4. Pharmacological properties of the Na$^+$/K$^+$/Cl$^-$ co-transport (main panel) and its role in Na$^+$ uptake (upper histogram) . Inset A : contribution of the Na$^+$/K$^+$/Cl$^-$ co-transport to K$^+$ entry into cardiac cells (measured by ^{86}Rb$^+$ influx). Inset B : increasing Cl$^-$ concentrations antagonize bumetamide inhibition. EIPA : ethylisopropyamiloride, a Na$^+$/H$^+$ exchanger blocker. Bu or B : Bumetanide. O : ouabain, a blocker of the (Na$^+$,K$^+$)ATPase.

The Na$^+$/K$^+$/Cl$^-$ co-transporter is less active for Na$^+$ entry than the Na$^+$/H$^+$ exchanger (Fig. 4) (12). Na$^+$ uptake _via_ the Na$^+$/K$^+$/Cl$^-$ co-transport represents about 50-60% of Na$^+$ uptake mediated by the Na$^+$/H$^+$ exchanger.

The voltage-dependent Na$^+$ channel and its cardiotonic effectors

This channel is essential for the generation of electrical signals by the cardiac cell. However, it does not represent an important Na$^+$ entry pathway in normal conditions since the opening time of the Na$^+$ channel is only of a few msec.

However it is well known that effectors of Na$^+$ channels that can prolong the open time - such as veratridine-like compounds, batrachotoxin, polypeptide toxins such as scorpion and sea anemone toxins - can transform the channel protein into a significant Na^+ entry pathway (14). These effectors when applied to cardiac cells are capable to work as cardiotonic agents.

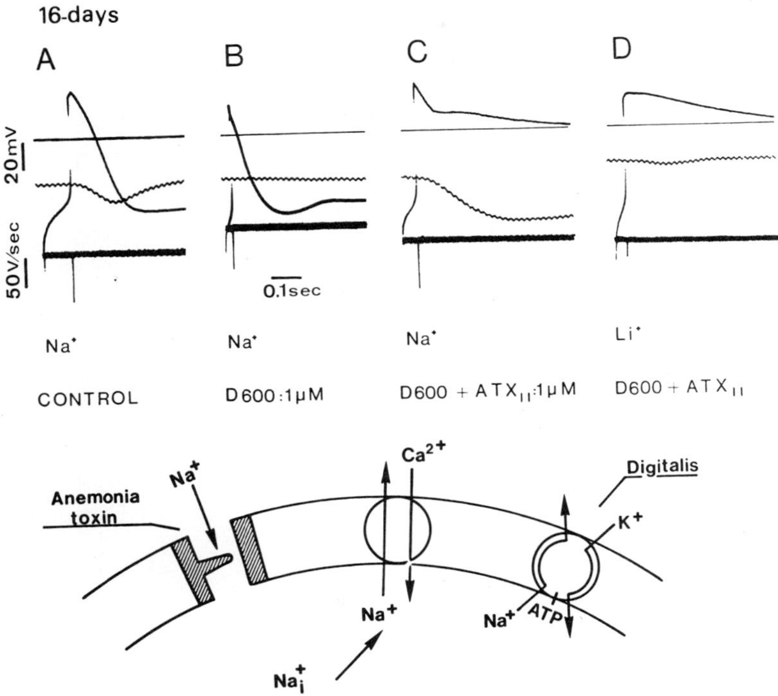

Fig. 5. Cardiotonic effects of sea anemone toxins. A. Action potential and contraction in 16-days chick ventricular cardiac cells in culture. B. D600 blocks the voltage-dependent Ca^{2+} channel and blocks contraction. C. With the Ca^{2+} channel blocked by D600, the sea anemone toxin ATX_{II} prolongs the action potential by slowing down Na^+ channel inactivation and provokes a strong contraction. D. Substitution of Na^+ by Li^+ in the external medium without changing other conditions keeps the prolonged action potential and abolishes contraction. Lower part : Sequence of events producing inotropic effects. $[Na^+]_i$ increases can be provoked by inhibition of the (Na^+,K^+)ATPase with ouabain, they can also be produced by inducing long open times of the Na^+ channel using adequate toxins. In both cases the rise of internal Na^+ triggers the Na^+/Ca^{2+} exchange system and provokes subsequent Ca^{2+} entry and contraction.

Fig. 5 shows the effects of a sea anemone toxin on chick cardiac cells in culture. In the presence of a Ca^{2+} channel blocker, i.e. without Ca^{2+} channel activity, the application of this sea anemone toxin provokes a large inotropic effect that is abolished when external Na^+ is replaced by Li^+. The sequence of events that explains this inotropic effect is (15, 16) **(i)** prolongation of the Na^+ channel open time by the sea anemone toxin, **(ii)** Na^+ accumulation, **(iii)** Ca^{2+} entry triggered by this Na^+ accumulation through the Na^+/Ca^{2+} exchange system **(iv)** more contraction.

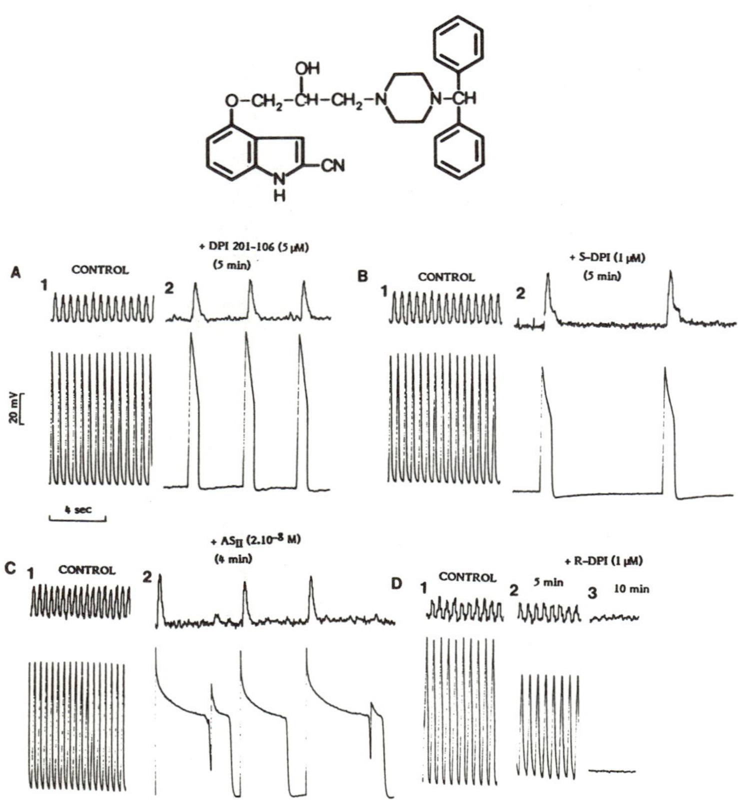

Fig. 6. The inotropic effect induced by DPI 201-106 and by S- and R-DPI. A. Contraction (upper part) and spontaneous electrical activity (lower part) of cultured cardiac cells. 1 - Control. 2 - Inotropic effect of the racemic mixture DPI 210-106. B. 1 - Control. 2 - With the optical enantiomer S-DPI. D. 1 - Control. 2 - Blocking effect of the other optical isomer R-DPI on both electrical activity and contraction. C - A comparison with cardiotonic effects produced by the sea anemone toxin from <u>Anemonia sulcata</u> (AS$_{II}$).

The sensitivity of mammalian cardiac cells to sea anemone and scorpion toxins is high and can be observed in the 0.1 nM to 10 nM range (16). However these toxins, similarly to ouabain, have a low therapeutic index. They have cardiotoxic (arythmogenic) effects at concentrations which are only a little higher than those required for an increased inotropy.

A new molecule has recently been synthesized by the pharmaceutical industry, DPI 201-106 (Sandoz). This small organic molecule, unlike polypeptide toxins is cardiotonic without being arythmogenic. Its effects are shown in Figs. 6 and 7. The molecule acts by slowing down Na^+ channel inactivation. Interestingly, the inotropic effect is due to the S optical isomer. The other optical enantiomer, R , blocks the Na^+ channel and of course blocks contraction. DPI 201-106 and its isomers bind to a new receptor site on the Na^+ channel structure, their receptor site is allosterically linked to the common batrachotoxin/veratridine site (17). DPI 201-106 appears to be, because of its lack of toxicity, one of the most promising cardiotonic molecules for the future.

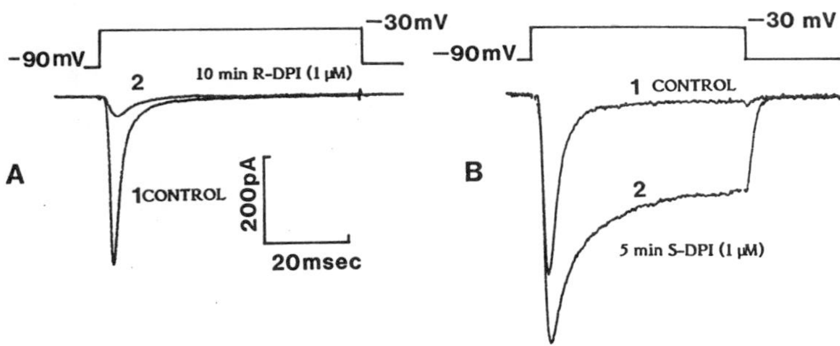

Fig. 7. Voltage-clamp experiments with the whole cell patch-clamp technique showing that R-DPI is a Na^+ channel blocker in cardiac cells whereas S-DPI is slowing down Na^+ channel inactivation (Na^+ channel against).

Acknowledgements

This work was supported by the 'Centre National de la Recherche Scientifique' and the 'Institut National de la Santé et de la Recherche Médicale' (grant n° 83 50 09). Thanks are due to C. Roulinat-Bettelheim for expert technical assistance.

REFERENCES

1. Kazazoglou, T., Renaud, J.F., Rossi, B. and Lazdunski, M. J. Biol. Chem. 258: 12163-12170, 1983.
2. Frelin, C., Vigne, P. and Lazdunski, M. J. Biol. Chem. 259: 8880-8885, 1984.
3. Lazdunski, M., Frelin, C. and Vigne, P. J. Moll. Cell. Cardiol. 17: 1029-1042, 1985.
4. Colquhoun, D., Neher, E., Reuter, H. and Stevens, C.F. Nature 294: 752-754, 1981.
5. Frelin, C., Vigne, P. and Lazdunski, M. Eur. J. Biochem. 149: 1-4, 1985.
6. Vigne, P., Frelin, C. and Lazdunski, M. J. Biol. Chem. 257: 9394-9400, 1982.
7. Green, R.D., Frelin, C., Vigne, P. and Lazdunski, M. FEBS Lett. 196: 163-166, 1986.
8. Piwnica-Worms, D. and Liberman, M. Am. J. Physiol. 244: C422-C428, 1983.
9. Piwnica-Worms, D., Jacob, R., Horres, C.R. and Liberman, M. J. Gen. Physiol. 85: 43-64, 1985
10. Vigne, P., Frelin, C., Cragoe, E.J. and Lazdunski, M. Mol Pharmacol. 25: 131-136, 1984.
11. Vigne, P., Frelin, C., Cragoe, E.J. and Lazdunski, M. Biochem. Biophys. Res. Commun. 116: 86-90, 1983.
12. Frelin, C., Chassande, O. and Lazdunski, M. Biochem. Biophys. Res. Commun. 134: 326-331, 1986.
13. Piwnica-Worms, D., Jacob, R., Horres, C.R. and Liberman, M. Am. J. Physiol. 249: C337-344, 1985.
14. Lazdunski, M. and Renaud, J.F. Ann. Rev. Physiol. 44: 463-473, 1982.
15. Romey, G., Renaud, J.F., Fosset, M. and Lazdunski, M. J. Pharm. Exp. Ther. 213: 607-615, 1980.
16. Renaud, J.F., Fosset, M., Schweitz, H. and Lazdunski, M. Eur. J. Pharmacol. 120: 161-170, 1986.
17. Romey, G., Quast, U., Pauron, D., Frelin, C., Renaud, J.F. and Lazdunski, M. Proc. Natl. Acad. Sci. USA in press, 1987.

6

NONDRIVEN ELECTRICAL ACTIVITY IN CARDIAC VENTRICULAR FIBERS

T.F.LIU, L.W.DONG and Z.M.WANG

Department of Biology, Peking University, Beijing 100871,
People's Republic of China

INTRODUCTION

Under normal conditions, there is no automaticity in
cardiac ventricular fibers. However, rhythmic activity may
occur in some circumstances, such as under stretch (1),
partial depolarization (2), and treated with chemical agent as
aconitine (3,4) or Ba^{2+} (5) etc. In 1977, Cranefield summarized
that triggered activity was an important mechanism in the genesis
of nondriven repetitive activity that arised from depolarizing
afterpotentials (6). Triggered activity could be divided into
two kinds, the early afterdepolarization (EAD) and delayed
afterdepolarization (DAD) depending on their occurrance before
or after the membrane potential had completely repolarized.
Since then, several reviews had been published (7,8,9).

Several factors may induce triggered activity: such as
catecholamine (10), aconitine (3,4,), hypoxia (11), Cs^+ (12),
reduction of K^+ (13) or Ca^{2+} (14) in the genesis of EAD ; cardiac
glycosides (15), Na^+-free and Ca^{2+}-rich solution (16), high
concentration of catecholamine (17), K^+-free and Ca^{2+}-rich
solution (18,19) and neuraminidase (20) in that of DAD.

In order to observe the genesis of nondriven action potential including sustained rhythmic activity in ventricular fibers,
the following treatments were used on guinea pig, rat, ground
squirrel and porcine hearts : reduction of K^+, application of
electrical stimulation on the early phase of repolarization
and long period of cold storage.

This study was supported in part by the Science Fund of the
Chinese Academy of Sciences.

RESULTS AND DISCUSSION

Nondriven action potentials in repolarizing phase of ventricular fibers

EAD induced by K$^+$-free solution after cold storage. Unlike the ventricular fibers of porcine (21) and rat hearts (S.Chang unpublished data), the papillary muscle fibers of guinea pig hearts could not tolerate long period of cooling (0-4°C). More than 10 hrs of cold storage, the ventricular fibers of guinea pig hearts could hardly respond to electrical stimulation after rewarming to 37°C and the membrane potential kept constantly at -20 mV level.

The papillary muscles of guinea pig hearts were treated in cold less than 6 hrs and rewarmed to 37°C with Tyrode solution. During the period of rewarming, hyperpolarization could be seen in these preparations. About 2 hrs later, the action potentials were similar to those of fresh preparations except the action potential duration was slightly prolonged. Under superfusion with K$^+$-free Tyrode solution and slow driving rate (0.2 Hz), EAD could be induced easily in all 15 preparations. At first, there was a small hump appearing in the middle of repolarizing phase about -50 mV level (Fig.1 B).Several seconds later, the small hump became a new plateau and could prolong to several handred of miliseconds (Fig.1C,D). Nondriven action potentials then appeared on the basis of the new plateau (Fig.1E,F) with typical characteristics of EAD (22).

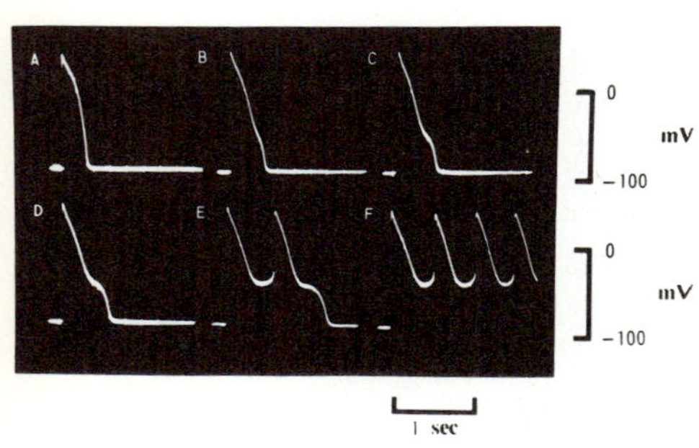

Fig.1　Induction of EAD in ventricular fiber of guinea pig heart under K$^+$-free superfusion of 10, 20, 40, 60, 65 and 70 sec respectively (A-F). A small hump in the middle of repolarizing phase can be seen in B and C. A new plateau is formed in D. EAD is induced in E and F.
All records were obtained in the same cell. The preparation had been stored in cold (0-4°C) for 5 hrs.

Two types of rhythmic activity might be found in the above EAD. One was rhythmic activity with high amplitude (50–70 mV) which could last for several minutes or more with regular frequency of 80–140/min (Fig.2A). The other was irregular oscillations with low amplitude(Fig.2B), which occurred following the first type and then stopped at –50 mV level. In this case, there appeared to exist two levels of resting potential in the ventricular fiber of guinea pig heart.

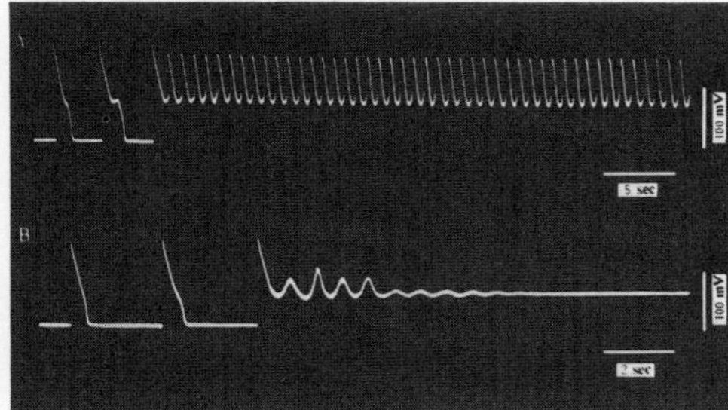

Fig.2 Two types of rhythmic activity induced in ventricular fiber of guinea pig heart after cooling under superfusion of K^+-free solution.
A) Rhythmic activity with high amplitude.
B) Irregular oscillations with low amplitude.

When K^+ was added to 3 mM in K^+-free superfusate, or Tl^+ to 1.5 mM, the EAD in low membrane potential stopped abruptly and concurrently the resting potential changed to high level (Fig.3).

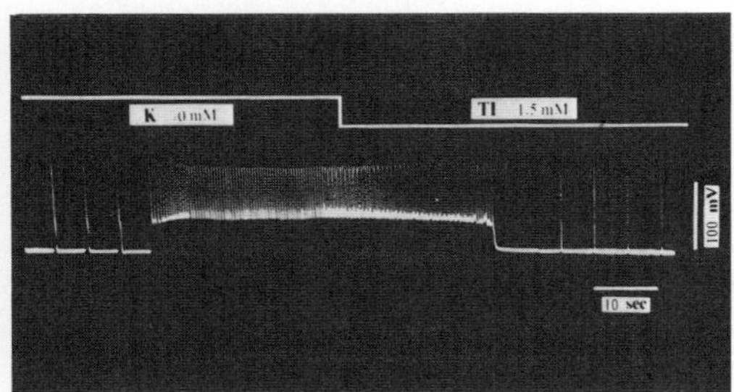

Fig.3 Inhibition effect of Tl^+ on EAD in ventricular fiber of guinea pig heart.

Under this condition, ventricular fibers are very similar to Purkinje fibers possessing two levels of resting potential and are sensitive to the activation of Na-K pump which can change the resting potential from the low level to high one.

Nondriven action potentials induced by single electrical stimulation on the early repolarizing phase of ventricular fibers. By definition, triggered activity is generated by the preceding action potential. Since in normal condition, it is difficult to get a stable EAD, we considered whether an action potential which induced by an electrical stimulation on the early phase of repolarization could generate nondriven action potentials or rhythmic activity.

In guinea pig (22) and rat ventricular fibers (23), nondriven action potentials could only occasionally be induced by single electrical stimulation in the early phase of repolarization. However, we found in ground squirrel, it was relatively easier to get such result (24). When a stronger stimulation was applied on the early repolarizing phase of action potential (at -40 to -60 mV level) in ventricular fiber of ground squirrel heart, in 6 out of 18 preparations, not only an action potential was evoked but also another one or even more reactions followed. Sometimes, a sustained rhythmic activity lasting for 2 to 3 sec was recorded (Fig.4). The interval in which the premature stimulation could trigger nondriven action potential was very short, only in about 5 to 10 msec.

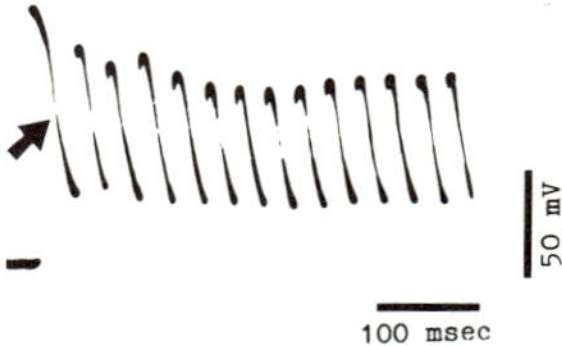

Fig.4 Sustained rhythmic activity induced by single stimulation on the early phase of repolarization in the ventricular fiber of ground squirrel heart. The artifact of the stimulation is demonstrated by arrow.

If the ventricular fibers treated with ouabain (2×10^{-7}M) or superfused with low K^+ (0 to 1.5 mM) tyrode solution, in all preparations (9 and 8 in number respectively), nondriven action potentials were induced by the premature stimulation in the early repolarizing phase. These kinds of nondriven activity could be inhibited by adding K^+ in the superfusate.

In guinea pig (22) and rat ventricular fibers (23), nondriven action potentials could also be induced easily by application of electrical stimulation on the early phase of repolarization under low K^+ or K^+-free superfusion, although it was difficult to generate such activity in normal condition (Fig.5). Sometimes, under K^+-free superfusion EAD which was similar to those induced by electrical stimulation might appear spontaneously in guinea pig ventricular fibers without any stimulation.

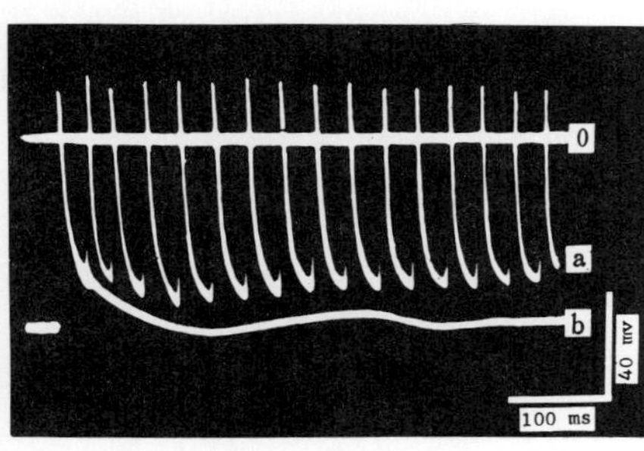

Fig.5 Rhythmic activity induced by single electrical stimulation on the early phase of repolarization in ventriaular fiber of guinea pig heart under K^+-free superfusion.
O) Zero line.
a) Rhythmic activity induced by electrical stimulation. The first premature reaction was evoked by stimulation.
b) Action potential of the same fiber without extra stimulation. Note, there is a remarkable DAD in the phase 4.

DAD induced in ventricular fibers

In rat (23), ground squirrel (24), pig (25) and some other mammalian ventricular fibers toxic concentration of cardiac glycosides did not evoke DAD and rhythmic activity under normal condition. However, in guinea pig ventricular fibers, things were different. Both ouabain and low K^+ superfusion could induce DAD very easily (22).

DAD induced in guinea pig ventricular fibers by low K^+.

Reduction of K^+ concentration in Tyrode solution caused shortening of the plateau and decreasing in the action potential

duration, but the 4th phase of the action potential still kept
quiescent as long as the K^+ concentration was not less than
0.75 mM under the driving rate of 1 Hz (Fig.6). Further reduction of K^+ concentration, DAD appeared and became more prominent
when the K^+ concentration decreased to zero mM.

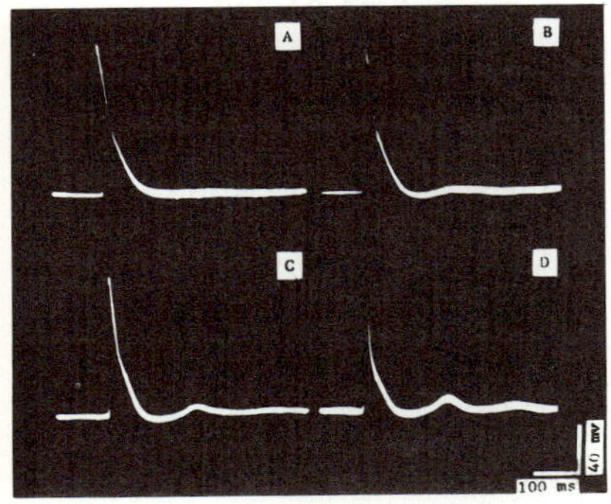

Fig.6 Different concentrations
of low K^+ induced DAD in ventri-
cular fibers of guinea pig heart.
A,B) K^+ concentration was 0.75mM,
     DAD sometimes appeared and
     sometimes not.
C) K^+ concentration was 0.38mM.
D) K^+ concentration was 0 mM.

Increasing the driving rate made the amplitude of DAD
heighten. For example, increasing in the rate from 1 to 2 Hz
the amplitude of DAD increased from 4.4 ± 3.0 to 6.7 ± 3.2 mV (n=8,
p<0.05) when K^+ was 0.38 mM; and from 9.0 ± 6.3 to 11.7 ± 5.6 mV
n=7, p<0.05) when K^+ was 0 mM.

When a train of stimulation was applied on the ventricular
fiber, the amplitude of DAD increased with increasing in the
pulse number of train stimulation and eventually nondriven action
potential was induced (Fig.7).

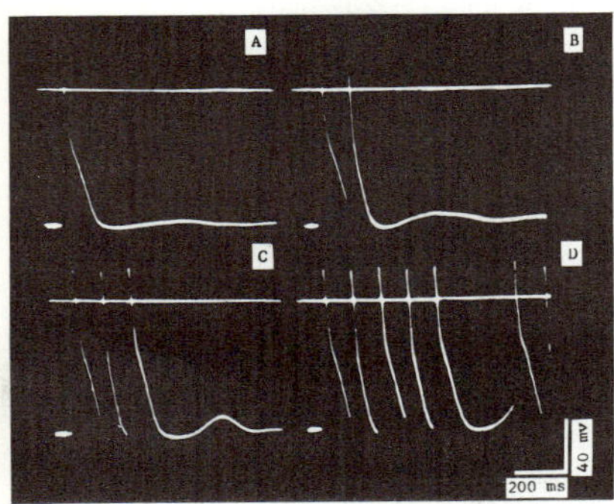

Fig.7 Nondriven action potential triggered by a train of
stimulation in guinea pig ventricular fiber under low K^+
superfusion. Increasing in
the number of impulse led to
enhancing the height of DAD
and eventually inducing nondriven activity.

Application of a train of stimulation with high frequency of impulses on the early phase of repolarization, the same result also could be obtained (Fig.8).

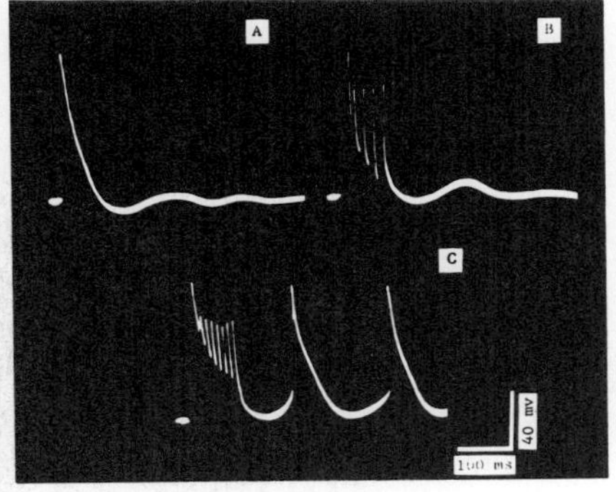

Fig.8 nondriven action potentials triggered by high frequency of train stimulation applied on the early phase of repolarization in ventricular fiber under low K^+ superfusion (K^+= 0.38 mM).

DAD generated in porcine ventricular fibers after cold

storage. In normal porcine fibers did not evoke DAD or oscillation by cardiac glycosides. However, after cold treatment for 24 hrs, DAD could be induced by ouabain in porcine ventricular fibers. Superfusion with low K^+, the oscillation induced by ouabain was enhanced and nondriven action potential or rhythmic activity could be triggered (25).

In rat papillary muscle, just like in porcine heart, did not respond to ouabain in ordinary condition. After cold treatment for 20 hrs, low K^+ could induce DAD which was enhanced by high Ca^{2+} or adrenaline.

Rhythmic activity evoked in porcine ventricular fibers after

long period of cold storage

Porcine ventricular fibers possess special ability to tolerate long period of cold storage (0 to $4°C$, 48-96 hrs). after 24 hrs of cold treatment, the preparations had normal reaction to electrical stimulation and hyperpolarization could be seen in the first hour of rewarming.

after 48 hrs of cooling, the resting potential of the ventricular fibers only kept in -20 mV level when the superfusion temperature rewarmed to $37°C$. The preparations could

respond to electrical stimulation with local response. At first,
the amplitude of the local responses was low about 5-10 mV.
Several minutes later, the amplitude of local responses grew
higher and higher, and an action potential bursted out when
the amplitude of the local response was higher than 15 mV(Fig.9).

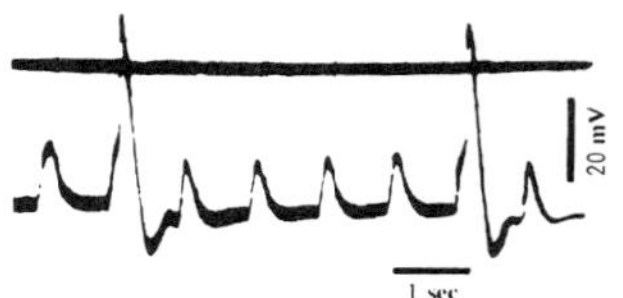

Fig.9 Local responses and action
potentials evoked by electrical
stimulation on the porcine ventricular fibers after cold storage
of 72 hrs. The 2nd and the 7th
are action potentials with afterpotentials.

Once the action potential appeared, the afterpotentials
followed. The first component was a hyperpolarization and immediately followed by a second component, a depolarization.
By the definition of Cranefield, they are typical early afterhyperpolarization and delayed afterdepolarization respectively.

As the action potentials driven by electrical stimulations
continued, the resting potential grew higher and higher, concurrently, the afterpotentials developed more markedly . When
the amplitude of the afterpotentials became higher than 15 mV,
rhythmic activity was induced (Fig.10).

Once the rhythmic activity appeared, it could last for
several hours. At first, the maximal diastolic potential (MDP)
was low (less than -60 mV), so, it was a low membrane potential
rhythmic activity (Fig. 11A). This kind of activity could keep
1-2 hrs, but it had a tendency to change to a high one with
MDP higher than -70 mV (Fig. 11B).

In the genesis of the rhythmic activity after long period
of cold storage, DAD was a major mechanism. However, as the
rhythmic activity going on, the characteristics of the triggered
activity was changed, especially in the high level membrane

potential rhythmic activity.

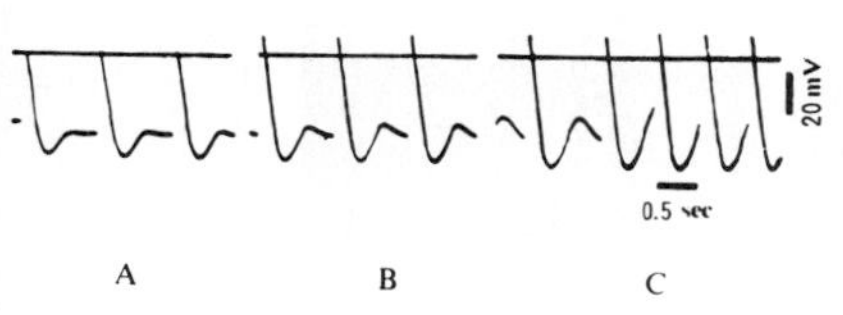

Fig.10 Genesis of rhythmic activity induced by electrical stimulation on the porcine ventricular fiber after 72 hr cold storage. A) at first, there is only afterhyperpolarization following each action potential. B) Later on, afterdepolarization is developed. C) Rhythmic activity is induced when the amplitude of afterdepolarization reaches a certain level.

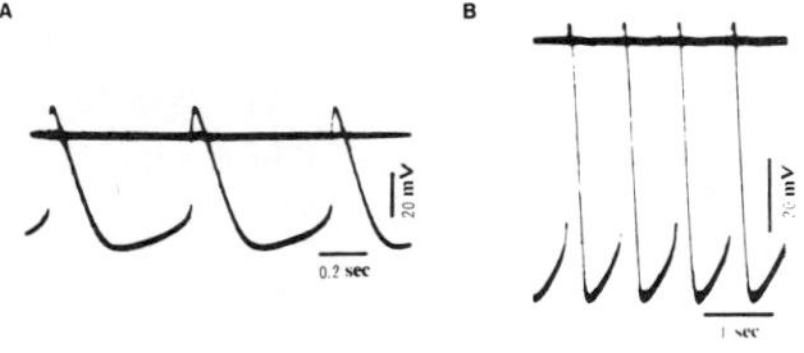

Fig.11 Two types of rhythmic activity in porcine ventricular fibers after cold storage. A) Low membrane potential rhythmic activity. B) High membrane potential rhythmic activity.

Application of overdrive stimulations on the preparation, there appeared typical overdrive suppression (26)which was much similar to that in pacemaker cell (Fig.12). Furthermore, when the MDP exceeded -80 mV, the frequency of the rhythmic activity became very low, sometimes less than 6/min. In these cases, the mechanism of the rhythmic activity could hardly be the triggerd one in nature. There was a definite pacemaker potential ahead of each action potential but far apart from the DAD of the preceding one (Fig.13).

As the MDP up to -90 mV, the rhythmic activity stopped and the ventricular fibers gave a typical ventricular action potential with a quiescent phase 4 to the stimulation.

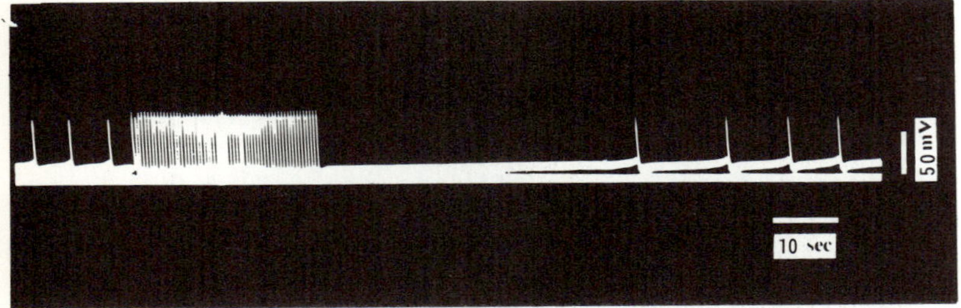

Fig. 12 Overdrive suppression occurred in rhythmic activity
of porcine ventricular fiber. Upper line: Action potential.
Lower line: V_{max} .

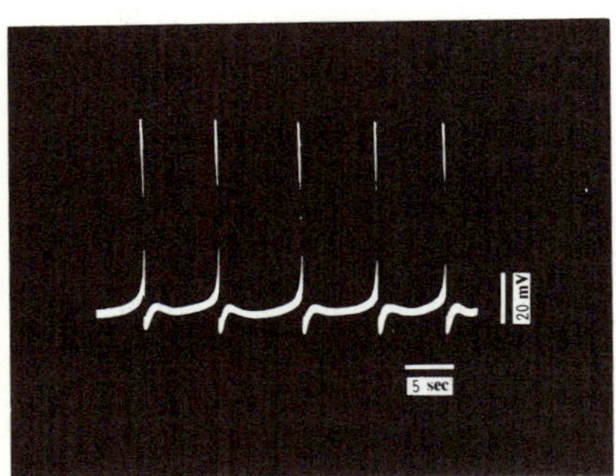

Fig.13 Slow rate of rhythmic
activity when the MDP was high.
Note: the afterdepolarization
and the pacemaker potential
were seperated far apart.

The reaction to low K^+ in cold treated porcine ventricular
fiber was also different from that of guinea pig ventricular
muscle (25,27). In porcine preparations low K^+ caused the appearance of diastolic depolarization in the quiescent phase 4
instead of DAD or EAD. In this respect, cold treated porcine
ventricular fibers were much similar to Purkinje fibers. Furthermore, high concentration of Ca^{2+} did not enhance the
'pacemaker potential' nor generate DAD in the cold treated
porcine ventricular fibers.

A possible explanation of the genesis of rhythmic activity
in porcine ventricular fiber after long period of cooling.

There was evidence showing that during hypothermia, the cardiac
cell gained Na^+ but lost K^+ and the resting potential was in

-20 mV level (28). This phenomenon was called " Na-loaded "
(29,30). The excessive loss of resting potential during deep
hypothermia was due to Na-pump arrest. The recovery of the
resting potential and the appearance of hyperpolarization after
rewarming from 24 hr cooling were contributed by electrogenic
Na-pump (31,32). When the period of cold treatment was more
than 24 hrs, the resting potential of porcine ventricular
fibers usually kept -20 mV level when rewarmed to $37°C$.
It meant that Na-pump could not work normally or it was inhibited
significantly.

After long period of cold storage, the characteristics of
porcine ventricular fibers changed markedly. It was much similar
to that of purkinje fiber, such as in response to low K^+ and
ouabain. It is worthy to note that there is an important difference between automatic fiber and working cell in the Na-pump
activity. The Na-pump activity of Purkinje fiber is less than
that of ventricular fiber (33).

There were lots of evidences showing that low K^+ could
suppress the activity of Na-pump (34,35,36). Lowering of the
K^+ concentration in superfusate gave rise to the appearance of
rhythmic activity and further reduction of the K^+ concentration
to zero mM depolarized the membrane potential to -20 mV in cold
treated ventricular fibers. Increasing in the K^+ concentration
made the membrane potential repolarize from -20 mV and rhythmic
activity recovered again. Further increasing in K^+ concentration
to 5.4 mM, the resting potential of ventricular fiber reached
to normal level and the rhythmic activity stopped immediately.
All of these suggested that the inhibition of Na-pump played
an important part in the genesis of rhythmic activity in the
porcine ventricular fiber after rewarming from long period of
cold treatment, although there was no direct evidence denoting
that the Na-pump was the only mechanism of the induction or
cessation of such activity.

SUMMARY

In guinea pig ventricular fibers EAD is easily induced
in K^+-free solution by cold storage for 5 hrs after the

preparation is rewarmed to 37°C. A new plateau which is the basis of EAD generation at the level of -50 mV of repolarization can be formed. It appears that guinea pig ventricular fibers possess two levels of resting potentials. Application of single electrical stimulation on the early phase of repolarization, in many mammalian ventricular fibers (guinea pig, rat, and ground squirrel hearts) can induce nondriven activity, especially under low K^+ or ouabain treatment, whose nature is identical with EAD.

DAD is easily induced in guinea pig ventricular fibers under low K^+ superfusion. It also can be induced in pig and rat ventricular fibers after rewarming from cold storage for 24 hrs under low K^+ or ouabain treatment.

Sustained rhythmic activity can be induced in porcine ventricular fibers after long period of storage. It seems to be automatic in nature, although its genesis is based on triggered mechanism. The mechanism involved in the generation of the rhythmic activity has been discussed.

REFERENCES

1. Kaufmann, R. and Theophile, U. Pflueg Arch 297:174-189, 1967.
2. Katzung, B. Life Sci 14:1133-1140, 1974.
3. Matsuda, K. et al. Jap J Physiol 9:419-429, 1959.
4. Schmidt, R.F. Pflueg Arch 271:526-536, 1960.
5. Antoni, H. and Oberdisse, E. Pflueg Aech 284:259-272, 1965.
6. Cranefield, P.F. Circ Res 41:415-423, 1977.
7. Hoffman, B.F. In: The Evaluation of New Antiarrhythmic Drugs. edited by Morganroth, J., Moore, E.N., Dreifus, L.S. and Michelson, E.L. Martinus Nijhoff Publishers, London 1981, pp. 5-15.
8. Cranefield, P.F. In: Slow Inward Current and Cardiac Arrhythmias. edited by Zppes, D.P., Bailey, J.C. and Elharrar pp.11-21, 1980. Martinus Nijhoff publishers London.
9. Cranefield, P.F. and Wit, A.L. Ann Rev Physiol 41:459-472, 1979.
10. Hoffman, B.F. and Cranefield, P.F. Electrophysiology of the Heart. McGraw-Hill Book Co., New York, 1960.
11. Trawtwein, W. et al. Pflueg Arch 260:40-60, 1954.
12. Damiano, B.P. and Rosen, M.R. Circulation 69:1013-1023, 1984.
13. Camelait, E.E. J Physiol 156:375-388, 1961.
14. Sano, T. and Sawanobori, T. Circ Res 31:158-164, 1972.

15. Ferrier, G.P. Prog Cardivasc Dis $\underline{19}$:459-490, 1977.
16. Wit, A.J. et al. $\underline{In}$: The Conduction System of the Heart, edited by Weldens, H.J.J., Lie, K.I. and Janse, M.J. PP. 163-181,1976, Leden, Stenfert Krose.
17. Yeh, B.K. and Lazzara, R. Fed Proc $\underline{36}$:586, 1977.
18. Hiraoka, M. Experientia $\underline{35}$:500-501,1979.
19. Hiraoka, M. and Kawano, S. J Mol Cell Cardiol $\underline{16}$:285, 1984.
20. Kimura, S. et al. Cardiovasc Res $\underline{18}$:294-301, 1984.
21. Liu, T.F. Acta Physiol Sinica $\underline{33}$:259-265, 1981.
22. Liu,T.F. et al. Chin J Cardiol $\underline{In Press}$.
23. Wang, Z.M. and Liu, T.F. Physiol Sci $\underline{5}$:180-185, 1985.
24. Liu, T.F. Kexue Tongbao $\underline{31}$:123-128, 1986.
25. Guo Y.E. et al. Acta Physiol Sinica $\underline{38}$:58-65,1986.
26. Liu, T.F. Acta Sci Nat Univ Pek $\underline{No.1}$:72-77,1981.
27. Liu, T.F. Physiol Sci $\underline{2}$:18, 1982
28. Glitch, H.G. J physiol $\underline{220}$:565-582, 1972.
29. Hiraoka, M. and Hecht, H.H. Pflueg Arch $\underline{339}$:25-36, 1973.
30. Sano, T. et al. $\underline{In}$: Developmental and Physiological Correlation of Cardiac Muscle. edited by Lieberman, M. and Sano, T. 1975,pp.299-310,Raven Press, New York.
31. Deleze,J. Circ Res $\underline{8}$:553-557, 1960.
32. Hiraoka, M. and Hecht, H.H. Proc Int Union Physiol Sci $\underline{9}$:249, 1971.
33. Kubler, W. and Von Smekal, P. Acta cardiol (Suppl) $\underline{17}$: 103-113, 1973.
34. Deitmer, J.W. and Ellis, D. J Physiol $\underline{284}$:241-259, 1978.
35. January, C.T. and Fozzard, H.A. Circ Res $\underline{54}$:652-665, 1984.
36. Glitch, H.G. et al. Pflueg Arch $\underline{391}$:28-34, 1981.

7

Regulation of Cl⁻ Activity in Ventricular Muscle: Cl^-/HCO_3^- Exchange and Na^+-dependent Cl⁻ Cotransport

C.M. BAUMGARTEN AND **S.W.N. DUNCAN**

Department of Physiology and Biophysics, Medical College of Virginia, Richmond, VA 23298

INTRODUCTION

Studies with ion-selective microelectrodes (ISE) have made it clear that Cl⁻ is actively accumulated in heart. Intracellular Cl⁻ activity (a_{Cl}^i) in quiescent mammalian Purkinje fibers (1,2) and ventricle (1,3-6) is 10-24 mM, while the expectation for a passive distribution is 4-6 mM. Cl⁻ is also accumulated in frog atrium, ventricle, and sinus venosus (7). The concept of active control of a_{Cl}^i receives further support from the modest response of a_{Cl}^i to variations in membrane potential (E_m) and extracellular K^+ ($[K^+]_o$) and Cl⁻ ($[Cl^-]_o$) concentrations (1-3,6-8).

Vaughan-Jones (2) provided evidence that a Cl^-/HCO_3^- exchanger mediates the uptake of Cl⁻ in Purkinje fibers and balances the passive leak of Cl⁻ out of the cell. As expected for such a system, a_{Cl}^i falls when Cl^-/HCO_3^- exchange is inhibited by either removal of extracellular HCO_3^- and CO_2 or by anion transport blockers (e.g., stilbene disulfonic acid derivatives, SITS and DIDS). To estimate the magnitude of the contribution of Cl^-/HCO_3^- exchange to Cl⁻ accumulation, the rate of reaccumulation of Cl⁻ after washout was studied (2). Uptake is slowed 18-fold in HCO_3^--free solution and 9-fold by SITS. Further evidence for the linkage of Cl⁻ and HCO_3^- transport comes from measurements of pH_i, which demonstrate SITS-blockable changes of pH_i associated with the movement of Cl⁻ (2).

The process responsible for accumulation of Cl⁻ in ventricular muscle is less clear, and evidence for the presence of Cl^-/HCO_3^- exchange is lacking. Removal of HCO_3^- and CO_2, even for a number of hours, does not cause a_{Cl}^i to fall and may cause it to increase (3-6). Based on these results, it was suggested that Cl^-/HCO_3^- exchange is not responsible for Cl⁻ accumulation in the myocardium. However, this conclusion is predicated on the assumption that Cl^-/HCO_3^- exchange is not maintained by metabolically produced HCO_3^-.

The present study more fully considers whether Cl^-/HCO_3^- exchange contributes to regulation of a_{Cl}^i in ventricle. Further, it investigates an alternative mechanism for Cl⁻ uptake, Na^+-dependent Cl⁻ cotransport, that has been found in other cells (e.g., 9-12).

The data indicate that while Cl^-/HCO_3^- exchange occurs, it does not physiologically control a_{Cl}^i in ventricle. On the other hand, Na^+-dependent Cl^- cotransport is important in regulating a_{Cl}^i and may operate as both Na^+/Cl^- and $Na^+/K^+/2Cl^-$ cotransport.

A brief report on some of these findings has appeared (13).

MATERIALS AND METHODS

Tissue preparation.

New Zealand white rabbits (1.5-2.5 kg) were killed by spinal dislocation. The heart was rapidly removed and washed in room temperature, oxygenated Tyrode solution. Papillary muscles were dissected from the right ventricular septum, pinned in a Sylgard-lined chamber, and suprafused at ~5 ml/min with oxygenated Tyrode solution warmed to 37 ± 0.5 °C. Muscles were stimulated initially at 1.4 Hz after isolation, but stimulation was discontinued at least 30 min before data was collected.

Solutions.

Two primary types of Tyrode solution were used. The first contained HCO_3^- and consisted of (in mM): 130 NaCl, 24 $NaHCO_3$, 5 KCl, 1.8 $CaCl_2$, 1.45 Na_2HPO_4, 0.3 NaH_2PO_4, 1.0 $MgCl_2$ and 10 glucose; it was equilibrated with 5% CO_2/95% O_2 (pH 7.4 at 37 °C). The second was nominally HCO_3^--free and had the following composition (in mM): 150 NaCl, 5 KCl, 1.8 CaCl2, 1.0 $MgCl_2$, 5 HEPES, and 10 glucose; or to keep $[Cl^-]_o$ constant, 130 NaCl and 20 Na methanesulfonate ($MeSO_3$) rather than 150 NaCl. These solutions were equilibrated with 100% O_2 (pH 7.4 at 37 °C). Cl^--free and low Cl^- Tyrodes were prepared by substituting the corresponding $MeSO_3$ salts, and low Na^+ solutions, by substituting N-methyl-d-glucamine Cl for NaCl. Where indicated, Ba^{2+} and Cs^+ were added as Cl^- salts with osmolarity kept constant by reduction of $NaMeSO_3$.

The anion transport blocker SITS (4-acetamido-4'-isothiocyano-stilbene-2,2'-disulfonic acid; Aldrich, St. Louis, MO) was added directly to the Tyrode solutions 10-15 min prior to use, giving a final concentration of 100 or 500 uM. Chlorothiazide (as base, courtesy of Merck Sharp & Dome, Rahway, NJ) was also dissolved just prior to use. Its final concentration was 100 or 400 uM.

Measurement of E_m and a_{Cl}^i.

Membrane potential (E_m) was recorded with conventional 3 M KCl-filled microelectrodes (15-25 MΩ). Cl^- ion-selective microelectrodes (ISE) were made as previously described (14,15) from Corning 477913 (Corning Glass, Medfield, MA) using trimethyl-silyldimethylamine (Fluka, Hauppauge, NY) for silanization. Signals from the electrodes were buffered by very high input impedance amplifiers (WP Instruments, New Haven, CT; models 750 and FD-223), were displayed on an oscilloscope and chart recorder (Gould, Cleveland, OH; model 2200), and were recorded on magnetic tape (Hewlett Packard, Palo

Alto, CA; model 3964A) for later analysis.

ISE were calibrated before and after the experiment by standard methods (15), and activities were calculated with a computer program (16). The slope of the ISE's response ranged from -48 to -56 mV/10-fold increase in Cl^- activity. A flowing 3 M KCl-filled flowing junction was used to ground the bath.

In the experiments reported here, a single pair of impalements were maintained for the duration of the experiment. a^i_{Cl} was calculated from the electronically obtained difference between the ISE and E_m voltages (14,15). However, multiple impalements were made with each electrode before and after the run to insure that the pair of impalements used to calculate a^i_{Cl} were typical. In control experiments, analogous results were obtained by calculating a^i_{Cl} from the averages of >5 ISE and E_m impalements.

Control experiments were also performed to evaluate the interference detected by the ISE (1,3,6,15). Papillary muscles were bathed in Cl^--free Tyrode for 1 hr, a time sufficient to completely wash out $^{36}Cl^-$ (3). The apparent a^i_{Cl} measured after total Cl^- washout was 4.2 ± 0.4 mM (n = 12), a level not significantly different in HCO_3^--buffered and HCO_3^--free solutions. This signal was attributed to interference, and consequently, 4.2 mM was subtracted from the apparent a^i_{Cl} (3,15).

Statistical methods.

Results are given as mean $\pm$ SE. Student's t-test was applied to paired data to determine statistical significance. Statistical analysis assumes that calculated values for a^i_{Cl} are precise determinations.

RESULTS

Regulation of a^i_{Cl} by Cl^-/HCO_3^- exchange.

The model proposed by Vaughan-Jones (2,8) for regulation of a^i_{Cl} in heart is illustrated in Fig. 1. Cl^- is taken up into the cell by Cl^-/HCO_3^- exchange and leaks out, moving down its electrochemical gradient. Consequently, inhibition of the exchanger is expected to cause a fall in a^i_{Cl}. Two procedures for inhibiting Cl^-/HCO_3^- exchange are available; removing HCO_3^- and CO_2 from the bathing media depletes the intracellular HCO_3^- necessary for exchange, and stilbene disulfonic acid derivatives, including SITS and DIDS, directly inhibit the exchanger in the presence of HCO_3^-. Both of these procedures for inhibiting Cl^-/HCO_3^- exchange have the expected effect in Purkinje fibers (1,2,8).

The same paradigms were used to evaluate the role of Cl^-/HCO_3^- exchange in ventricular muscle. Fig. 2 shows continuous recordings of a^i_{Cl} and E_m during an experiment in which HCO_3^-/CO_2-buffered Tyrode solution was replaced with HEPES-

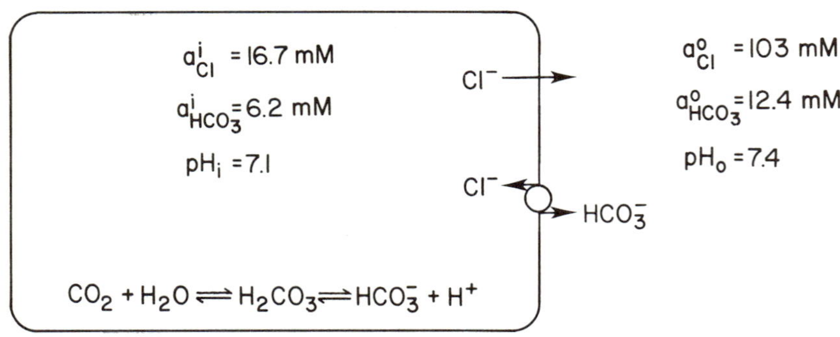

Fig. 1. Model of a^i_{Cl} regulation in heart proposed by Vaughan-Jones (2,8). a^i_{Cl} is determined by balance between uptake of Cl^- by electroneutral Cl^-/HCO_3^- exchange and its passive efflux. The magnitude of inward-directed chemical gradient for Cl^- is normally greater than that for HCO_3^-, and the exchanger operates to accumulate Cl^-. Removing extracellular HCO_3^- and CO_2 lowers $[HCO_3^-]_i$ as CO_2 leaves the cell. Typical ionic activities and pH values for heart are given.

buffered solution. In HCO_3^--buffered Tyrode, a^i_{Cl} was 13.8 mM and gradually *increased* to 18.0 mM on switching to HCO_3^--free solution. This finding was confirmed in 8 additional experiments. On removing HCO_3^-, a^i_{Cl} increased by 4.8 ± 0.8 mM (n = 9, p < 0.001), from 14.7 ± 0.6 to 19.5 ± 0.5 mM. These results are distinctly different than those of Vaughan-Jones (1,2) in Purkinje fibers where a^i_{Cl} decreased by 5.7 mM on removal of HCO_3^-. On the other hand, they are consistent with previous reports in ventricular muscle that suprafusion with HCO_3^--free media fails to lower a^i_{Cl} (3-6).

The simplest interpretation of Fig. 2 is that Cl^-/HCO_3^- exchange is not the primary means of Cl^- uptake in ventricle. Such an interpretation is based on the commonly made assumption that removal of extracellular HCO_3^-/CO_2 is sufficient to deplete intracellular HCO_3^- and stop Cl^-/HCO_3^- exchange (1-6). This may not be the case, however. Ventricular muscle is capable of producing substantial amounts of CO_2

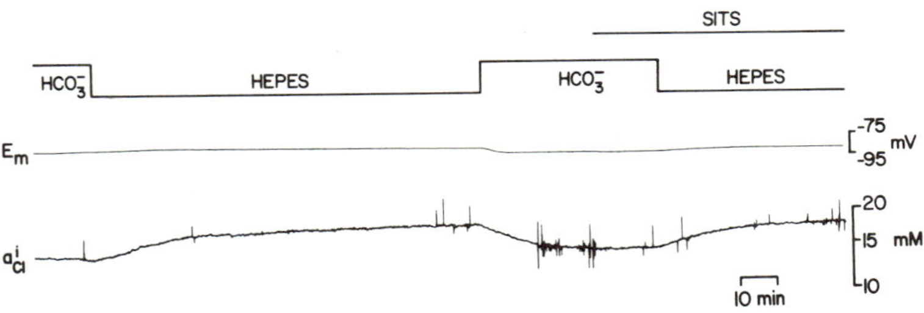

Fig. 2. Effect of removal of extracellular HCO_3^- and CO_2 on a^i_{Cl}. Switching from HCO_3^-/CO_2 to HEPES-buffered Tyrode solution caused a^i_{Cl} to increase from 13.8 to 18.0 mM. This Cl^- accumulation was not inhibited by 100 uM SITS. In the presence of SITS, a^i_{Cl} increased from 14.1 to 18.3 mM. SITS also had no effect on a^i_{Cl} in the presence of HCO_3^-. E_m was not significantly altered by any of these maneuvers. These data demonstrate that Cl^-/HCO_3^- exchange does not regulate a^i_{Cl} in ventricle.

metabolically, and lowering $[HCO_3^-]_i$ to negligible levels is not accomplished simply. A metabolic production yielding only 0.1% CO_2 would give about 1 mM $[HCO_3^-]_i$, and such levels have been suggested for barnacle skeletal muscle (17), mammalian smooth muscle (18) and crayfish neurons (19) in the nominal absence of HCO_3^-/CO_2. The difficulty in depleting $[HCO_3^-]_i$ implies that under nominally HCO_3^--free conditions, the HCO_3^- chemical gradient will still favor Cl^- accumulation, and in fact, the magnitude of the gradient will be larger than under control conditions. Without detailed knowledge of the kinetics of Cl^-/HCO_3^- exchange in ventricle, prediction of the effect of removal of $[HCO_3^-]_o$ on the rate of Cl^-/HCO_3^- exchange is uncertain at best. For example, if the rate limiting step in Cl^-/HCO_3^- exchange in heart is the unloading of HCO_3^- at the external membrane surface, removal of $[HCO_3^-]_o$ might even increase the rate of Cl^- accumulation. This could explain the observed increase in a_{Cl}^i. Alternatively, the increase in a_{Cl}^i could result from the inhibition of a Na^+-HCO_3^-/H^+-Cl^- exchanger in heart muscle, similar to those described in erythrocytes (20), snail neuron (21), squid giant axon (22,23) and barnacle skeletal muscle (17,24). The Na^+-HCO_3^-/H^+-Cl^- exchanger normally functions to *extrude* Cl^- from the cell (i.e., it physiologically transports Cl^- in the opposite direction as the Cl^-/HCO_3^- exchanger of Purkinje fiber), and it is inhibited by removal of HCO_3^- and by SITS.

These possibilities were tested by examining the response of ventricular muscle to removal of extracellular HCO_3^- in the presence of 100 uM SITS. In the example in Fig. 2, a_{Cl}^i increased from 14.1 to 18.3 mM, nearly the same change as observed without SITS. To compare Cl^- accumulation more precisely under the two conditions, the initial rates of Cl^- uptake were determined. SITS had no effect on a_{Cl}^i accumulation. Under control conditions, a_{Cl}^i increased by 0.51 $\pm$ 0.02 mM/min on $[HCO_3^-]_o$ removal and by 0.54 $\pm$ 0.04 mM/min in the presence of 100 uM SITS (n = 7, p > 0.2). These data imply that Cl^-/HCO_3^- exchange is not involved in the accumulation of a_{Cl}^i on $[HCO_3^-]_o$ removal. Furthermore, they also exclude a role for the Na^+-HCO_3^-/H^+-Cl^- exchanger in the regulation of a_{Cl}^i in heart.

A final point can be made from the experiment shown in Fig 2. Blocking Cl^-/HCO_3^- exchange with SITS in the continued presence of $[HCO_3^-]_o$ does not significantly alter a_{Cl}^i. Overall, a_{Cl}^i initially was 18.9 $\pm$ 1.0 mM and was increased by 0.2 $\pm$ 0.2 mM after 15-30 min in HCO_3^- Tyrode with 100 uM SITS (n = 7, p > 0.3). This finding is also contrary to expectations for a system where Cl^- accumulation is mediated by Cl^-/HCO_3^- exchange (see Fig. 1).

Is Cl^-/HCO_3^- exchange present in ventricle?

Failure to observe a decrease in a_{Cl}^i with both HCO_3^- removal and SITS and the lack of effect of SITS on Cl^- uptake under these conditions argues strongly that

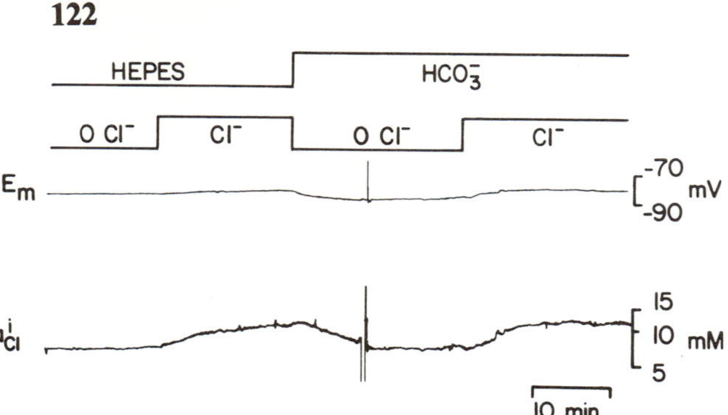

Fig. 3. Effect of HCO_3^- and CO_2 on Cl$^-$ reaccumulation after washout. After 1 hr in HEPES-buffered, Cl$^-$-free Tyrode (substituted with methanesulfonate), apparent a_{Cl}^i was 6.1 mM. On admission of Cl$^-$, a_{Cl}^i increased to 12.5 mM in 15 min. Cl$^-$ was then washed out for 30 min in HCO_3^-/CO_2-buffered Tyrode, and the rate of reaccumulation was measured again. This time, the initial rate of increase was 2.38-times faster. These data suggest Cl$^-$/HCO_3^- exchange contributes to Cl$^-$ reaccumulation.

Cl$^-$/HCO_3^- exchange is not important in the regulation of a_{Cl}^i under physiological conditions. Nevertheless, Fig. 3 demonstrates that HCO_3^--dependent Cl$^-$ uptake occurs in ventricle. First, muscles were Cl$^-$ depleted by exposure to Cl$^-$-free Tyrode for at least 30 min, and then, Cl$^-$ was readmitted. In the presence of HEPES-buffered Tyrode, a_{Cl}^i increased 6.4 mM in 15 min. When the experiment was repeated in the presence of HCO_3^-, a_{Cl}^i increased 7.4 mM over the same interval. Analysis of the initial rates of Cl$^-$ accumulation in this group of experiments showed that Cl$^-$ uptake was 1.61 ± 0.09 times faster (n = 7, p < 0.005) in the presence of $[HCO_3^-]_o$ than in its absence, 0.75 ± 0.25 and 0.49 ± 0.18 mM/min, respectively. This slowing of Cl$^-$ reaccumulation in the absence of HCO_3^- suggests that Cl$^-$/HCO_3^- exchange plays a role in Cl$^-$ uptake under these conditions.

To verify that Cl$^-$/HCO_3^- exchange was involved, the effect of SITS on Cl$^-$ reaccumulation after its washout in Cl$^-$-free Tyrode was studied. Fig. 4 compares reaccumulation under control conditions with that in the presence of 500 uM SITS. Under control conditions, a_{Cl}^i increased 7.0 mM in 15 min. SITS slowed reaccumulation substantially. In this example, a_{Cl}^i increased only 1.9 mM in the same interval, and analysis of the initial rates of accumulation showed a nearly 2-fold slowing of Cl$^-$ uptake from 1.4 to 0.71 mM/min. In 3 experiments, the ratio of the initial rate of a_{Cl}^i accumulation in control/500 uM SITS was 1.42 ± 0.14 (p < 0.05). In 6 additional experiments, 100 uM SITS slowed uptake by the same amount; the control/100 uM SITS ratio was 1.49 ± 0.18 (p < 0.005). Taken together, the effects of removal of $[HCO_3^-]_o$ and SITS on a_{Cl}^i reaccumulation indicate that Cl$^-$/HCO_3^- exchange occurs in ventricle and

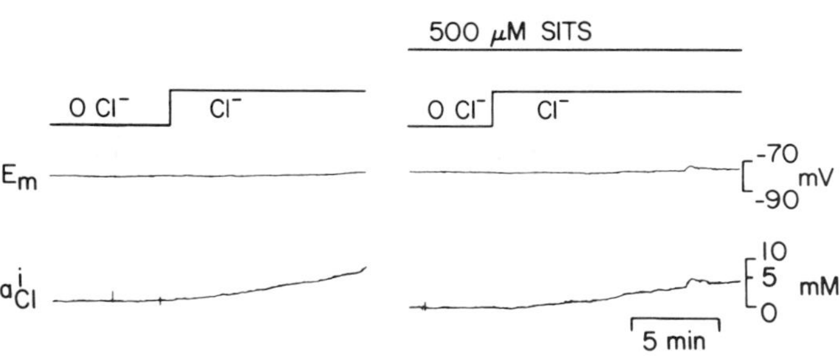

Fig. 4. Effect of SITS on Cl⁻ reaccumulation after washout. Cl⁻ was washed out in HCO_3^-/CO_2-buffered Tyrode (see Fig. 3 for details). On readmitting Cl⁻, apparent a_{Cl}^i increased from 2.8 mM to 9.8 mM in 15 min. Procedure was then repeated, except in the presence of 500 uM SITS. SITS was added to solutions 15 min before Cl⁻ was increased. This time, apparent a_{Cl}^i increased from 3.0 to 4.9 mM after 15 min. These data confirm that Cl^-/HCO_3^- exchange contributes to Cl⁻ reaccumulation. Continuous impalements were maintained throughout the experiment; a portion of the record is omitted for clarity.

can mediate the influx of Cl⁻. Our inability to reduce steady state a_{Cl}^i by inhibiting Cl^-/HCO_3^- exchange implies, however, that this process does not regulate a_{Cl}^i.

Na⁺-dependent Cl⁻ accumulation.

If Cl^-/HCO_3^- exchange is not responsible for the maintenance of high a_{Cl}^i in ventricle under physiological conditions, what is? In a variety of cells, electroneutral Na⁺-dependent Cl⁻ cotransport moves Cl⁻ into cells (e.g., 9-12). Cl⁻ and Na⁺ uptake occur together with a 1:1 stoichiometry (Na⁺/Cl⁻ cotransport), or 1 Na⁺, 1 K⁺ and 2 Cl⁻ enter the cell together (Na⁺/K⁺/2Cl⁻ cotransport; in some cases, the stoichiometry is different but still electroneutral, e.g., 25). In both systems, the Na⁺ gradient helps drive the accumulation of Cl⁻, and the rate of Cl⁻ uptake is slowed if the extracellular Na⁺ concentration ($[Na^+]_o$) is lowered.

Fig. 5 suggests that Na⁺-dependent Cl⁻ cotransport occurs in heart. To eliminate any contribution from Cl^-/HCO_3^- exchange, HCO_3^--free Tyrode containing 100 uM SITS was used as the basic solution. When $[Na^+]_o$ in this solution was successively reduced from 100% to 75 and 50% of normal, a_{Cl}^i fell from 19.6 mM to 17.4 and 13.8 mM, respectively. On restoring 100% $[Na^+]_o$, a_{Cl}^i rapidly increased to very close to its initial value. Similar results were seen on switching directly from 100% to 50% $[Na^+]_o$. The average decrease of a_{Cl}^i was 2.7 ± 0.6 mM in 75% $[Na^+]_o$ (n = 5, p < 0.005) and was 4.1 ± 0.3 mM in 50% $[Na^+]_o$ (n = 10, p < 0.005). These data strongly argue that a Na⁺-dependent Cl⁻ transport system helps regulate a_{Cl}^i.

In an attempt to identify the Na⁺-dependent process as Na⁺/Cl⁻ cotransport, chlorothiazide (CTZ) was employed. CTZ is a distal tubule diuretic and inhibits Na⁺/Cl⁻ cotransport (26-28a) but not Na⁺/K⁺/2Cl⁻ cotransport (29,30). Fig. 6 shows the effect

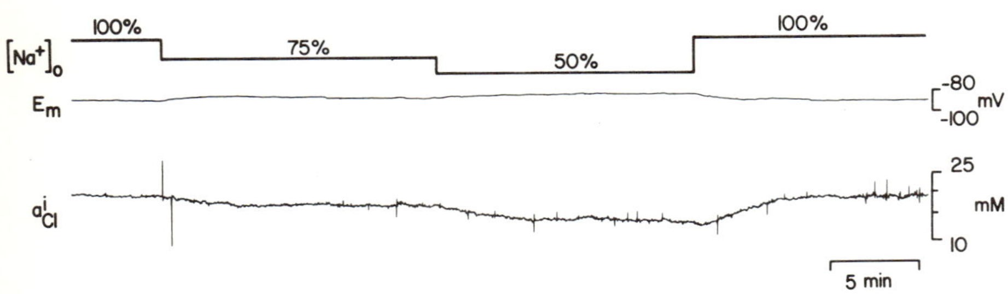

Fig. 5. Effect of $[Na^+]_o$ on a^i_{Cl}. $[Na^+]_o$ was reduced from 100% to 75 and 50% and then returned to 100% (equimolar substitution of N-methyl-d-glucamine). On lowering $[Na^+]_o$, a^i_{Cl} decreased from 19.6 mM to 17.4 and 13.8 mM, respectively. On restoring 100% $[Na^+]_o$, a^i_{Cl} increased rapidly to 18.6 mM. E_m was not significantly affected. The results suggest that Na^+-dependent Cl^- cotransport modulates a^i_{Cl}.

of 100 and 400 uM CTZ on Na^+-dependent Cl^- uptake stimulated by switching from 50 to 100% $[Na^+]_o$. Again, all solutions were HCO_3^--free and contained 100 uM SITS. While CTZ did not abolish the uptake of Cl^- on increasing $[Na^+]_o$, and eventually nearly the same increase in a^i_{Cl} was observed, analysis of the initial rates of a^i_{Cl} accumulation showed a marked effect of CTZ. In Fig. 6, the initial rates of Cl^- uptake were 0.48 mM/min under control conditions and 0.29 and 0.28 mM/min in the presence of 100 and 400 uM CTZ, respectively. In 5 trials, 100 uM CTZ slowed Cl^- uptake by 46%, from 0.48 $\pm$ 0.03 to 0.26 $\pm$ 0.03 mM/min (p < 0.005). Lack of further inhibition on raising the dose of CTZ from 100 to 400 uM was confirmed in one additional experiment. Additionally, 100 uM CTZ caused a significant decrease in a^i_{Cl} in 100% $[Na^+]_o$ Tyrode, 2.4 $\pm$ 0.1 mM (n = 4, p < 0.005).

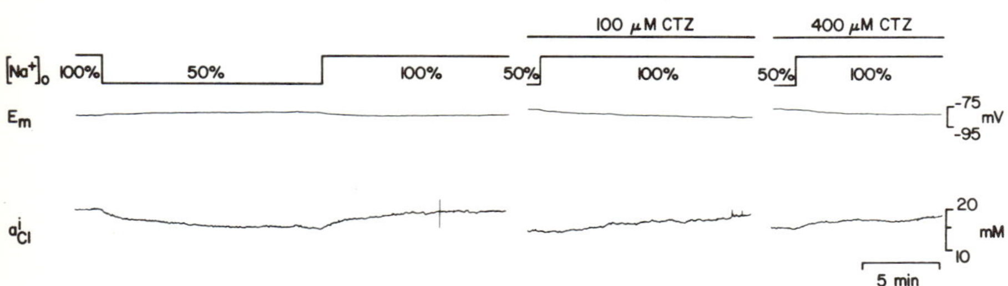

Fig. 6. Effect of chlorothiazide (CTZ), a Na^+/Cl^- cotransport blocker, on Na^+-dependent Cl^- uptake. $[Na^+]_o$ was lowered to 50%, and after a^i_{Cl} reached a steady-state, Na^+-dependent Cl^- cotransport was stimulated by returning $[Na^+]_o$ to 100%. Under control conditions, a^i_{Cl} increased from 20.4 to 24.3 mM in 15 min. In the presence of 100 and 400 uM CTZ, a^i_{Cl} increased in 15 min from 20.6 to 23.9 mM and from 19.5 to 22.5 mM, respectively. While Cl^- accumulation was not blocked, CTZ reduced the initial rate of Cl^- uptake. E_m was unaffected. The CTZ sensitivity of Cl^- uptake suggests Na^+/Cl^- cotransport. Continuous impalements were maintained throughout the experiment; portions of the record during exposure to low $[Na^+]_o$ Tyrode are omitted for clarity.

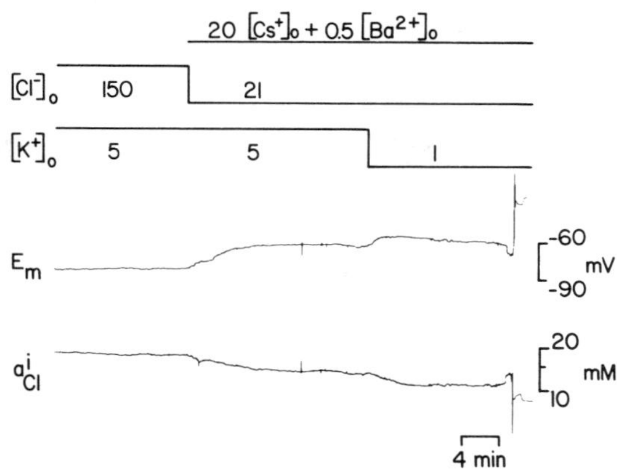

Fig. 7. [K$^+$]$_o$-dependence of a$^i_{Cl}$ was studied in 21 mM [Cl$^-$]$_o$ with 0.5 mM [Ba^{2+}]$_o$ and 20 mM [Cs$^+$]$_o$ added to block K$^+$ conductance. In low Cl$^-$, 5 mM [K$^+$]$_o$ Tyrode, a$^i_{Cl}$ was 13.3 mM and decreased to 11.2 mM when [K$^+$]$_o$ was reduced to 1 mM. The 4-6 mV depolarization of E$_m$ cannot explain the decrease in a$^i_{Cl}$. Sensitivity of a$^i_{Cl}$ to [K$^+$]$_o$ suggests K$^+$-dependent Cl$^-$ cotransport.

The inability of CTZ to fully abolish Na$^+$-dependent Cl$^-$ accumulation may suggest that Cl$^-$ uptake is mediated, at least in part, by Na$^+$/K$^+$/2Cl$^-$ cotransport. Support for this idea was obtained by showing that a$^i_{Cl}$ can be altered by [K$^+$]$_o$, independent of its effect on E$_m$. To maximize the effect of [K$^+$]$_o$ on the putative Na$^+$/K$^+$/2Cl$^-$ cotransporter, [Cl$^-$]$_o$ was lowered to 21 mM, reducing the Cl$^-$ gradient. Further, 0.5 mM [Ba^{2+}]$_o$ and 20 mM [Cs$^+$]$_o$ were used to minimize changes in E$_m$ on varying [K$^+$]$_o$. Fig. 7 illustrates the experimental results. a$^i_{Cl}$ decreased from 17.1 to 13.3 mM on reducing [Cl$^-$]$_o$, and simultaneously, E$_m$ depolarized because of the K$^+$ channel blockers. The critical observation is the additional reduction in a$^i_{Cl}$ to 11.2 mM when [K$^+$]$_o$ was lowered to 1 mM. This fall in a$^i_{Cl}$ cannot be explained by increased passive Cl$^-$ efflux; a small depolarization occurred and, if anything, should have increased a$^i_{Cl}$ by reducing passive Cl$^-$ efflux.

DISCUSSION

Several important conclusions can be drawn from these experiments. Cl$^-$/HCO$_3^-$ exchange does not control a$^i_{Cl}$ in ventricle, although evidence for its presence was obtained. Further, Na$^+$-dependent Cl$^-$ transport was identified and found to regulate a$^i_{Cl}$, at least in part. The sensitivity of Na$^+$-dependent Cl$^-$ uptake to chlorothiazide and [K$^+$]$_o$ suggests the process may reflect Na$^+$/Cl$^-$ and Na$^+$/K$^+$/2Cl$^-$ cotransport, systems described in numerous other cells (9-12,25,28-29,31). These findings are incorporated in Fig. 8, a revised model of the control of a$^i_{Cl}$ in ventricle.

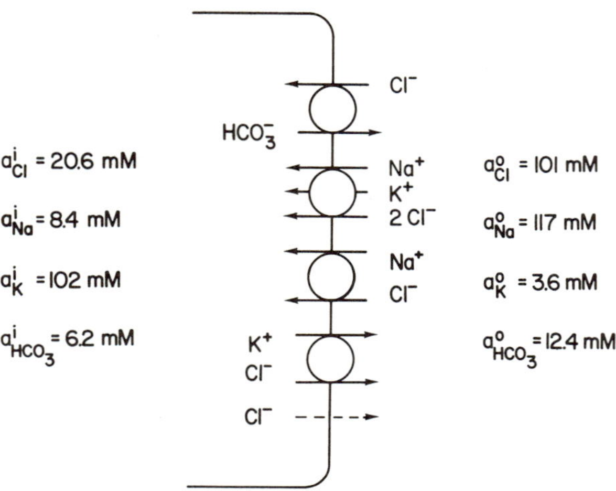

$a^i_{Cl} = 20.6$ mM

$a^i_{Na} = 8.4$ mM

$a^i_K = 102$ mM

$a^i_{HCO_3} = 6.2$ mM

$a^o_{Cl} = 101$ mM

$a^o_{Na} = 117$ mM

$a^o_K = 3.6$ mM

$a^o_{HCO_3} = 12.4$ mM

Fig. 8. A new model for a^i_{Cl} regulation in ventricle. Include are: (1) Cl^-/HCO_3^- exchange, which moves Cl^- into the cell in exchange for HCO_3^-; (2) Na^+-dependent Cl^- cotransport as Na^+/Cl^- and $Na^+/K^+/2Cl^-$ cotransport, which move Cl^- into the cell concomitantly with Na^+ and K^+; (3) K^+/Cl^- cotransport, which moves Cl^- *out* of the cell with K^+; and (4) an outward-directed passive Cl^- leak. Typical intra-and extracellular ionic activities for heart are given.

Differences in regulation of a^i_{Cl} in ventricle and Purkinje fibers.

In Purkinje fibers, the resting level of a^i_{Cl} is sensitive to HCO_3^- and CO_2 and falls by 5.7 mM when they are removed (1); the rate of Cl^- reaccumulation in Cl^- depleted fibers is dramatically reduced to 5-10% of its value in HCO_3^-/CO_2-buffered solution by removing and HCO_3^- and CO_2 or by the Cl^-/HCO_3^- exchange blocker SITS (2); the rate of Cl^- depletion in Cl^--free solutions is slowed by HCO_3^--free solution or by SITS (2); and changes in pH_i are associated with simultaneous movements of Cl^- and are blocked by SITS and DIDS (2,8). Vaughan-Jones (1-2,8) concluded from these data that a^i_{Cl} was regulated in Purkinje fibers by Cl^- uptake via a reversible Cl^-/HCO_3^- exchanger. This system is somewhat unusual in that HCO_3^--dependent Cl^- transport in several other tissues acts to *reduce* a^i_{Cl} and is stimulated by acidosis (24,32). On the other hand, Cl^-/HCO_3^- exchange in smooth muscle appears similar to that in Purkinje fibers both in its transport of Cl^- and lack of response to acidosis (18).

The present results establish that regulation of a^i_{Cl} in ventricle is very different from that in Purkinje fibers. a^i_{Cl} does not fall on removal of HCO_3^- and CO_2; rather, continuous impalement experiments show that it rises by 5 mM. This confirms observations that a^i_{Cl} remains much higher than expected from a passive distribution in ventricular muscle perfused with HCO_3^--free Tyrode (3-6). Based on comparisons of a^i_{Cl} in different muscles, it was previously suggested that on removal of HCO_3^-, a^i_{Cl} may increase (5,6) or may not be affected (4). Interpretation of data under nominally HCO_3^--

free conditions is complicated by uncertainty regarding continued function of Cl^-/HCO_3^- exchange, either supported by metabolically produced HCO_3^- (17-19) or during the washout of $[HCO_3^-]_i$ (5). However, the finding that SITS has no effect on the initial rate of Cl^- uptake or final a^i_{Cl} on switching to HCO_3^--free Tyrode rules out a contribution of Cl^-/HCO_3^- exchange to the accumulation of Cl^- under nominally HCO_3^--free conditions. Further, the lack of SITS sensitivity also suggests Na^+-HCO_3^-/H^+-Cl^- exchange, which mediates a SITS-sensitive efflux of Cl^- in other tissues (21,22), is not involved. These data together with the failure of SITS to cause a decrease of a^i_{Cl} in the continued presence of HCO_3^- argue persuasively that Cl^-/HCO_3^- exchange does not have a significant role in controlling a^i_{Cl} at physiological levels in ventricle.

Despite the unimportance of Cl^-/HCO_3^- exchange under physiological conditions in ventricle, a Cl^- uptake attributable to Cl^-/HCO_3^- exchange was demonstrated, as in Purkinje fibers (2,8). Reaccumulation of Cl^- in Cl^--depleted papillary muscles was slowed by about 1.5-fold by both removal of HCO_3^- and CO_2 and by SITS. This implies about 1/3 of the Cl^- influx was mediated by Cl^-/HCO_3^- exchange. The contribution of Cl^-/HCO_3^- exchange under these conditions also appears to be less important in ventricle than in Purkinje fibers, where these maneuvers slowed reaccumulation by 18- and 9-fold, respectively (2). Other evidence suggesting Cl^-/HCO_3^- exchange in ventricle comes from experiments on the effect of hypoxia on a^i_{Cl} (33). Hypoxia in HCO_3^--free Tyrode caused a fall in a^i_{Cl}, but a^i_{Cl} remained constant in the presence of HCO_3^-. Apparently, Cl^-/HCO_3^- exchange is relatively more important under hypoxic conditions.

Na^+-dependent Cl^- cotransport.

Evidence was obtained supporting the idea that Na^+-dependent Cl^- cotransport mediates an accumulation of Cl^- under physiological conditions and regulates a^i_{Cl}. Both reducing $[Na^+]_o$ and exposure to CTZ, a Na^+-dependent Cl^- cotransport blocker (26-28a), cause a fall of a^i_{Cl}, and CTZ slows the rate of Cl^- uptake on increasing $[Na^+]_o$ by nearly 50%. The k_m with respect to $[Na^+]_o$ of this process in some other systems (12) appears to be appropriate to qualitatively explain the decreased Cl^- uptake in the present study. Although conductive Cl^- fluxes were not rigorously excluded, the underlying process is likely to be electroneutral because significant changes in E_m did not occur. The Na^+-dependent Cl^- uptake cannot be attributed to Cl^-/HCO_3^- nor Na^+-HCO_3^-/H^+-Cl^- exchange because these experiments were done in HCO_3^--free Tyrodes containing SITS (2,8,21,22). Consistent with Na^+-dependent Cl^- cotransport, a^i_{Na} in heart also falls when $[Na^+]_o$ is reduced (34); however, other Na^+ transport processes involved in the regulation of a^i_{Na} contribute to the fall of a^i_{Na}. These processes and Na^+ binding would seriously confound attempts to directly measure the stoichiometry of the transport mechanism.

It is tempting to speculate that Na^+-dependent Cl^- cotransport may be involved in the accumulation of Cl^- on removing HCO_3^-. For example, if HCO_3^- and Cl^- compete for a binding site on the exchanger, removal of HCO_3^- would increase occupancy of the site by Cl^- and might increase the rate of Cl^- uptake. Binding constants and kinetics of the transport process, details not presently available, are required to evaluate this idea. Nevertheless, it is interesting that rabbit gall bladder apparently absorbs HCO_3^- and some other anions in a Na^+-dependent, electrically silent manner (35). Such lack of anion specificity may not be universal, however (12).

Stilbene-insensitive, Na^+-dependent Cl^- cotransport occurs in other tissues including erythrocytes (9,12), epithelia (10,28-29), Ehrlich cells (11), nerve (25), and smooth muscle (31) as either Na^+/Cl^- or $Na^+/K^+/2Cl^-$ cotransport, and it is not surprising that it also operates in heart muscle. It does not appear to be present in Purkinje fibers, however. Vaughan-Jones (8) claimed Cl^- uptake in Purkinje fibers is insensitive to removal of $[Na^+]_o$ and $[K^+]_o$, although details of the experiments were not presented.

Na^+/Cl^- cotransport. Based on the inhibition Na^+/Cl^- (26-28a) but not $Na^+/K^+/2Cl^-$ (29,30) cotransport in epithelia by CTZ, it seems reasonable to suggest that part of the Na^+-dependent Cl^- uptake in ventricle is Na^+/Cl^- cotransport. Hints of a linkage between Na^+ and Cl^- fluxes were obtained in early flux studies on Purkinje fibers (36). Nevertheless, this suggestion must be regarded cautiously. A linkage between Cl^- and Na^+ *transport* was not rigorously demonstrated in the present experiments, and the effect of $[K^+]_o$ on the CTZ-sensitive Cl^- uptake was not evaluated.

$Na^+/K^+/2Cl^-$ cotransport. CTZ slowed the Na^+-stimulated Cl^--uptake by only about 50% and did not substantially decrease the final a_{Cl}^i attained. This suggests that another Na^+-dependent process operates in ventricle. The sensitivity of a_{Cl}^i to $[K^+]_o$ under conditions where changes in the passive Cl^- efflux were not important are consistent with $Na^+/K^+/2Cl^-$ cotransport. In other systems, the k_m with respect to $[K^+]_o$ is 5-6 mM (9,12). Decreasing $[K^+]_o$ from 5 to 1 mM is therefore expected to significantly reduce the rate of Cl^- uptake. A furosemide-sensitive Rb^+ influx in cultured embryonic chick heart previously has been attributed to a $Na^+/K^+/2Cl^-$ cotransporter (37). However, neither a Cl^- nor Na^+ dependence was demonstrated, and K^+/Cl^- cotransport in heart (38), the sodium pump and adenyl cyclase (9) are also among the furosemide-sensitive membrane processes.

An alternative explanation for the fall in a_{Cl}^i on lowering $[K^+]_o$ is the behavior of K^+/Cl^- cotransport, a system recently demonstrated in cultured embryonic chick heart by Piwnica-Worms et al. (38). Lowering $[K^+]_o$ is expected to increase the rate of coupled KCl efflux by this mechanism and could also result in a fall in a_{Cl}^i. However, a_{Cl}^i in mammalian preparations is insensitive to increased $[K^+]_o$ unless it is raised to high levels. Then, a^i_{Cl} increases, an effect attributed to decreased passive efflux or passive influx when E_m exceeds the Cl^- equilibrium potential, E_{Cl} (1-3,8; cf., 38). Piwinica-Worms et al. (38) also argued $Na^+/K^+/2Cl^-$ cotransport was not present in their preparation; Cl^- transport was insensitive to Li^+ which can substitute for Na^+ in the $Na^+/K^+/2Cl^-$ cotransport process in other tissues.

A physiological role for Cl^- regulation.

The maintenance of a^i_{Cl} above the level for passive distribution in the face of the substantial Cl^- permeability of ventricle (39) requires the expenditure of energy. What is the benefit to the cell? Cl^- appears to have a very minor direct role in electrical and mechanical activity of heart. The Cl^- gradient is important, however, in electro-neutral exchange and cotransport processes. Cl^--dependent pH_i regulation is important in other tissues (17,20-24,32), and Cl^-/HCO_3^- exchange has been shown to assist recovery from alkalosis but not acidosis in cardiac Purkinje fibers (2,8,40). While Cl^-/HCO_3^- exchange is relatively less important in ventricle than Purkinje fiber, it may still have a role in pH_i regulation. If that is the case, Na^+-dependent Cl^- cotransport would indirectly contribute to pH_i regulation by setting a^i_{Cl}.

Another potentially important role for a^i_{Cl} is in volume regulation. Both Na^+/Cl^- and $Na^+/K^+/2Cl^-$ cotransport normally present an osmotic load to the cell and should be accompanied by the influx of H_2O. In contrast, K^+/Cl^- cotransport normally reduces intracellular osmolarity (38). Modulation of the rates of these processes could be used by the heart to regulate cell volume, and both Na^+-dependent Cl^- cotransport and K^+/Cl^- cotransport have been implicated in volume regulation (9,38,41-43). It would not be surprising for Cl^- to have a central role in maintaining osmotic balance. Cl^- is the predominant intra- and extracellular mobile anion, and its movement can be linked with cation fluxes to maintain electroneutrality while doing osmotic work. Little is presently known about cellular volume regulation in the heart. That Cl^- is not passively distributed implies that the mechanism underlying volume regulation is very different than in a Donnan equilibrium system (cf., 44). Nevertheless, Cl^- may have a still have a fundamental role.

SUMMARY

In contrast to results in Purkinje fibers (1,2,8), Cl^-/HCO_3^- exchange does not regulate a^i_{Cl} in ventricular muscle. Inhibiting Cl^-/HCO_3^- exchange by removal of HCO_3^- and CO_2 from the bathing media or by SITS failed to cause a fall in a^i_{Cl}. However, a Cl^-/HCO_3^- exchange that mediates Cl^- uptake was identified. Both HCO_3^--free Tyrode and SITS slowed reaccumulation of a^i_{Cl} in Cl^--depleted muscle by about 35%, far less than in Purkinje fibers. In ventricular muscle, regulation of a^i_{Cl} at physiological levels appears to be accomplished predominantly by Na^+-dependent Cl^- cotransport that accumulates Cl^-. Lowering $[Na^+]_o$ resulted in a rapid but reversible decrease of a^i_{Cl}. Based on the sensitivity of Cl^- accumulation to CTZ about half of the Na^+-dependent Cl^- uptake was attributed to Na^+/Cl^- cotransport. Demonstration of a $[K^+]_o$-sensitivity of a^i_{Cl} that was independent of E_m suggests the rest of the Na^+-dependent Cl^- uptake may be $Na^+/K^+/2Cl^-$ cotransport.

ACKNOWLEDGEMENTS

We thank Drs. M. Desilets and L.S. Costanzo for helpful discussions, Dr. L.S. Costanzo for suggesting the use of chlorothiazide, and Ms. K.E. Cress and the staff of the Biomedical Instrumentation Facility for technical support.

Supported by a grant from the National Heart, Lung and Blood Institute (HL-24847). C.M.B. is an Established Investigator of the American Heart Association.

REFERENCES

1. Vaughan-Jones, R.D. *J. Physiol. Lond.* **295**:83-109, 1979.
2. Vaughan-Jones, R.D. *J. Physiol. Lond.* **295**:111-137, 1979.
3. Baumgarten C.M. and Fozzard, H.A. *Am. J. Physiol.* **241**:C121-C129, 1981.
4. Caille, J.P., Ruiz-Ceretti, E. and Schanne, O.F. *Am. J. Physiol.* **240**:C183-C188, 1981.
5. Fong, C.N. and Hinke, A.M. *Can. J. Physiol. Pharmacol.* **59**:479-484, 1980.
6. Spitzer, K.W. and Walker, J.L. *Am. J. Physiol.* **238**:H487-H493, 1980.
7. Ladle R.O. and Walker, J.L. *J. Physiol. Lond.* **251**:549-559, 1975.
8. Vaughan-Jones, R.D. *Phil. Trans. Roy. Soc. Lond. B* **299**:537-548, 1982.
9. Ellory, J.C., Dunham, P.B., Logue, P.J. and Stewart, G.W. *Phil. Trans. Roy. Soc. Lond. B* **299**: 483-495, 1982.
10. Frizzel, R.A., Field, M. and Schultz, S.G. *Am. J. Physiol.* **236**:F1-F8, 1979.
11. Geck, P., Pietrzyk, C., Burkhardt, B.C., Pfeiffer B. and Heinz, E. *Biochem. Biophys. Acta.* **600**: 432-447, 1980.
12. Palfrey, H.C. and Rao, M.C. *J. Exp. Biol.* **106**: 43-54, 1983.
13. Duncan, S.W.N. and Baumgarten, C.M. *Circulat.* **70**:II-271, 1984.
14. Baumgarten, C.M. *Am. J. Physiol.* **241**:C258-C263, 1981.
15. Baumgarten, C.M. In: *Methods in Studying Cardiac Membranes, Vol. II.* (Ed.: N.S. Dhalla), CRC Press, Boca Raton, 1984, pp. 213-237.
16. Baumgarten, C.M. *Comput. Biol. Med.* **11**:189-196, 1981.
17. Boron, W.F., McCormick, W.F. and Roos A. *Am. J. Physiol.* **240**:C80-C89, 1981.
18. Aickin, C.C. and Brading, A.F. *J. Physiol. Lond.* **349**:587-606, 1984.
19. Moody, W.J. *J. Physiol. Lond.* **316**:293-308, 1981.
20. Becker, B.F. and Duhm, J. *J. Physiol. Lond.* **282**:149-168, 1978.
21. Thomas, R.C. In: *Intracellular pH: Its Measurement, Regulation and Utilization in Cellular Function.* (Ed.: R. Nuccitelli and D.W. Deamer) Alan R. Liss, New York, 1982, pp. 189-204.
22. Boron, W.F. and Russel, J.M. *J. Gen. Physiol.* **81**:373-399, 1983.
23. Boron, W.F. *J. Gen. Physiol.* **85**:325-345, 1985.
24. Russell, J.M., Boron, W.F. and Brodwick, M.S. *J. Gen. Physiol.* **82**:47-78, 1983.
25. Russell, J.M. *J. Gen. Physiol.* **81**:909-925, 1983.
26. Kunau, R.T., Weller, D.R. and Webb, H.L. *J. Clin. Invest.* **56**:401-407, 1975.
27. Costanzo, L.S. and Windhager, E.E. *Am. J. Physiol.* **235**:F492-F506, 1978.
28. Stokes, J.B. *J. Clin. Invest.* **74**:7-16, 1984.
28a. Velazquez, H. and Wright, F.S. *Am. J. Physiol.* **250**:F1013-F1023, 1986.
29. Schlatter, E., Greger, R. and Weidtke, C. *Pfluegers Arch.* **396**:210-217, 1983.

30. Burg, M. personal communication, cited in ref. 27.
31. Brading, A.F. *Brit. Med. Bull.* **35**:227-234, 1980.
32. Roos, A. and Boron, W.F. *Physiol. Rev.* **61**:296-434, 1981.
33. Duncan, S.W.N. and Baumgarten, C.M. *Proc. Soc. Exp. Biol. Med.* **176**:216, 1983.
34. Sheu, S.-S. and Fozzard, H.A. *J. Gen. Physiol.* **80**:325-351, 1982.
35. Whitlock, R.T. and Wheeler, H.O. *Am. J. Physiol.* **213**:1199-1204, 1967.
36. Carmeliet, E.E. and Bosteels, S. *Arch. Int. Physiol. Biochem.* **77**:57-72, 1969.
37. Aiton, J.F., Chipperfield, A.R., Lamb, J.F., Ogden, P. and Simmons, N.L. *Biochim. Biophys. Acta* **646**:389-398, 1981.
38. Piwnica-Worms, D., Jacob, R., Horres, C.R. and Lieberman, M. *Am. J. Physiol.* **249**:C337-C344, 1985.
39. Fozzard, H.A. and Lee, C.O. *J. Physiol. Lond.* **256**:663-689, 1976.
40. Vanheel, B., de Hemptinne, A. and Leusen, I. *Am. J. Physiol.* **246**:C391-C400, 1984.
41. Hoffman, E.K. *Phil. Trans. Roy. Soc. Lond.* B **299**:519-535, 1982.
42. Geck, P. and Pfeiffer, B. *Ann. N.Y. Acad. Sci.* **456**:166-182, 1985.
43. McManus, T.J., Haas, M., Starke, L.C. and Lytle, C.Y. *Ann. N.Y. Acad. Sci.* **456**:183-197, 1985.
44. Jakobsson, E. *Am. J. Physiol.* **238**:C196-C206, 1980.

C. SARCOLEMMAL FUNCTIONS

8

PARASYMPATHETIC CONTROL OF THE HEART: SUBCELLULAR MECHANISMS

P.V. SULAKHE, J.E. MACKAY, D.G. ROKOSH, T. MORRIS AND T.D. PHAN

Department of Physiology, University of Saskatchewan, Saskatoon, Sask.
Canada S7N 0W0

INTRODUCTION

The well-established control of the heart by autonomic nerves
involves the action of two neurotransmitters, acetylcholine and
norepinephrine, with the specific receptors located postsynaptically in
the heart.   Depending on whether the region harbors pacemaker, conducting or contractile tissue, the well-known reciprocal effects on
excitability, automaticity, conductivity and contractility of parasympathetic and sympathetic nerves are expressed within the appropriate
regions of the heart (1,2).   How neurotransmitter action at the cell
surface locale, irrespective of the heart region, influences selectively
the main functions of these specialized heart regions remains an enigma.
It is becoming apparent that the influence of receptor activation on
coupled effector systems vicinally located within the surface membrane
matrix sets in motion subcellular and metabolic processes within the
cellular interior that subserve appropriate responses of the heart
regions to autonomic transmitters (1-3). From the stand-point of innervation the mammalian heart (notwithstanding species specificity) shows a
diffuse regional pattern for sympathetic innervation with slightly
greater density in the pacemaker or nodal regions.   By comparison the
parasympathetic innervation shows greater specificity in that nodal
regions are highly innervated and left ventricle free wall sparsely
innervated (3).   This alone is indicative of greater control of chrono-
tropy by parasympathetic nerves over the inotropy.   In fact it is often
difficult to document direct actions of cholinergic stimuli on mammalian
ventricular contractility.   On the other hand cholinergic stimuli
potently antagonize beta-adrenergically induced positive inotropic state
of the ventricular myocardium (1-3).   Rarely one can envisage an _in vivo_
situation showing the altered activity of only one division of the

autonomic nervous system innervating the heart (ventricles). It is commonly observed that the efficacy of cholinergic antagonism increases with the increased sympathetic drive to the ventricle. This intriguing phenomenon, called accentuated antagonism by Professor M. Levy (4,5), might involve at the level of ventricular contractile cell accentuated antagonism in the interaction between agonist occupied cholinergic receptor and beta-adrenergic receptor and various effector systems coupled to and regulated by these receptors. It may also involve the expression of effector system-generated messengers acting on a finite number of proteins (some possessing enzymatic machinery) participating in contraction and relaxation as well as in energy metabolism linked to mechanical events. The observed resting heart rate and parasympathetic tone show an intriguing parallel relation and this has led to the possibility that parasympathetic tone is a dominant determinant "at rest" setting the level of the heart's performance _in vivo_ (4). Altered sympathetic tone then can be thought to modulate the heart's pumping action in relation to the varying demands imposed in situations like exercise, fright and flight etc. Simultaneous alterations in the peripheral vasculature, both neurally and humorally, along with those in the heart's pumping action form the highly integrative cardiovascular system serving the bodily needs in terms of the tissues receiving appropriate energy supply for their proper functioning. The main emphasis of this article is to describe briefly the subcellular basis of the parasympathetic control of the myocardium and will include recent evidence implicating the roles that various effector systems play in this control. We will describe the results from our laboratory obtained by examining the phosphorylation of critical myocyte proteins and the metabolism of phosphoinositides in isolated, intact, rat ventricular cardiomyocytes. We also present the influence of autonomic receptor agonists on these biochemical events. The likely physiological signif-icance of our findings is discussed. Further, based on these observa-tions and those published by others we propose a working hypothesis involving the contributions of phospho-dephosphorylation of myocyte proteins in the autonomic control of the myocardium. A brief review of current state of knowledge is presented prior to the description of our findings.

<u>Cholinergic Receptor and Associated Effectors in the Heart:</u>

Physiological and pharmacological investigations carried out in isolated mammalian hearts or heart regions clearly document that chronotropic as well as inotropic alterations evoked by cholinergic stimuli result from the activation of plasma membrane-bound cholinergic receptors that are of the muscarinic type (1-3,6). Recent availability of subtype-specific agonists and antagonists has provided information for the presence of M_1 and M_2 subtypes of cholinergic receptors in the heart with the latter subtype being the most predominant (2,6,7). The available evidence is consistent with the view that the cholinergic regulation of such effector systems as adenylate cyclase, phosphoinositol phosphodiesterase, slow calcium channels and specific potassium channels (in the case of the SA node and atria) is M_2-receptor mediated in mammalian heart (2,8). Recent investigations document an obligatory role of GTP binding coupling proteins in the regulation of effector system(s) by agonist-occupied M_2 receptors (1,2,9,10). How agonist binding to the M_2 receptor leads to alterations in one or more effector systems remains a topic of considerable interest. Several possibilities have been considered. First the knowledge that more than one type of coupling protein is detected in the heart (9,10) has led to the suggestion of selective recruitment of each type in a specific effector response; for example Ni is believed to be involved in the adenylate cyclase regulation (2). Alternatively the "activation" of specific coupling proteins is believed to depend on the concentration of the physiological agonist, acetylcholine, such that there may be a sequential participation of coupling proteins regulating specific effector systems; for example, adenylate cyclase regulation (by Ni) occurring at lower agonist concentration than that of phosphoinositol phosphodiesterase regulation (by another coupling protein tentatively termed Np) (11). It is also likely that there exists kinetic difference in the onset or duration of specific effector response which in turn may depend on the kinetic difference in the interaction between the agonist-occupied receptor and a coupling protein specific for a particular effector system.

Recent investigations have witnessed the intriguing nature of coupling proteins in terms of their structure and amounts (12). These show considerable structural homologies in their subunit structures (and particularly in beta/gamma subunits) with minor differences in the alpha subunits which possess guanine nucleotide binding domains, enzymatic machinery as GTPase, effector interaction domains, receptor interaction domains, and domains for interaction with beta/gamma subunits. There is evidence that "inhibitory" receptor linked coupling proteins are present in higher amounts relative to a GTP binding coupling protein called Ns linked to a "stimulatory" receptor like beta-adrenergic receptor and which plays an obligatory role in stimulation of adenylate cyclase by beta-receptor agonists (2,12). While the precise stoichiometric relation among receptors/coupling proteins/effectors is of considerable interest, so far only rough estimates have been made based on (many) assumptions. They indicate much greater amounts of coupling proteins than receptors or effectors and perhaps the rank order may be coupling proteins > receptors > effectors. It needs to be determined whether the amounts of each component of receptor/effector systems provide any pertinent insights to the issue of reciprocal control of myocardial function by autonomic receptors. The idea that these components must be vicinal within the membrane matrix suggests the influence of beta-adrenergic receptor activation may involve the specific coupling protein Ns but will not exclude some influence on other coupling proteins like Ni and vice versa may occur following muscarinic receptor activation. A supporting evidence (13) for this view is available, although very much inconclusive at present. On the other hand beta-receptor activation evokes specifically alterations in adenylate cyclase and calcium channels (2,14,15) but not in phosphoinositol phosphodiesterase (16) indicates higher level of specificity within the effector systems. The accentuated antagonism defined physiologically is in essence a response phenomenon and thus at the level of plasma membrane it is not surprising it might also be expressed as a response of a particular effector. As will be discussed later in this article, such type of antagonism may be evident at the level of proteins (response elements) involved in the regulation of intracellular actions of calcium or membrane-linked fluxes of calcium.

<u>Adenylate Cyclase/Cyclic AMP Involvement:</u>

The first indication that cholinergic stimuli influence cardiac adenylate cyclase activity was seen now nearly 25 years back (17). This was followed by the observed decrease in cyclic AMP concentration in atrial slices exposed to acetylcholine in 1971 (18). Numerous studies, especially in late seventies and in eighties, have consistently shown the coupling of cardiac cholinergic receptor of M_2 type to adenylate cyclase of myocardial plasma membrane and the action of agonist binding is to decrease the activity of this enzyme (2). It is now almost established that such coupling involves an obligatory role of a GTP binding protein termed Ni which has the potential of regulating both the receptor as well as the catalytic unit of adenylate cyclase (12,19). An implication of decreased cyclic AMP formation by decreasing the catalytic reactivity of adenylate cyclase by cholinergic stimuli is that there is decreased functioning of intracellular cyclic AMP receptor called protein kinase A. The documented actions of this enzyme include the phosphorylation occuring on serines or threonine residues of such proteins as inhibitory subunit of troponin (TN I,), a myofibrillar regulatory protein, phospholamban (PLN,), a sarcoplasmic reticulum regulatory protein, and perhaps plasma membrane calcium channel (slow channel) protein or regulatory proteins closely associated with the channel (20-23). The result of such phosphorylation on serine or threonine residues of these polypeptides is to alter their functions that include control of calcium affinity (TNI,) at the level of myofibrills, calcium sequestration (PLN,) at the level of sarcoplasmic reticulum and calcium influx through plasma membrane slow channels (20-23). Thus by decreasing cyclic AMP formation it is anticipated that cholinergic stimuli "slow down" the heart's pumping action especially if it were to be operating at higher level by sympathetic nerve stimulation that augment myocardial cyclic AMP concentration. While supporting evidence for such view is available (1,2), it is by no means complete or accounts for all alterations evoked by cholinergic stimuli in the heart. For example the well-known negative chronotropic action on the nodal, pacemaker, tissue which involves the regulation of specific potassium channels appears to be "cyclic AMP independent" (24,25). The possibility that cholinergic stimuli via stimulating cyclic AMP phophodiesterase might bring about the decrease in cytosolic cyclic AMP level has not been ruled out either. There exists evidence, albeit indirect, that has been interpreted to postulate (26) the activation of dephosphorylation mechanism being central to the cholinergic control rather than decreased kinase A catalyzed phosphorylation of above mentioned proteins. This does not necessarily rule out the contribution of "cyclic AMP response" to the cholinergic control of the myocardium or other regions of the heart but perhaps indicates the need to seriously consider the actions of other intracellular signals along with those of cyclic AMP.

Guanylate Cyclase/Cyclic GMP Involvement:

The intriguing observation (27) that acetylcholine increased cyclic GMP concentration, besides decreasing cyclic AMP concentration, in perfused rat heart has never been fully explained in terms of whether cyclic GMP participates in the cholinergic control of the myocardium. At the same time there are observations reported by many, some in seventies and in eighties as well, that strongly implicate as yet un-clarified role for this nucleotide (1,28,29). The presence of guanylate cyclase in the myocardium is unequivocally documented (1,28-31) and this is also true for cyclic GMP phophodiesterase (32-33) and cyclic GMP sensitive protein kinase (34-36). Although a significant portion of myocardial guanylate cyclase is plasma membrane bound (31), there is no clear-cut evidence that it is coupled to cholinergic receptors. On the other hand, there is evidence that kinase G is modulated by agonist binding to the receptor (34), although the physiological substrates for kinase G remain to be identified. Some results point out that cyclic GMP antagonizes the actions of cyclic AMP (1). This may include an intriguing possibility of cyclic GMP promoting the dephosphorylation mechanisms (26) or catalyzing the phosphorylation of sites other than those by kinase A as a means for such antagonism. Such speculative, albeit interesting, proposals demand rigorous experimental scrutiny prior to their acceptance.

Phosphoinositide Metabolism:

The results of the past several years have raised the possibility that agonist binding to cholinergic receptor stimulates the activity of phosphodiesterase (phospholipase C-type) that acts on the plasma membrane polyphophoinositides, a minor phospholipid fraction, to generate diacylglycerol (DG) and water-soluble inositolphosphates (IPs) (37). DG has been shown to activate a newly discovered protein kinase called kinase C, whose activity depends on phospholipids and calcium (38). While by no means exhaustive, there is now evidence that myocardium contains this enzyme, mostly in cytosolic compartment (39), and perhaps a portion of this translocates to other regions of the cell, particularly membranes, following the exposure of the tissue to cholinergic stimuli. It is also believed that by analogy to the kinase A system there exist specific substrates for kinase C that undergo phosphorylation at amino acid residues likely distinct from those for kinase A. The presence of endogenous substrates for kinase C, both soluble and membrane-bound, has been described in vitro (40-42). It is remarkable that amongst these TN I and PLN have been shown to undergo kinase C-dependent phosphorylation, although the significance of this in the context of cholinergic control of the myocardium is entirely speculative at present. An intriguing link between the kinase A and kinase C is evident in the studies carried out on non-cardiac tissues and this shows the phosphorylation of alpha-subunit of Ni by kinase C with the attendant "uncoupling" between the receptor and adenylate cyclase (43). Inositolphosphates, particularly inositoltriphosphate (IP_3), have been shown to cause the release of calcium from the endoplasmic reticulum of non-contractile cells (44), although there is no documentation of this effect in cardiac muscle in studies using the fragments of cardiac sarcoplasmic reticulum or isolated cardiomyocytes (45). In some preliminary investigations phorbol esters like PMA have been shown to influence myocardial contractility (46) and it is known that PMA acts as potent DG substitute to stimulate protein kinase C in many tissues including cardiac tissue (39). This and other recent evidence that cholinergic receptor agonists like carbachol increase the formation of IPs in isolated cardiac cells (16,47) lend support to the notion that kinase C pathway may participate in the parasympathetic control of the myocardium.

METHODS

Isolation of myocytes from rat heart ventricles:

This was essentially carried by the method described by Severson and Associates (48). Briefly rat (male, Wistar, 150-250 g body weight) heart was perfused retrograde for a few min in calcium-free KRB at $37^{o}C$ and then switched to perfusion containing Joklik medium supplemented with collagenase type II (Worthington, 300 units/ml, 100 ml per heart, perfusion rate of 5 ml/min). The ventricles were cut into small pieces and further incubated in Joklik medium containing collagenase. Dissociated cells were recovered by low gravitational centrifugation and their viability checked by trypan blue exclusion. Detailed methodology can be found in reference 48 and will be reported by us elsewhere. The recovery of myocytes was about 20 million cells per heart. Isolated myocytes were immediately used in the subsequently described assays.

Isolated myocytes were predominantly rod-shaped and quiescent and showed overall viability of at least 75% (most often 85-90% viability of isolated cells was noted); non-viable cells of rod and round shape constituted less than 20%. Elsewhere we will describe that these cells showed the presence of muscarinic cholinergic receptors, and beta- & alpha-adrenergic receptors. Also these myocytes showed the presence of autonomic receptor sensitive adenylate cyclase system and calcium channel supported calcium influx which was sensitive to autonomic receptor agonists and calcium channel agonists and antagonists. Thus isolated myocytes represented a useful preparation for investigating the phosphorylation of intact myocyte proteins relevant to contraction and relaxation of the myocardium and how it may be influenced by autonomic receptor agents and other stimuli that influence the generation of "second messengers" and myocardial contractility.

<u>Phosphorylation of myocytes:</u>

Isolated myocytes suspended in phosphate-free KRB buffer supplemented with 1% BSA (fatty acid free) were incubated under 95% O_2/5% CO_2 atmosphere at 30^0C for 60 min in the presence of $[^{32}P]$-Na_2HPO_4 (inorganic) (50 μCi/million cells). The cells were then transferred to assay mixture containing KRB/BSA and various agents (as described in appropriate figures) and incubated for 15 min; generally each assay contained 100,000 myocytes. Following this, cells were centrifuged and washed twice by suspending in KRB buffer and low gravitational centrifugation. The cells were then dissolved in the electrophoresis buffer containing SDS. Solubilized myocyte proteins were electrophoretically fractionated on a 7%-15% polyacrylamide gradient slab by the Laemmli's method. The slabs were stained with Coomassie Blue, destained with acetic acid, dried and then exposed to x-ray films at -70^0C with amplifying screens for 1 to 3 days. In some instances, autoradiograms were scanned and the phosphorylation results are expressed as arbitrary units (relative absorbance).

<u>Phospholipid labelling experiments:</u>

<u>Myocytes in KRB/BSA buffer were incubated either with [3-H]</u>

myoinositol (l0 uCi/million cells) or ^{32}-P (inorganic) for 60 min as described above and then were further incubated in the presence of various agents as described in Figure legends; 20 mM LiCl was included to inhibit inositolphosphatase(s) (49). Myocytes were sedimented and lipids were extracted (50). Phosphoinositides were extracted with acidified chloroform/methanol subsequent to the extraction of neutral lipids and other phospholipids. Extracted phospholipids and phospho-inositides were fractionated by TLC on oxalate-impregnated Silica gel plates (50) and dried plates were exposed to x-ray films at -70°C with amplifying screens for up to 3 days. In the case of tritium incorporation, the TLC plates were treated with 7% PPO in diethylether (51) prior to exposure to x-ray films.

<u>Inositol phosphate determination:</u>

Inositol phosphates released in the aqueous extracts of myocytes were fractionated essentially by the method of Berridge (52) involving Dowex-formate anion exchange chromatography. In some instances, labelled ^{32}-P (inorganic) was first removed as phosphomolybdate complex by isobutanol extraction prior to chromatographic separation of inositol phosphates.

RESULTS AND DISCUSSION

<u>Phosphorylation of Cardiomyocyte Proteins:</u>

Isolated myocytes were first incubated for 60 min at 30°C in phosphate-free, oxygenated KRB buffer supplemented with ^{32}P (inorganic) in order to label intracellular ATP stores. Subsequently cells were exposed to various stimuli that are known to (a) increase (isoproterenol, forskolin) or decrease (carbachol, oxotremorine) intracellular cyclic AMP, (b) increase calcium influx and or release (isoproterenol, ouabain, phenylephrine), (c) increase the formation of diacylglycerol and inositol phosphates (carbachol), (d) activate kinase C (phorbol ester PMA) and (e) increase cyclic GMP (dibutyryl derivative of cyclic GMP).

Figs. 1 & 2 summarize the main observations. First while several polypeptides, high and low molecular weight, underwent phosphorylation (i.e. showed ^{32}-P incorporation), a few bands labelled C protein and TN-I displayed marked alterations in myocytes exposed to above mentioned stimuli. These bands showed increased incorporation under the conditions that are known to increase either intracellular concentration of cyclic AMP (isoproterenol, forskolin) or diacylglycerol (carbachol) but not that increase cyclic GMP (dibutyryl cyclic GMP) or calcium (ouabain, phenylephrine in the presence of propranolol).

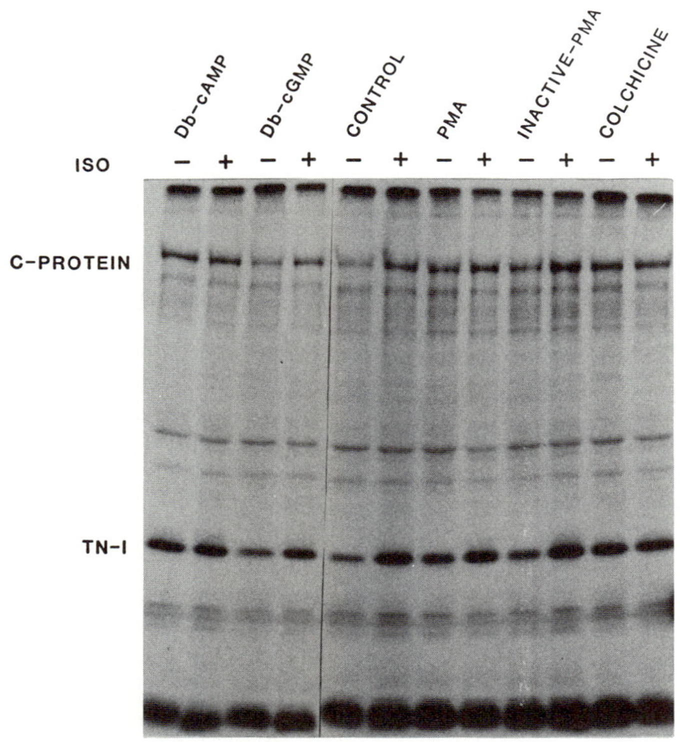

Fig. 1. Phosphorylation of rat ventricular myocytes. This figure shows an autoradiogram of phosphorylation of electrophoretically fractionated myocyte proteins following exposure of myocytes to various conditions as indicated in the fugure. Note that while several high and low molecular weight polypeptides underwent phosphorylation the bands labelled C-protein and TN-I showed marked alterations.

Kinase A Phosphorylation:

That the increase in the phosphorylation of these proteins due either to isoproterenol or forskolin was in fact the results of kinase A action was clearly suggested from the observed increase in myocytes incubated with dibutyryl derivative of cyclic AMP and that this was not

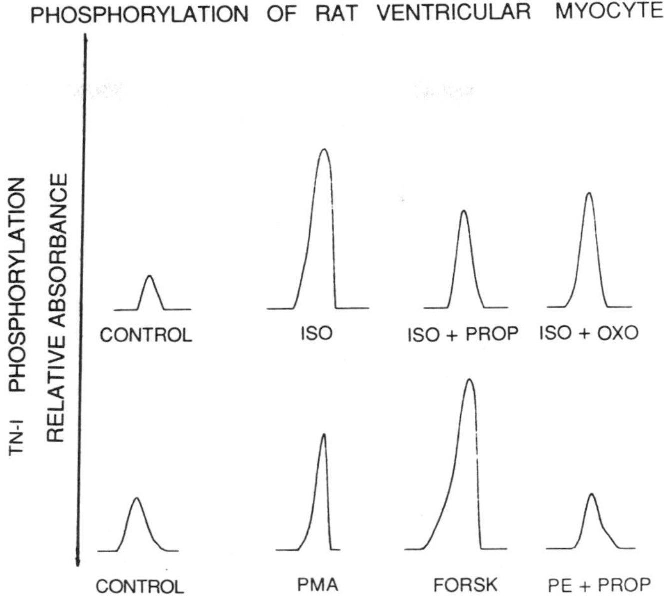

Fig. 2. Phosphorylation of rat ventricular myocytes. This figure describes (densitometric scans) TN-I phosphorylation in myocytes exposed to various conditions as shown in the figure.

further increased by the subsequent exposure to isoproterenol or forskolin. This suggested that kinase A catalyzed the phosphorylation of a "fixed" amount of "A sites" in these proteins and thus one would not expect additivity of effects by those stimuli that augment intra-cellular cyclic AMP or perhaps recruit the same compartment of kinase A subsequent to elevation of cyclic AMP. The works by others show that serine-20 of cardiac TN-I (20) and serine-16 of PLN (53) are phosphory-lated by kinase A. Which of the serine or threonine residues of C protein is attacked by kinase A has yet to be reported. However, the fact that the phosphorylation of C protein showed identical response (increase, decrease or no effect) to that seen in the TN-I band is highly indicative of the same functional kinase A compartment being responsible for the phosphorylation of both polypeptides. In view of the intriguing location of C protein within thick filament structure (present in the overlap region between thick and thin filament), and the observed parallel response among TN-I and C protein bands in terms of their phosphorylation, it is extremely attractive to consider that TN-I

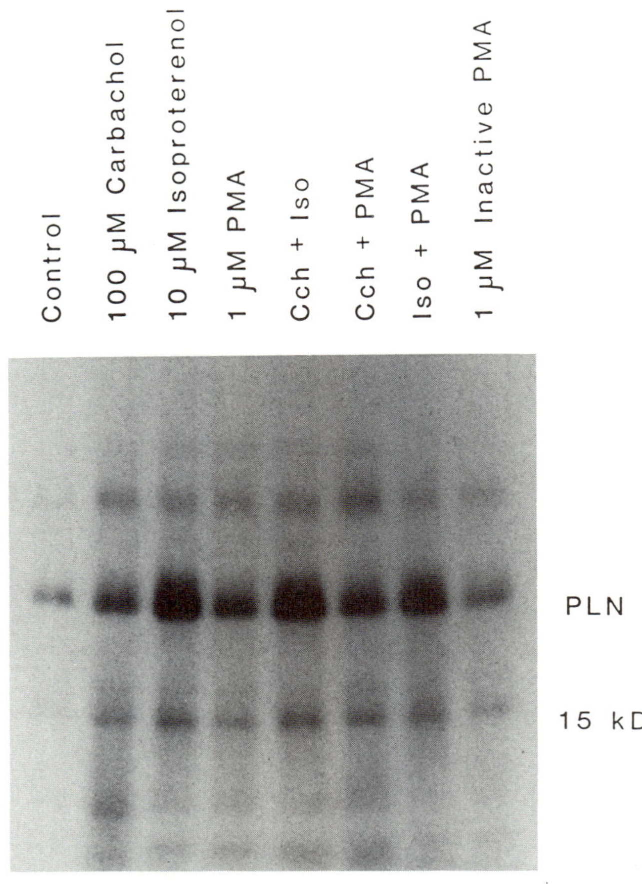

^{32}P Incorporation into Acidified C:M
Extractable Polypeptides   in Rat
Ventricular Myocytes

Fig. 3. Phosphorylation of Phospholamban (PLN). Following phosphorylation of myocytes (exposed to various conditions) myocytes were extracted
with acidified chloroform methanol (C:M). The C:M extract were electrophoretically fractionated prior to exposure of dried gels to X-ray
films.

located on thin filament regions overlapping with thick filament
undergoes initial or preferential phosphorylation following activation
of kinase A compartment that also must be vicinal to these regulatory
proteins. The likely implication of the result will be accelerated
dissociation of calcium from TN-C caused by cyclic AMP stimulants that
abbreviate cardiac systole (i.e. augment rate of relaxation). Little is

known about the role of C-protein in contraction or relaxation of the myocardium. Perhaps C protein phosphorylation ("A site" phosphorylation) assists the known action of TN-I phosphorylation ("A site") in decreasing TN-C affinity for calcium (54). Alternatively C protein phosphorylation may regulate actomyosin ATPase dependence on calcium and thus assist TN-I in evoking faster rate of relaxation.

Since under the electrophoretic conditions both TN-I and PLN migrated very similarly, it was necessary to examine the phosphorylation of either protein following additional manipulation of myocyte homogenate prior to electrophoresis. Several approaches were considered in this regard. First acidified chloroform/methanol (C/M) extract contained PLN, but not TN-I, since the former, but not the latter, is a proteolipid. We examined the phosphorylation in several fractions - unextracted homogenate, acidified C/M extract and residue following acidified CM extraction; these contained TN-I plus PLN, PLN, and TN-I respectively along with other polypeptides. It is clear from Fig. 4 that both TN-I and PLN are excellent substrates for kinase A. Second TN-I along with C protein were recovered quantitatively in washed myofibrills and, PLN, in microsomes enriched in sarcoplasmic reticulum fragments. PLN present in acidified C/M extract was depolymerised to its monomeric form following boiling of SDS solubilized C/M extract prior to electrophoresis. Thus it is clear that the kinase A-catalyzed phosphorylation of both TN-I and PLN accounts for the observed phosphorylation in the TN-I band seen in myocyte homogenate (Figs. 1 & 2). The well-documented role of PLN phosphorylation ("site A" phosphorylation) in stimulation of sarcoplasmic reticulum calcium sequestration via stimulating calcium pump is thought to increase the rate of lowering of myoplasmic calcium and thus participate in augmented rate of myocardial relaxation evoked by cyclic AMP stimulants (55). The _in situ_ site A phosphorylation of PLN described here is consistent with this view.

<u>Kinase C Activation:</u>

Many studies document the activation of cardiac muscarinic receptor to decrease or attenuate the beta-adrenergic increase in intracellular cyclic AMP (2). It was thus anticipated that muscarinic receptor agonists like carbachol and oxotremorine via attenuating cyclic AMP response will influence the A site phosphorylation of PLN, TN-I and

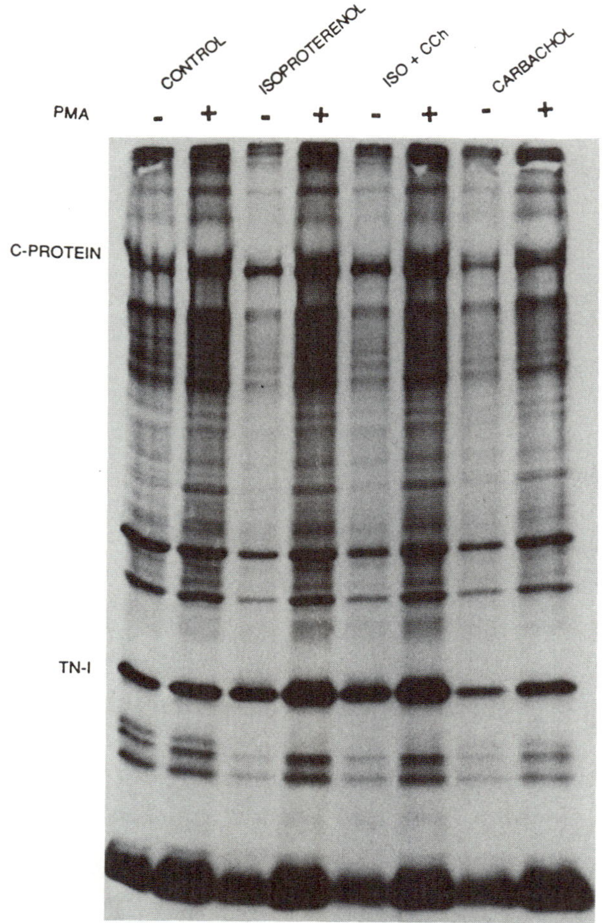

PHOSPHORYLATION OF RAT VENTRICULAR MYOCYTES

Fig. 4.   Phosphorylation of rat ventricular myocytes.   Phosphorylation
patterns of control and phorbol ester (PMA) treated myocytes are shown.
Phosphorylation was conducted in the presence of autonomic receptor
stimuli as shown.

C-protein. The results shown in Figs. 1 & 2 are consistent with this

idea. At the same time it was somewhat puzzling that only 60 to 70%

attenuation was noted following oxotremorine and even lesser by

carbachol. It is becoming apparent now that muscarinic receptor

activation evokes alterations in effector systems besides adenylate cyclase and, amongst these, enzymes related to the "Hokin and Hokin PI response" (56), and guanylate cyclase have attracted considerable attention. As shown by the results in Figs. 1 & 2 incubation of cardiomyocytes with dibutyryl derivative of cyclic GMP failed to show any (significant) effect on the phosphorylation of TN-I, PLN and C-protein. Thus it is apparent that these proteins are not substrates for kinase G and muscarinic receptor action might instead utilize the newly discovered kinase C whose stimulation requires the formation of diacylglycerol. Isolated cardiomyocytes indeed showed the formation of inositol phosphates as well as turnover of ^{32}-P in phosphoinositides (see later section). This raised the possibility of kinase C activation in myocytes exposed to carbachol. The results in Fig. 4 document the evidence supporting this possibility. Carbachol exposure increased the phosphorylation of PLN, a finding observed for the first time and is of considerable interest. The direct activation of kinase C by active phorbol ester, PMA, which is obtained by exposing myocytes to PMA, increased the phosphorylation of PLN, besides that of TN-I and C-protein. 4-beta phorbol, which does not activate kinase C, failed to influence the phosphorylation of these proteins.

The question arises whether the same amino acid residues underwent phosphorylation by the action of kinase C as that by kinase A. If it were to be the case, one may not observe increased phosphorylation in the PMA treated myocytes subsequently incubated in the presence of cyclic AMP stimulants like isoproterenol. The results (Fig. 4) in fact showed the opposite i.e. there was further increase by isoproterenol in such treated cells. This raises a strong possibility that the amino acid residue(s) phosphorylated by kinase A is(are) separate from those phosphorylated by kinase C. This will then account for the observed additivity or interaction in the ^{32}-P incorporation in PLN, TN-I and C protein in the PMA treated cells subsequently exposed to isoproterenol or forskolin that elevate intracellular cyclic AMP. In fact two simultaneous alterations will have to be considered in the presence of isoproterenol and carbachol. First, carbachol binding to muscarinic receptors via attenuating the beta-adrenergic increase in cyclic AMP formation will decrease the site A phosphorylation of these proteins and at the same time via promoting the degradation of polyphosphoinositides raises diacylglycerol formation, which via activating kinase C promotes the phosphorylation of the C site of these proteins. This view may account for the differences in the attenuation of phosphorylation response with isoproterenol by carbachol versus oxotremorine. While both muscarinic agonists decrease cyclic AMP formation, only carbachol appears to augment the "PI response" (57) in terms of eventual kinase C recruitment. It is tempting to consider the influence of site C phosphorylation is to attenuate the effect of Site A phosphorylation on the functioning of these proteins. For example, the site A phosphorylation decreases the affinity of TN-C towards calcium and site C phosphorylation might attenuate this effect. It remains to be elucidated whether site C phosphorylation in the absence of site A phosphorylation has any effect of its own. _In vitro_ studies indicate that sarcoplasmic reticulum PLN phosphorylation by kinase C augments calcium pumping activity (58-59). However in view of rather large amounts of kinase C required to document this effect it is unclear whether it is of physiological significance (41).

Ca/Calmodulin Kinase Activation:

Numerous _in vitro_ studies, document Ca/calmodulin to augment the SR calcium pumping via phosphorylation of PLN (60). The phosphorylation by this mechanism is additive to that catalyzed by kinase A (60). However, _in vivo_ studies have failed to provide supportive evidence for the phosphorylation of PLN under the conditions that augment calcium influx into the myocardium. They include alpha-adrenergic activation and digitalis evoked inotropy (61). In isolated cardiomyocytes, phenylephrine failed to alter the phosphorylation of PLN, TN-I and C-protein; this was also true when myocytes were exposed to ouabain. The only reported evidence that implicated in vivo phosphorylation by Ca/calmodulin kinase of PLN is based on the action of trifluoperazine (TFP) in perfused rat heart, which assumed that TFP selectively blocked the action of calmodulin (60). However it is also known that TFP decreases the activity of kinase C and further there is not much difference in the concentrations of TFP required to decrease either kinase (62). While our results to-date tend to negate the involvement of Ca/calmodulin kinase action on the proteins, they do not rule out the possibility that this kinase might play as yet unclarified role(s) in myocardial contractility.

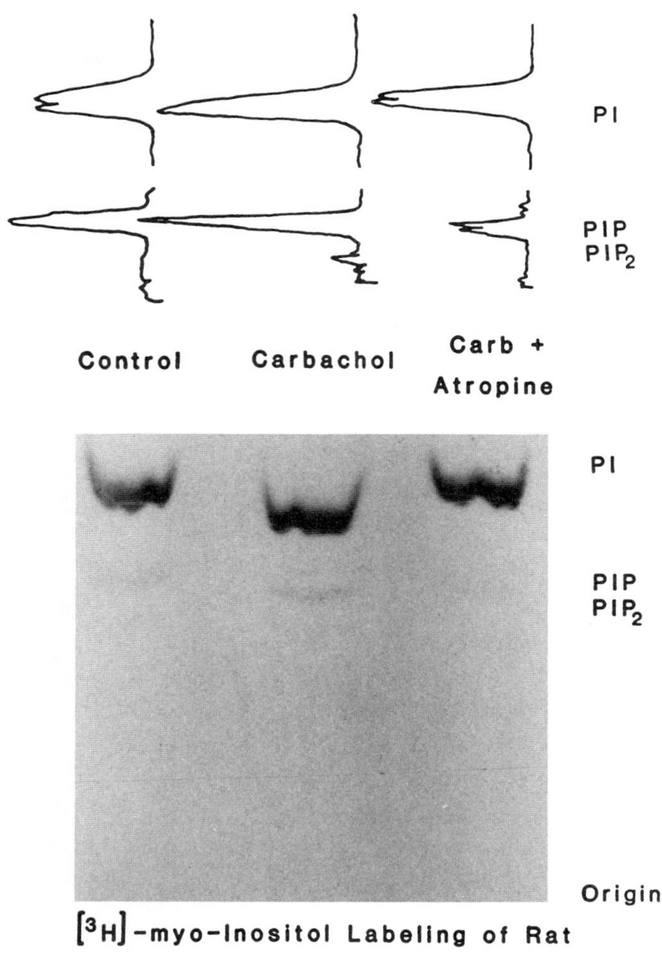

Fig. 5. [^{3}H] myoinositol incorporation in rat ventricular myocytes. Myocytes were treated with carbachol in the absence and presence of atropine. Labelled phospholipids were extracted, separated by TLC and plates exposed to X-ray films. Autoradiogram and densitometric scans are shown in the figure. PI; phosphatidylinositol; PIP, phosphatidylinositol-1,4-bisophosphate; PIP$_2$, phosphatidylinositol-1,4,5-trisphosphate.

<u>Evidence For The Presence Of Phosphoinositide Turnover:</u>

It is evident that, in tissues examined for the presence of enzymes relevant to the synthesis and degradation of phosphoinositides, several

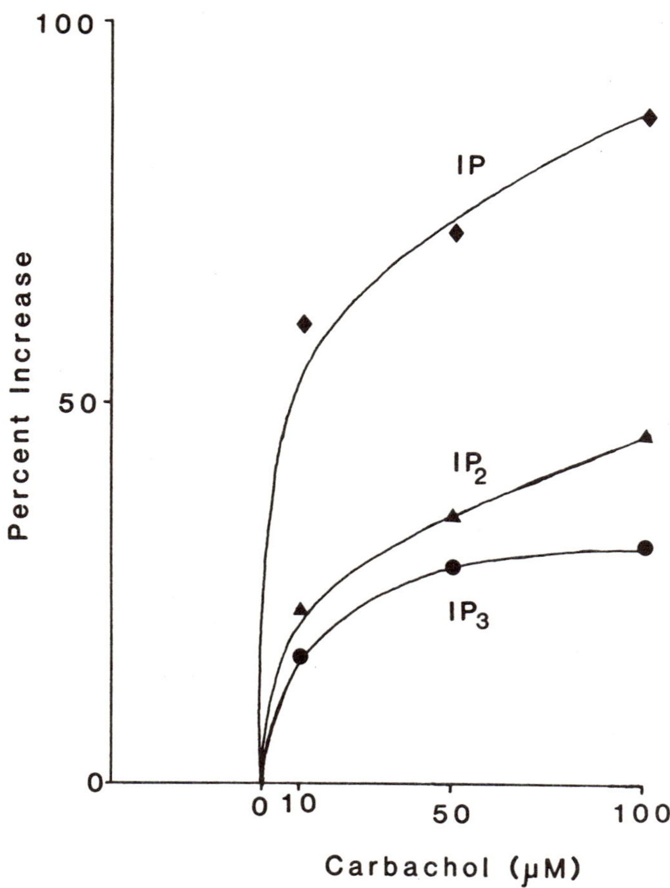

Fig. 6. Formation of inositol phosphates. Myocytes were exposed to [^{32}P] in the presence of varying amounts of carbachol and subsequently inositol phosphates from the aqueous extracts were separated by an ion exchange chromatography. IP, inositol-1-monophosphate; IP$_1$, inositol-1,4-bisphosphate; IP$_3$,-inositol-1,4,5-trisphosphate.

experimental approaches have been considered to document the existence of the "PI turnover system" (37). They include (a) assessment of [^{3}H] myoinositol incorporation into phosphoinositides (b) assessment of ^{32}P-incorporated into phosphoinositides and (c) assessment of degradation of phosphoinositides by determining the formation of inositol phosphates and diacylglycerol by the action of phosphomono- and diesterases on phosphoinositide stores. We have employed these approaches to examine the presence of PI turnover in isolated cardiomyocytes and the effect of various stimuli, notably autonomic receptor ligands, on the synthesis and degradation of phosphoinositides.

Incorporation Of [3H]-Myoinositol:

Isolated myocytes were incubated in KRB buffer supplemented with radiolabelled inositol and LiCl and in the presence of carbachol, atropine or both; Lithium was included since it is known to inhibit dephosphorylation of inositolphosphate(s). Subsequently phospholipids were extracted and separated by TLC and plates were exposed to x-ray films to detect incorporation of inositol. Radiolabelled PI, PIP and PIP_2 were run along with samples to identify labelled myocyte phosphoinositides. It was evident that carbachol augmented inositol incorporation into PI, PIP and PIP_2 and this effect involved the interaction of carbachol with the muscarinic receptor since atropine antagonized the stimulatory action of carbachol. On a quantitative basis the incorporation into PI was much greater than into PIP which in turn was much greater relative to that in PIP_2 (Fig.5).

Release Of Inositol Phosphates:

Incubation of myocytes in the presence of carbachol also augmented the formation of labelled inositol phosphates, IP, IP_2 and IP_3. This effect required the action of carbachol via muscarinic receptor as can be judged from the blockade of carbachol stimulation by atropine. Further the results showed a requirement of extracellular calcium for muscarinic stimulation of the formation of inositol phosphates which were recovered in the soluble fraction prepared from cardiomyocytes. Isoproterenol, unexpectedly, augmented the formation of IP, albeit to a lesser extent relative to carbachol action. Phorbol ester PMA decreased the muscarinic increment in inositol phosphates. This may indicate that activated kinase C exerts a feedback inhibitory action in PI turnover cycle. The enzymatic site(s) influenced by kinase C and the likely underlying mechanisms remain to be clarified (Fig. 6).

Incorporation Of ^{32}P Into Phosphoinositides:

When incubated in the presence of radiolabelled phosphorous, it was anticipated that phospholipids besides phosphoinositides would show the incorporation of radioactivity. This was indeed the case (Fig. 7). However, the results clearly documented the alterations in the PIP and

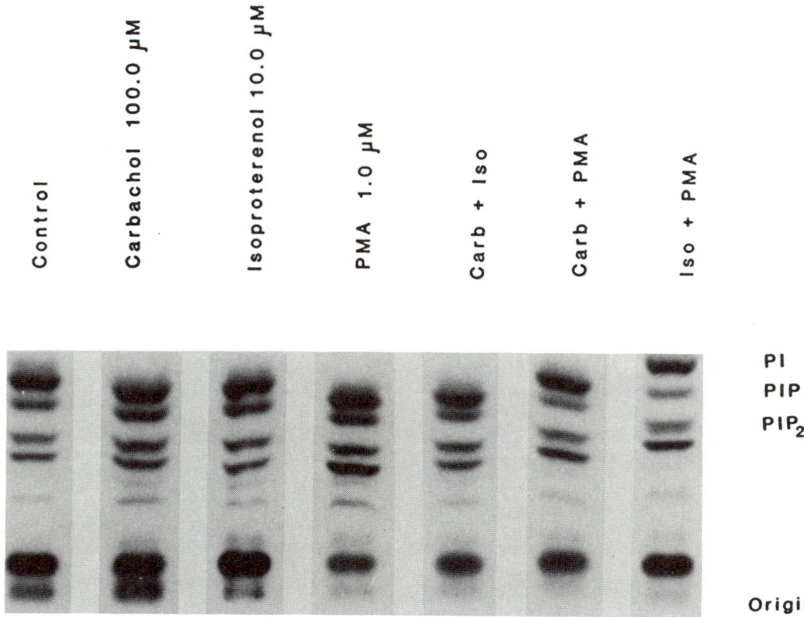

^{32}P Incorporation into Rat Ventricular Myocyte Phospholipids

Fig. 7.   [^{32}P] incorporation into rat ventricular myocytes phospholipids.   Labelled phospholipids were extracted from myocytes treated with various agents and labelled phospholipids separated by TLC were identified by autoradiography.   Incorporation into phosphatidylserine, phosphotidycholine, phosphatidylethanolamine and phosphatidic acid were not shown as there were no discernable changes in incorporation; these phospholipids migrated ahead of PI.

PIP$_2$ and not in other phospholipids caused by the activation of muscarinic receptor. For example, carbachol, but not isoproterenol, augmented the incorporation in PIP and PIP$_2$. Phorbol ester, PMA, antagonized the muscarinic stimulation of radiolabel incorporation into PIP and PIP$_2$. At the same time PMA significantly increased the incorporation into an unidentified phospholipid that showed a lower R_f value than PIP$_2$. Isoproterenol, on the other hand, markedly increased incorporation into an unidentified phospholipid that migrated with the lowest R_f amongst the resolved phospholipids in the solvent system employed. It would be rewarding to identify this phospholipid since PMA decreased radiolabelled phosphate incorporation into this lipid fraction. Both these phospholipids were present in minute quantities.

Two Possible Mechanisms for Autonomic Control of Myocardial Performance: Phospho-Dephosphorylation and Multisite Phosphorylation.

The results reported by many laboratories utilizing physiological, electrophysiological and biochemical approaches in investigations have provided considerable support to the notion that A-site phosphorylation of such critical myocyte proteins as TN I & PLN evokes functional alterations in these and somehow dephosphorylation restores their functions towards the "prestimulated state". The in vivo and in vitro evidence that TN I and PLN undergo site A phosphorylation attendant with contractile and calcium flux alterations following beta-adrenergic stimulation provides a major thrust to this view, despite the document- ation that dephosphorylation occured rather sluggishly (1,14,15,20-22, 26,55,60,61,63-65). Nevertheless, this idea has now been extended to the beta-adrenergic control of plasma membrane "slow channel" as well, a supportive evidence for which is provided primarily through a patch clamp analysis of single channel activity in whole cell or inside-out membrane patch preparations. While the much slower dephosphorylation rates does not invalidate the role for this mechanism, it need not be considered a priory as the sole mechanism for restoration. In fact electophysiological observations on calcium channel regulation by "cyclic AMP independent stimuli" might indicate the need for considering non-A site phosphorylation as an opposing signal controlling the site A-evoked functional changes in proteins like PLN or TN I or even slow channel. A circumstantial evidence suggests G-site phosphorylation controls calcium channel activity in a manner opposite to that by site A phosphorylation. However, as was stated earlier, the role of cyclic GMP in the control of myocardial performance, while not being ruled out, remains entirely elusive. But the idea that multisite phosphorylation controls the function of rate-limiting enzymes, frequently in opposing fashion, has gained wide acceptance, since a good deal of evidence supporting it is now available. The results described by us dealing with the phosphorylation of TN I, PLN and C-protein, by kinase A and kinase C, have led us to propose the alternate hypothesis of functional antagonism in the effects of site A versus site C on these critical proteins. At the outset it must be made clear the "garden variety" hypothesis of phospho-dephosphorylation is not ruled out in our thinking but instead our proposal suggests, besides this, there is a strong likelihood that multisite phosphorylation mechanism participates in the overall control of the myocardium by autonomic nerves. The following briefly elaborates this view.

Several minimum aspects need to be considered from the stand-point of physiological significance or relevance of the postulated site A / site C antagonism. (a) The generation of two signals, cyclic AMP and diacylglycerol, by their appropriate synthetic enzymes must show kinetic differences in terms of their dependence on the concentration of appropriate agonist-occupied receptors linked to effectors and on the onset of changes in these effectors. While the effect on the adenylate cyclase system is now known to be sufficiently rapid, there is incomplete evidence for the rate of phosphodiesteratic cleavage of polyphosphoinositide stores in myocyte plasma membranes. On the other hand there is preliminary data suggesting higher concentrations of cholinergic agonists are required for the "PI response" relative to the "cyclic AMP response". This might indicate perhaps the site C phosphorylation follows the site A phosphorylation and this is of physiological relevance. For example it will allow the site A phosphorylation effect being expressed prior to its antagonism by the site C phosphorylation.

(b) As the phosphorylation is a consequence of recruitment of appropriate kinase activated by two signals, both the amounts and their locations assume important consideration. While the functional compartmentation of these kinases is an obviously critical issue, little experimental evidence can be cited. On the other hand, it is interesting, albeit intriquing, that kinase A and kinase C appear to translocate within the cellular interior in the myocytes challenged with autonomic receptor agonists. What is perhaps interesting that while kinase A exists in cytosolic and particulate compartments of myocytes, kinase C is predominently a cytosolic activity. Thus for the action of kinase C on particulate proteins like PLN and TN I there will be a need for its translocation. A likely implication of this is that site C phosphorylation will occur after site A phosphorylation and this consideration is consistent with sequential and opposing regulation of the functions of these target proteins by multisite phosphorylation. As far as amounts are concerned in cardiac tissue, kinase A is much greater than kinase C based on the _in vitro_ evidence. Whether this is also responsible for sequential phosphorylation is clearly speculative. It could perhaps indicate limited number of substrates for kinase C relative to that for kinase A.

(c) An equally important question arises as to why the activiation of "stimulatory" receptor leads to the generation of only two messengers-cycle AMP and Ca^{2+}-whereas the "inhibitory" receptor activation not only influences cyclic AMP and calcium signals but additionally provokes changes in diacylglycerol and cyclic GMP signals as well. In the answer to this question perhaps lies the "missing" clues whose understanding is central to the appreciation of underlying subcellular mechanisms responsible for integrative and coordinate regulation of the myocardium by the autonomic nervous system. One such missing clue deals with the issue of dephosphorylation whose control may depend on the generation of "inhibitory" signals like cyclic GMP. It is thus not surprising that some investigators have postulated that "somehow" cyclic GMP participates in the cholinergic control of the myocardium from such a perspective. A logical extension of such view will be that inhibition of site A phosphorylation (decreased cyclic AMP signal), antagonism of site A phosphorylation by site C phosphorylation (diacylglycerol signal) and increased dephosphorylation (perhaps cyclic GMP signal) are necessary for the muscarinic opposition of intracellular calcium actions promoted by the cyclic AMP signal generated by beta-adrenergic receptor activation. In essence the multiplicity of signals is required to "fine tune" the actions of the main signal which is undoubtedly calcium ion in the contractile myocardium. While calcium ion via calmodulin may exert phospho-dephosphorylation related actions, there is as yet little evidence implicating such a role of calcium in the regulation of myocardial contractility. Instead if it were to play role, it may be in the metabolic and energy adjustments of the myocardium whose _in vivo_ pumping function is indeed subjected to varying demands.

The above discussion is relevant to the cholinergic antagonism subsequent to the beta-adrenergically stimulated state of the myocardium. In view of the strong likelihood that _in vivo_ parasympathetic tone maintains the "resting" state of the heart and this is modulated by alterations in sympathetic discharge it is necessary to consider the following. It may be in the resting myocardium low amount of C site phosphorylation is present on proteins such as TN I, PLN, C-protein and perhaps calcium channel and this is required to maintain their respective "inhibitory" functions or "low activity states". The beta-adrenergic increase in site A phosphorylation then can be viewed to overcome the site C-imposed inhibition and thus leading to the expression of the roles played by these critical polypeptides in beta-adrenergically stimulated state of the myocardium. It is equally possible the "vacant" (i.e. non-phosphorylated) C sites exert inhibitory action and the phosphorylation of these modifies such inhibition. It is considered now the "vacant" A site on PLN maintains the low activity state of sarcoplasmic reticulum calcium pumping ATPase and its phosphorylation transiently overcomes this inhibitory effect leading to augmentated rate of calcium sequestration, an event critical to he beta-adrenergically evoked abbreviation of cardiac systole. Similar situation may well exist with regard to the action of "vacant" A sites on calcium channels, TN I and C protein. The role of dephosphorylation enzymes is then to render the low activity states on these proteins. In essence this implies the greater the ratio of site A / site C in terms of their phosphorylation greater will be the efficacy with which sympathetic nerve stimulation evokes positive inotropic state of the myocardium and of course the reverse is to be expected in the case of parasympathetic modulation of the heart's performance. Thus the observed accentuated antagonism in the physiological response of the myocardium seen when both sympathetic and parasympathetic nerves are stimulated is expressed intracellularly as varying ratios in the site A / site C phosphorylation of such proteins as TN I, C-protein, PLN and perhaps calcium channel related polypeptide(s) which regulate both calcium actions and distribution within the myocardial cell. This in essence represents a 1986 modification of the Goldberg's Yin Yang hypothesis of the seventies (28) for the autonomic control of the myocardium and incorporates cyclic AMP and diacylglycent as opposing signals instead of cyclic GMP and cyclic AMP regulating Ca^{2+} mediated intracellular processes that subserve evoked physiological responses of the heart.

SUMMARY

The phosphorylation of myocyte proteins and phosphlipids was investigated in intact, isolated rat ventricular cardiomyocytes. While many polypeptides showed ^{32}P-incorporation, polypeptide bands containing inhibitory subunit of troponin (TN-I), myofilorillar C protein and sarcoplasmic ventricular phospholarnban (PLN) showed marked alterations in ^{32}P-incorporation in myocytes exposed to autonomic receptor agonists and other agents. The stimuli known to increase myocardial cyclic AMP concentration increased the phosphorylation of TN-I, C protein and PLN catalyzed by kinase A. On the other hand these proteins were not found to be the substrates for kinase G or Ca^{2+}/calmodulin protein kinase. Activation of kinase C by phorbol esters (like PMA) increased the phosphorylation of TN-I, C protein and PLN (site C phosphorylation). The turnover myocytes phosphoinostides (PI, PIP and PIP_2) was also influenced by autonomic receptor agonists. For example, carbachol augmented both synthesis and degradation of phosphoinositides. Activation of kinase C by PMA appeared to decrease the stimulation by carbachol of phosphoinositide turnover. B-adrenergic receptor agonist, isopronenol, and phorbol ester, PMA, increased ^{32}P-labelling of unidentified minor phosphohpids. From these results and those available in the literature, a hypothesis is presented that incorporates the roles for site A and site C phosphorylation of myocyte proteins in the autonomic control of the myocardium.

ACKNOWLEDGEMENTS

This work was supported by a grant received from the Medical Research Council of Canada (PVS). Ms. MacKay was a recipient of a graduate studentship from the Saskatchewan Heart Foundation. We thank Mr. A. P. Braun and Dr. M. Desautels and V. Gopalkrishnan for critical reading of this manuscript.

REFERENCES

1.   Watanabe, A.M. In: Cardiac Therapy (Eds. M.R. Rosen and B.F. Hoffman), Martinus Nijhoff Publishers, Boston, 1983, pp 95-144.
2.   Sulakhe, P.V., Jagadeesh, G. and Braun, A.P. In: The Regulation of Heart Function (Eds. H. Rupp), George Thieme Verlag, Stuttgart, 1986, pp. 71-94.
3.   Lottelholz, K. and Pappano, A.J. Pharmacol. Rev. 37:1-24, 1985.
4.   Levy, M.N. The Physiologist. 26:115-118, 1983.
5.   Levy, M.N. Circ. Res. 29:437-445, 1971.
6.   Braun, A.P. and Sulakhe, P.V. In: Neuro Methods. Vol. 4 Receptor Binding (Eds. A.A. Boulton, G.B. Baker and P.D. Hrdina), Humana Press, Clifton, New Jersey, 1986, pp 139-170.

7. Hammer, R. and Giachetti, A. Life Sciences 31:2991-2998, 1982.

8. Brown, J.H., Goldstein, D. and Brown-Masters, S. Mol. Pharmacol. 27:525-531, 1985.

9. Malbone, C.C., Mangano, D.J. and Watkins, D.C. Biochem. Biophys. Res. Comm. 128:809-815, 1985.

10. Braun, A.P. and Sulakhe, P.V. In: G. Proteins and Signal Transduction, Cold Spring Harbour Laboratory Publications, 1986, p 26 (Abstract).

11. Gomperts, B.D. In: G. Proteins and Signal Transduction, Cold Spring Harbour Laboratory Publications, 1986, p 47 (Abstract).

12. Gilman, A.G. Cell 36:577-579, 1984.

13. Cerione, R.A., Staniszewski, C., Caron, M.G., Lefkowitz, R.J., Codina, J. and Birnbaumer, L. Nature 318:293-295, 1985.

14. Osterriden, W., Bruan, G., Hescheler, J., Trautwin, W., Flockerzi, V. and Hofmann, F. Nature 298:576-578, 1982.

15. Reuter, H. Nature 301:569-573, 1983.

16. Rokosh, G., Morris, T., Phan, T.D. and Sulakhe, P.V. FEBS Letters, Submitted 1986.

17. Murad, F., Chi, Y.M., Rall, T.W. and Sutherland, E.W. J. Biol. Chem. 237:1233-1238, 1962.

18. La Raia, P.J. and Sommenblick, E. Circ. Res. 28:377-384, 1971.

19. Smigel, M., Katada, T., Northrup, J.K., Bokoch, G.M., Vi, M. and Gilman, A.G. Adv. Cyclic Nucleotide Res. 17:1-18, 1984.

20. England, P.J. In: The Regulation of Heart Function (Eds. H. Rupp) Georg Thieme, Verlag, Stuttgart, 1986, pp 223-233.

21. Tada, M. and Katz, A.M. Ann. Rev. Physiol. 44:401-423, 1982.

22. Bkaily, G. and Sperelakis, N. Amer. J. Physiol. 266:H630-H634, 1984.

23. Curtis, B.M. and Catterall, W.A. Proc. Natl. Acad. Sci. U.S.A. 82:2528-2532, 1985.

24. Pfaffinger, P.J., Martin, J.M., Hunter, D.D., Nathanson, N.M. and Hille, B. Nature 317:536-538, 1985.

25. Noma, A. and Trautwein, W. Pflingers Arch. 377:193-200, 1978.

26. Winegrad, S. Circ. Res. 55:565-574, 1984.

27. George, W.J., Willerson, R.D. and Kadowitz, P.J. J. Pharmacol. Exp. Ther. 184:228-235, 1973.

28. Goldberg, N.D., Haddox, M.K., Nicol, S.E., Glass, D.B., Sanford, C.H., Kucnl, F.A., Jr., and Estensen, R. Adv. Cyclic Nucleotide Res. 5:307-330, 1970.

29. Murad, F., Anrold, W.P., Mittal, C.K. and Braughler, J.M. (1979). Adv. Cyclic Nucleotide Res. 11:175-204, 1979.

30. Kimura, H., and Murad, F., J. Biol. Chem. 249:6910-6916, 1974.

31. Sulakhe, P.V., Sulakhe, S.J., Leung, N.L., St. Louis, P.J. and Hickie, R.A. Biochem. J. 157:705-712, 1976.

32. Beavo, J.A., Hardman, J.G. and Sutherland, E.W. J. Biol. Chem. 245:5649-5655, 1970.

33. St. Louis, P.J. and Sulakhe, P.V. Biochem. J. 158:535-541, 1976.

34. Lincoln, T.M. and Keely, S.L. Biochim. Biophys. Acta 676:230-244, 1981.

35. Lohmann, S.M. and Walter, U. Adv. Cyclic Nucleotide Res. 18:63-118, 1984.

36. St. Louis, P.J. and Sulakhe, P.V. Archives Biochem and Biophys. 198:227-240, 1979.

37. Hokin, L.E. Annual Rev. Biochem. 54:205-235.

38. Kishimoto, A., Takai, Y., Mori, T. Kikkawa, U. and Nishizuka, Y. J. Biol. Chem. 255:2273-2276, 1980.
39. Kikkawa, U. Kaibuchi, K., Takai, Y and Nishizuka, Y. In: Phospholipids and Cellular Regulation (Eds. J.F. Kao) CRC Press, Bocha Raton, Florida, 1985, pp 111-126.
40. Turner, R.S. and Kuo, J.F. In: Phospholipids and Cellular Regulation (Eds. J.F. Kuo) CRC Press, Boca Raton, Florida, 1985, pp 75-110.
41. Presti, C.F., Scott, B.T. and Jones, L.R. J. Biol. Chem. 260:13879-13889, 1985.
42. Yuan, S. and Sen, A.K. Biochim, Biophis, Acta. 886:152-161, 1986.
43. Sibley, D., Nambi, P., Peters, J.R. and Lefkowitz, R.J. Biochem. Biophy. Res. Commun. 121:973-979, 1984.
44. Berridge, M.J. and Irvine, R.F. Nature 312: 315-321, 1984.
45. Movsevian, M.A., Thompson, A.P. Selah, M. and Williamson, J.R. FEBS 185:328-332, 1985.
46. Yuan, S., Durante, W., Sunahara, F.A. and Sen, A.K. Proc. Can. Fed. Biol. Soc. 29:101, 1986 (Abstract).
47. Brown, S.L. and Brown, J.H. Mol. Pharmacol. 24:351-356, 1983.
48. Kryski, A.,Jr., Kenno, K.A. and Severson, D.L. Amer. J. Physiol. 248:H203-H216, 1985.
49. Berridge, M.J., Downes, C.P. and Hanley, M.R. Biochem. J. 206:587-595, 1982.
50. Goswami, S.K. and Gould, R.M. J. Neurochemistry 44:941-946, 1985.
51. Randerath, K. Analytical Biochem. 34:188-205, 1970.
52. Berridge, M.J. Dawson, C.P. Heslop, J.P. and Irvine, R.F. Biochem. J. 212:473-482, 1983.
53. Tada, M., Kadoma, M. and Fujii, J. This volume.
54. Holroyde, M.J., Howe, E. and Soluro, R.J. Biochim. Biophys. Acta. 586:63-69, 1979.
55. Katz, A.M., Tada, M. and Kirchberger, M.A. Adv. Cyclic Nucleotide Res. 5:453-472, 1975.
56. Hokin, L.E. and Hokin, M.R. Can. J. Biochem. Physiol. 34:349-358, 1956.
57. Brown, J.H. and Brown S.L. Journ. Biol. Chem. 259:3777-3781, 1984.
58. Iwasa, Y. and Hosey, M.M. J. Biol. Chem. 259:1834-1841, 1984.
59. Movsevian, M.A., Nighikawa, M. and Adelstein, R.S. J. Biol. Chem. 259:8029-8032, 1984.
60. LePeuch, C.J. and Demaille, J.G. In: The Regulation of Heart Function (Eds. H. Rapp) Georg Thieme Verlag, Stuttgart, 1986, pp 137-144.
61. Lindeman, J.P. J. Biol. Chem. 261:4860-4867, 1986.
62. Wise, B.C. and Kuo, J.F. Biochem. Pharmachol. 32:1259-   , 1983.
63. Lindemann, J.P. and Watanabe, A.M. J. Biol. Chem. 260:4516-4525, 1985.
64. Onorato, J.J. and Rudolf, S.A. J. Biol. Chem. 256:10697-10703, 1981.
65. Blackshear, P.J. Nemenoff, R.A., Bonourtre, J.V., Cheung, J.Y. and Aurach, J. Amer. J. Physiol. 246:C439-C449, 1984.

9

ROLE OF PHOSPHATIDYLETHANOLAMINE N-METHYLATION ON Ca^{2+} TRANSPORT IN CARDIAC MEMBRANES

V. PANAGIA, K. OKUMURA, N. MAKINO, D. ZHAO and N.S. DHALLA

Laboratory of Membrane Biology, Department of Anatomy and Experimental Cardiology Section, Department of Physiology, Faculty of Medicine, University of Manitoba, Winnipeg, Canada R3E OW3

INTRODUCTION

Evidence is accumulating that lipid composition of the membrane plays an important role in a variety of membrane-mediated functions of the myocardial cell, including the activities of membrane-bound enzymes and ion transport systems (1-6). The intramembranal rearrangement of the two major membrane phospholipids, phosphatidylethanolamine (PE) and phosphatidylcholine (PC), can occur through three successive N-terminal methylations of PE where S-adenosyl-L-methionine (AdoMet) is the physiological methyl donor (7). In previous studies we have described the characteristics of three methyltransferase catalytic sites (I, II and III) for PE N-methylation in cardiac subcellular membranes which can be readily identified at 0.055 - 0.1, 10 and 150 μM concentrations of AdoMet (8). Under optimal conditions, predominant synthesis of specific phospholipid molecules, namely phosphatidyl-N-monomethylethanolamine (PMME), phosphatidyl-N, N-dimethylethanolamine (PDME) and PC was found to occur in heart membranes at sites I, II and III, respectively. The methyltransfer scheme is illustrated in Figure 1. Since the physical state of the cell membrane is determined by several chemical modulators including the methylation of PE polar head group (9), it is plausible that PE N-methylation may participate in regulating different membrane functions.

It is now well established that calcium ions are essential for supporting the cardiac contractile activity and several biochemical mechanisms have been implicated in Ca^{2+} movements at the level of sarcolemmal and sarcoplasmic reticular membranes in cardiac cell (10,11). Electrogenic Na^+-Ca^{2+} exchange is known to act in heart sarcolemma as a major mechanism for extruding Ca^{2+} ions (12). However, it is becoming evident that Na^+-Ca^{2+} exchange system may operate in both directions at the plasma membrane and it may be involved in both contraction and relaxation processes in the myocardium (12). Because of its dependence on the Na^+

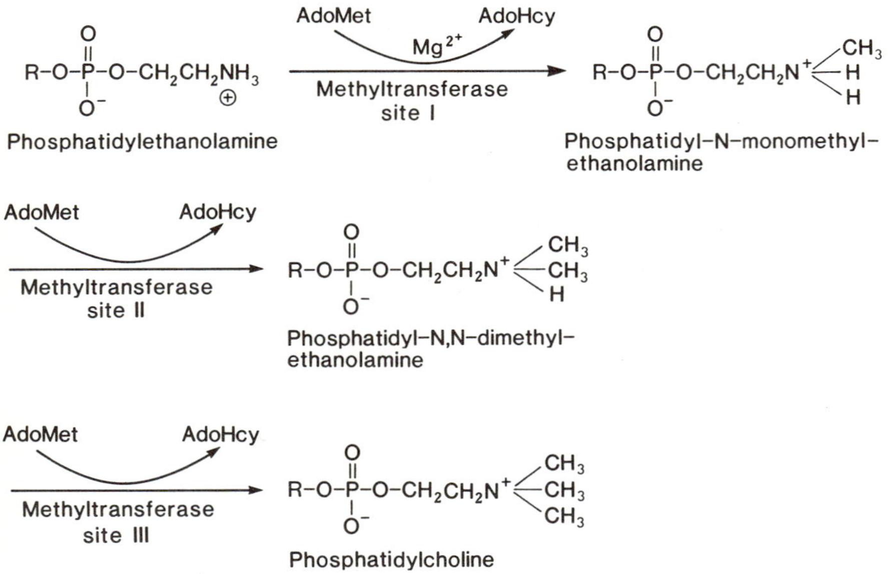

Phosphatidylethanolamine

AdoMet → AdoHcy, Mg^{2+}

Methyltransferase site I

Phosphatidyl–N–monomethyl–ethanolamine

AdoMet → AdoHcy

Methyltransferase site II

Phosphatidyl–N,N–dimethyl–ethanolamine

AdoMet → AdoHcy

Methyltransferase site III

Phosphatidylcholine

Figure 1. Enzymatic N-methylation of phosphatidylethanolamine to phosphatidylcholine in cardiac membranes. R = α, β-diacylglycerate; AdoMet = S-adenosyl-L-methionine; AdoHcy = S-adenosyl-L-homocysteine.

gradient, the exchanger depends on sarcolemmal Na^+, K^+-ATPase activity which determines that gradient. Another important factor for the exchanger activity is the intracellular Ca^{2+} concentration, which in turn is regulated by other membrane-bound transport mechanisms. In fact, ATP-dependent Ca^{2+} uptake and Ca^{2+}-stimulated ATPase of the sarcolemmal membrane are concerned with Ca^{2+} efflux from the myocardial cell, while the active transport of Ca^{2+} in sarcoplasmic reticulum is primarily achieved by the sarcoplasmic reticular Ca^{2+}-stimulated ATPase (10,11). Since the role of PE N-methylation process in regulating membrane-related Ca^{2+} transport systems of the heart is not known at present, it was the object of this study to investigate the influence of PE N-methylation on the Na^+-Ca^{2+} exchange, Ca^{2+}-pump and Na^+, K^+-ATPase activities of cardiac sarcolemma. The effect of PE N-methylation was also tested on the sarcoplasmic reticular Ca^{2+}-pump activity.

METHODS

Male Sprague-Dawley rats weighing approximately 250-300 g were employed in this study. Animals were sacrificed by decapitation, hearts were

immediately excised and ventricular tissue was then processed in pooled
samples of three or more hearts for the isolation of subcellular organelles.
All procedures were carried out at 0 to 5°C. Purified sarcolemmal (SL)
vesicles were prepared by the method of Pitts (13) and cardiac microsomes
containing predominantly sarcoplasmic reticular (SR) vesicles were obtained
according to the procedure described by Sulakhe and Dhalla (14). In agreement
with previous observations (8), marker enzyme activities revealed that both
SL and SR membrane preparations had minimal cross contamination by other
subcellular organelles.   For Na^{+}-Ca^{2+} exchange studies, sarcolemmal
vesicles were methylated with non-radioactive AdoMet and the incubation was
carried out under conditions optimal for catalytic sites I, II and III (8).
The reaction was stopped by three volumes of ice-cold buffer and the assay
mixture was immediately centrifuged. The pellet was resuspended in the same
buffer used for the measurement of Na^{+}-Ca^{2+} exchange, which was performed
essentially as described by Reeves and Sutko (15) with some modification.
For studies involving Na^{+}-dependent Ca^{2+} uptake, sarcolemmal vesicles
suspended in 160 mM NaCl- 20 mM Mops, pH 7.4, were incubated at 37°C for 30
min. NaCl-loaded vesicles (Na^{+}-vesicles) were then added (10 µl) to a
series of tubes containing an incubation mixture (at 37°C) consisting of 160
mM KCl, 20 mM Mops (pH 7.4) and 40 µM $^{45}CaCl_{2}$ (50 µCi/nmol of Ca^{2+}) in a
final volume of 500 µl to induce Na^{+}-Ca^{2+} exchange. The reaction was
terminated at desired times by the addition of 100 µl of 160 mM KCl, 5 mM
$LaCl_{3}$, 20 mM Mops, pH 7.4. Aliquots (100 µl) were withdrawn, immediately
filtered through Millipore filters (0.45 µm) and then washed with 1 ml
aliquots of 160 mM KCl, 20 mM Mops, 1 mM $LaCl_{3}$, pH 7.4 to displace
externally bound Ca^{2+}. To obtain control blanks, the membrane vesicles
suspended in 160 mM KCl - 20 mM Mops were also incubated for 30 min at 37°C
with KCl/Mops to load K^{+} (K^{+}-vesicles), and then nonspecific (Na^{+}-
independent) Ca^{2+} uptake was determined in a manner similar to that
described for Na^{+}-vesicles. The net Ca^{2+} influx activity was calculated as
the difference between the Ca^{2+} uptake activities of the Na^{+}-vesicles and
the K^{+}-vesicles. For studies on Na^{+}-induced Ca^{2+} release, Na^{+} loaded
vesicles were allowed to accumulate $^{45}Ca^{2+}$ for 2 min in KCl/Mops, following
the procedure outlined for the Ca^{2+}-uptake study. Ca^{2+} release was then
assayed upon exposure to 40 mM Na^{+} (16).

For the Ca^{2+}-stimulated ATPase assay in SL vesicles 25 µg protein were
preincubated at 37°C in a medium (pH 7.4) containing 160 mM KCl, 5 mM $MgCl_{2}$,

5 mM NaN_3 and 20 mM Mops with varying concentrations of non-radioactive AdoMet for 10 min and then the total $(Mg^{2+} + Ca^{2+})$-ATPase and Mg^{2+}-ATPase activities were determined for 5 min by measuring the hydrolysis of ATP (2 mM) in the presence and absence of 10 µM free Ca^{2+}, respectively. When Mg^{2+}-ATPase was measured, 0.2 mM EGTA was also added in the incubation medium. The Ca^{2+} stimulated ATPase activity reported here is the difference between total ATPase and Mg^{2+}-ATPase activities. ATP-dependent Ca^{2+} uptake of SL vesicles was determined in the presence of 10 µM free Ca^{2+} as previously described (16). Na^+, K^+-ATPase was measured according to the procedure outlined elsewhere (16) in the presence or absence of varying concentrations of non-radioactive AdoMet. To test the Ca^{2+}-stimulated ATPase activity in cardiac SR, membranes (30 µg/ml) were preincubated at $37^{o}C$ in a medium containing 100 mM KCl, 5 mM $MgCl_2$ and 20 mM Tris-HCl (pH 6.8) with varying concentrations of non-radioactive AdoMet for 10 min and then the total $(Mg^{2+} + Ca^{2+})$-ATPase and Mg^{2+} ATPase activities were determined for 5 min by measuring the hydrolysis of ATP (5 mM) in the presence and absence of 10 µM free Ca^{2+}, respectively. When Mg^{2+} ATPase was measured 0.2 mM EGTA was also added in the incubation medium. The Ca^{2+}-stimulated ATPase activity was calculated as the difference between the total ATPase and Mg^{2+} ATPase activities. The patterns of $[^3H]$ methyl group incorporation into individual membrane phospholipids (PMME, PDME and PC) were followed under all the experimental conditions of this study by using $[^3H]$ methyl labeled AdoMet. The detailed procedure for the measurement of intermediate methylated phospholipids has been reported earlier (8). The results were analyzed statistically by the Student's 't'-test and P values < 0.05 were considered to reflect significant differences.

RESULTS

As reported previously (8), the activities of three catalytic sites involved in the methylation process were manifested by the major synthesis of specific phospholipid molecules, namely PMME, PDME and PC at 0.1 µM (site I), 10 µM (site II) and 150 µM (site III) $[^3H]$-AdoMet respectively. Results representing the effect of PE N-methylation on sarcolemmal Na^+-Ca^{2+} exchange are shown in Table 1. Na^+-dependent Ca^{2+} uptake was significantly inhibited at sites II and III as compared with control preparations, whereas no significant changes were seen in Na^+-induced Ca^{2+} release, nonspecific Ca^{2+} uptake and nonspecific Ca^{2+} release. To confirm the decreased Na^+-dependent Ca^{2+} uptake after methylation, we examined the time course of Ca^{2+} uptake in control and experimental membranes methylated at site II, where maximal inhibition was observed. As it can be seen in Table 2, the methylation reaction involved a strong inhibition of Na^+-dependent Ca^{2+} uptake at all the time points studied. Time course of Ca^{2+} release from control and site II methylated sarcolemmal vesicles was also studied and the results show that Na^+-induced Ca^{2+} release was unaltered as a function of time after methylation treatment (Table 3). The experiments in Tables 2 and 3 further indicate no differences between control and methylated preparations with respect to the patterns of nonspecific Ca^{2+} uptake and release. These results seem to exclude that the effect of PE N-methylation on Na^+-Ca^{2+} exchange is indirectly mediated through changes in membrane permeability. Since the degree of Ca^{2+} influx

Table 1. Effect of phosphatidylethanolamine N-methylation on Na^+-Ca^{2+} exchange in cardiac sarcolemma.

	Control	Catalytic sites		
		I	II	III
Na^+-dependent Ca^{2+} uptake	26.1 ± 1.9	25.4 ± 2.3	12.3 ± 1.1*	15.8 ± 1.6*
Na^+-induced Ca^{2+} release	22.3 ± 0.5	20.2 ± 0.5	21.5 ± 0.8	21.9 ± 1.5
Nonspecific (Na^+-indep.) Ca^{2+} uptake	2.39 ± 0.16	2.55 ± 0.19	2.45 ± 0.26	2.23 ± 0.15
Nonspecific (Na^+-indep.) Ca^{2+} release	1.60 ± 0.04	1.47 ± 0.09	1.45 ± 0.05	1.66 ± 0.05

Values are means ± S.E. of 5 experiments and are expressed as nmoles/mg/15 sec. Methylation at catalytic sites I, II and III was performed for 30 min in the presence of 0.1, 10 and 150 μM AdoMet, respectively (8). Na^+-Ca^{2+} exchange activities were measured as indicated in Methods. Nonspecific Ca^{2+} uptake and Ca^{2+} release activities were measured in the K^+-vesicles.
* Significantly (P < 0.05) different from control.

Table 2. Time course of Ca^{2+} uptake in control and methylated heart sarcolemmal vesicles.

Time (sec)	Na^+-dep. Ca^{2+} uptake		Nonspecific (Na^+-indep.) Ca^{2+} uptake	
	Control	Methylated	Control	Methylated
	(nmoles/mg)			
5	13.5	4.5	1.7	1.6
15	22.4	10.9	2.1	1.9
30	30.7	18.7	2.3	2.4
60	38.5	20.4	3.1	2.9
180	41.9	21.7	4.1	4.3

Values are averages of 2 experiments. Methylation at site II was carried out as indicated in Table 1. Na^+-Ca^{2+} exchange was measured as indicated in Methods.

Table 3. Time-course of Ca^{2+} release in control and methylated heart sarcolemmal vesicles.

Time (sec)	Residual Ca^{2+} in the K^+-vesicles		Residual Ca^{2+} in the Na^+-vesicles			
			In the presence of 40 mM Na^+		In the absence of Na^+	
	Control	Methylated	Control	Methylated	Control	Methylated
	(nmol/mg)					
0	4.2	3.9	44.3	26.6	45.6	26.2
10	3.0	3.0	33.8	17.5	41.9	23.0
20	2.5	2.4	25.3	9.0	38.6	20.2
60	2.3	2.3	21.5	5.8	36.5	19.1
180	1.8	2.1	19.7	4.5	35.4	17.8

Values are averages of 3 experiments. Na^+- or K^+-vesicles were incubated with 40 µM $^{45}CaCl_2$ for 2 min for Ca^{2+} uptake as described in Methods. Na^+-vesicles were then diluted with the medium containing either 40 mM NaCl and 120 mM KCl or 160 mM KCl in 1 mM EGTA and 20 mM Mops, pH 7.4, to initiate Ca^{2+} release. Ca^+ release was also tested in K^+-vesicles with 160 mM KCl, 1 mM EGTA and 20 mM Mops, pH 7.4. Na^+-induced Ca^{2+} release from Na^+-vesicles may be calculated as the difference between net residual Ca^{2+} in Na^+-vesicles at 0 time and at various time intervals. Methylation at site II was carried out as indicated in Table 1.

via the exchanger is altered by methylation, one may argue that efflux experiments may be affected by different Ca^{2+} loading conditions. Therefore, in two experiments, vesicles were loaded with Ca^{2+} by ATP-dependent Ca^{2+} pump. Na^+-induced Ca^{2+} release was then examined (17) and found to be similar in control (18.2 nmol/mg/15 sec) and membrane methylated at site II (21.4 nmol/ mg/15 sec).

In a different set of experiments, the effect of methylation on the heart sarcolemmal Ca^{2+}-pump and Na^+, K^+- ATPase activities was studied. Results in Table 4 show that both Ca^{2+}-stimulated ATPase and ATP-dependent Ca^{2+} uptake activities, which are functional expression of the pump mechanism (10,11), were significantly enhanced at 10 μM (site II) and 150 μM (site III) AdoMet; these AdoMet concentrations are typical for the major synthesis of PDME and PC, respectively (8). In contrast, Na^+, K^+-ATPase and Mg^{2+}-ATPase activities were unaffected by the methylation reaction (Table 4). In an attempt to expose all sites of the Na^+, K^+-ATPase enzyme system accessible to methylation process, sarcolemmal vesicles were mildly pretreated with sodium deoxycholate (0.2 mg/mg SL protein) (18). However, no positive results were obtained. The sensitivity of Na^+, K^+-ATPase to ouabain was also similar in control and methylated membranes (data not shown).

Table 4. Effect of phosphatidylethanolamine N-methylation on heart sarcolemmal Ca^{2+}-pump and Na^+, K^+-ATPase activities.

	Control	AdoMet (μM)		
		0.1	10	150
Ca^{2+}-stimulated ATPase[a]	7.1 ± 0.5	8.1 ± 0.7	14.5 ± 1.1*	13.1 ± 1.0*
ATP-dependent Ca^{2+} uptake[b]	19.6 ± 1.4	20.3 ± 1.4	36.9 ± 2.9*	35.3 ± 2.1*
Na^+, K^+-ATPase[a]	25.9 ± 2.0	27.1 ± 1.9	25.6 ± 1.5	23.8 ± 1.6
Mg^{2+}-ATPase[a]	196.1 ± 12.3	196.1 ± 11.5	201.3 ± 10.9	202.7 ± 12.9

Values are means ± S.E. of 4 to 6 experiments. Sarcolemmal activities were assayed as indicated in Methods and in the presence or absence of 0.1, 10 and 150 μM AdoMet. Specific activities are expressed as: a = μmoles Pi/mg/ h; b = nmoles/mg/min. * Significantly (P < 0.05) different from control.

Table 5. Effect of phosphatidylethanolamine N-methylation on ATPase
activities of cardiac sarcoplasmic reticulum.

Enzyme	Control	AdoMet (μM)		
		0.1	10	150
		μmoles Pi/mg/5 min		
Ca^{2+}-stimulated ATPase	1.1 ± 0.1	1.1 ± 0.1	1.3 ± 0.1	1.9 ± 0.2[*]
Mg^{2+}-ATPase	12.3 ± 0.9	12.4 ± 1.0	11.6 ± 1.0	12.0 ± 0.8

Values are the means $\pm$ S.E. of 5 experiments. Sarcoplasmic reticular
activities were assayed as indicated in Methods and in the presence or
absence of 0.1, 10 and 150 μM AdoMet. [*] Significantly (P < 0.05) different
from control.

As it can be seen in Table 5, Ca^{2+}-stimulated ATPase activity of
sarcoplasmic reticular membranes was enhanced upon methylation and maximal
stimulation occurred at a concentration of AdoMet (150 μM) that synthesized
PC and comparatively smaller amounts of other N-methylated phospholipids
such as PMME and PDME. The Mg^{2+}-ATPase activity remained unaltered.   The
ATP-supported Ca^{2+} uptake activity of SR in the presence of 5 mM oxalate
(19) was increased by approximately 45% by methylating with 150 μM AdoMet.
It should be pointed out that methylation-induced alterations of SL and SR
Ca^{2+} transport functions were prevented by inhibitors of PE N-methylation
such as S-adenosyl-L-homocysteine (20) and methyl acetimidate hydrochloride
(21). Therefore, it is likely that PE N-methylation process is responsible
for the above observed alterations.

DISCUSSION

Phosphatidylethanolamine (PE) N-methylation is a reaction in which
ethanolamine phospholipids are converted to choline-phospholipids. This
activity has been shown to exist in a variety of tissues (22). In fact, it
has been shown that this methyl transfer reaction starts on the cytoplasmic
side of the cell membrane while its final product, PC, is located on the
outside of the membrane (22). This enzyme-mediated movement of methylated
phospholipids across the bilayer has been implicated in changing
membrane-associated functions including alteration of membrane fluidity,

receptor-mediated signal transduction and Ca^{2+} influx (22). Previous
reports from our laboratory (8,20,23) have shown the existence in cardiac
subcellular membranes of three methyltransferase catalytic sites for PE
N-methylation, each exhibiting different kinetic parameters, pH profile,
sensitivity to divalent cations as well as major synthesis of a specific
N-methylated phospholipid. Results of this study indicate that PE
N-methylation influences several membrane-related Ca^{2+} transport systems of
the myocardial cell. In this regard, it should be noted that the Na^{+}-
dependent Ca^{2+} uptake of purified cardiac sarcolemmal (SL) vesicles was
inhibited upon N-methylation at catalytic sites II and III, whereas it was
unaltered in site I methylated membranes. These changes seem to be
specifically due to PE N-methylation because the inhibitory effect was
prevented by pretreating sarcolemma with methyl acetimidate, which blocks
the amino group of intramembranal PE and its subsequent methylation (21).
Furthermore, nonspecific Ca^{2+} uptake was not affected by PE N-methylation
under different experimental conditions. It was interesting to observe that
methylation at site II was more effective in inhibiting the Na^{+}-dependent
Ca^{2+} uptake than at site III. Since methylation of site III produces high
levels of both PDME and PC in comparison with those at site II condition
(8), one may expect a greater inhibition of Na^{+}-dependent Ca^{2+} uptake upon
methylation at site III. However, the ratio of PDME/PC at site II is about
3 fold that at site III (8) and thus it is possible that it is the ratio
rather than the absolute concentrations of methylated phospholipids which
may be responsible for altering the microdomain of the exchanger and thereby
determining the observed inhibition. This view is supported by earlier
observations (24) in which the ratio of PMME/PC was found to be closely
related to changes in membrane fluidity of synthetic liposomes.
Methylation-induced inhibition of Ca^{2+} uptake through the exchanger is
consistent with previous data (25) showing a decrease, upon methylation at
sites II and III, of the ATP-independent Ca^{2+}-binding at the low affinity-
high capacity sarcolemmal sites. This ATP-independent Ca^{2+}-binding seems to
represent a superficial, rapidly exchangeable calcium pool that enters the
cardiac cell upon depolarization and is responsible for maintaining the
cardiac contractile function (10). At any rate, alteration of Na^{+}-Ca^{2+}
exchange mechanism by PE N-methylation appears to be restricted to
inhibition of Ca^{2+} uptake since the Na^{+}-induced Ca^{2+} release was unaffected

in the methylated membranes. Such a type of alteration in Ca^{2+} transport by the Na^+-Ca^{2+} exchange has been demonstrated in a previous study (25), where it was seen that diltiazem (0.1 - 10 μM) depressed Ca^{2+}-uptake but had little effect on Ca^{2+}-release in this system. In addition, Trosper and Philipson (27) observed that divalent and trivalent cations inhibited Ca^{2+}-uptake in this system whereas the trivalent cations inhibited Ca^{2+}-release and the divalent cations stimulated Ca^{2+} release in the same vesicular preparation. Such results are consistent with the view that mechanisms controlling Ca^{2+}-uptake via the Na^+-Ca^{2+} exchange system in the sarcolemmal preparations may be different from those involved in Ca^{2+}-release (12). A more detailed account of the interaction of Ca^{2+} with Na^+-Ca^{2+} exchange system must await molecular description of the exchanger itself in addition to its characteristics at both surfaces of the cell membrane.

Under our experimental conditions, N-methylation of sarcolemmal vesicles did not induce any changes in Na^+, K^+-ATPase activity. Earlier studies have shown an activation of liver plasma membrane Na^+, K^+-ATPase after _in vivo_ administration of AdoMet (28), but an inhibition of the brain microsomal enzyme upon _in vitro_ treatment with AdoMet (29). These conflicting observations may be due to tissue-specificity of the Na^+, K^+-ATPase system with respect to its organization in the membrane. On the other hand, membrane PE N-methylation was associated with approximately 100% stimulation of the sarcolemmal Ca^{2+}-pump. From a functional viewpoint, this activation can be seen to promote Ca^{2+} efflux and thus exhance the rate of cardiac relaxation (10,11). Since in the activity of the sarcoplasmic reticular (SR) Ca^{2+}-ATPase was also activated by PE N-methylation, and since there is a close relationship between SR Ca^{2+} transport activity and muscle relaxation, the observed augmentation in SR Ca^{2+}-ATPase activity can also be seen to enhance the rate of cardiac relaxation. In this regard it should be noted that catecholamines, which are known to increase SR Ca^{2+} transport activity and shorten the diastole (10), have also been reported to stimulate membrane PE N-methylation in myocardium (30). The results of this study suggest that, at the sarcolemmal level, inhibition of Na^+-dependent Ca^{2+} uptake activity of the Na^+-Ca^{2+} exchanger and activation of Ca^{2+}-pump upon methylation would tend to prevent the occurrence of intracellular Ca^{2+} overload, which is considered to represent an important mechanism in the pathogenesis of cardiac contractile failure (10). The augmentation of Ca^{2+} pump activities in the heart sarcolemmal and sarcoplasmic reticular membranes confirms our earlier reports (31,32).

SUMMARY

In this study we have shown that the Na^+-dependent Ca^{2+} uptake of purified cardiac sarcolemmal vesicles was depressed upon phosphatidylethanolamine (PE) N-methylation whereas Na^+-induced Ca^{2+} release and Na^+, K^+-ATPase activity were not affected in the methylated membranes. On the other hand, methylation process increased the Ca^{2+}-pump activities of both sarcolemmal and sarcoplasmic reticular membranes. The observed alterations were prevented by inhibitors of PE N-methylation such as S-adenosyl-L-homocysteine and methyl acetimidate hydrochloride. These results suggest that N-methylation of intramembranal PE molecules may modify either directly or indirectly the localized phospholipid domains of cardiac Na^+-Ca^{2+} exchange and Ca^{2+}-pump systems which may influence their functions.

ACKNOWLEDGEMENTS

This research was supported by a grant from the Manitoba Heart Foundation. Dr. V. Panagia is a scholar of the Manitoba Heart Foundation and Dr. K. Okumura was a postdoctoral fellow of the Canadian Heart Foundation.

REFERENCES

1. Caroni, P., Zurini, M., Clark, A. and Carafoli E. Further characterization and reconstitution of the purified Ca^{2+}-pumping ATPase of heart sarcolemma. J. Biol. Chem. <u>258</u>: 7305-7310, 1983.
2. Lentz, B.R., Clubb, K.W., Alfort D.R., Hochli, M. and Meissner, G. Phase behavior of membrane reconstituted from dipentadecanoylphosphatidylcholine and the Mg^{2+}-dependent Ca^{2+} stimulated adenosine triphosphatase of sarcoplasmic reticulum: evidence for a disrupted lipid domain surrounding protein. Biochemistry <u>24</u>: 433-442, 1985.
3. Karli, J.N., Karikas, G.A., Hatzepavlou, P.K., Lewis, G.M. and Moulopoulos, S.N. The inhibition of Na^+ and K^+ stimulated ATPase activity of rabbit and dog heart sarcolemma by lysophosphatidylcholine. Life Sci. <u>24</u>: 1869-1876, 1976.
4. Matsuda, T. and Iwata, H. Phospholipid composition of cardiac (Na^+ + K^+)-ATPases from various species. Experientia <u>42</u>: 405-407, 1986.
5. Panagia, V., Michiel, D.F., Dhalla, K.S., Nijjar, M.S. and Dhalla, N.S. Role of phosphatidylinositol in basal adenylate cyclase activity of rat heart sarcolemma. Biochim. Biophys. Acta <u>792</u>: 245-253, 1984.
6. Philipson, K.D. and Nishimoto, A.Y. Stimulation of Na^+-Ca^{2+} exchange in cardiac sarcolemmal vesicles by phospholipase D. J. Biol. Chem. <u>259</u>: 16-19, 1984.

7. Bremer, J. and Greenberg, D.M. Methyltransferring enzyme system of microsomes in the biosynthesis of lecithin (phosphatidylcholine). Biochem. Biophys. Acta 46: 205-216, 1961.

8. Panagia, V., Ganguly, P.K., Okumura, K. and Dhalla, N.S. Subcellular localization of phosphatidylethanolamine N-methylation activity in rat heart. J. Mol. Cell. Cardiol. 17: 1151-1159, 1985.

9. Shinitzky, M. Membrane fluidity and cellular functions. In: Physiology of Membrane Fluidity, vol. 1, (edited by M. Shinitzky). CRC Press, Boca Raton, 1984, pp. 1-51.

10. Dhalla, N.S., Pierce, G.N., Panagia, V., Singal, P.K. and Beamish, R.E. Calcium movements in relation to heart function. Basic Res. Cardiol. 77: 117-139, 1982.

11. Carafoli, E. The homeostasis of calcium in heart cells. J. Mol. Cell. Cardiol. 17: 203-212, 1985.

12. Reeves, J.P. The sarcolemmal sodium-calcium exchange system. In: Current Topics in Membranes and Transport, Vol. 25, Regulation of Calcium Transport across Muscle Membranes, (edited by A.E. Shamoo), Academic Press, Orlando, 1985, pp. 77-127.

13. Pitts, B.J.R. Stoichiometry of sodium-calcium exchange in cardiac sarcolemmal vesicles. J. Biol. Chem. 254: 6232-6235, 1979.

14. Sulakhe, P.V. and Dhalla, N.S. Excitation-contraction coupling in the heart. VII. Calcium accumulation in subcellular particles in congestive heart failure. J. Clin. Invest. 50: 1019-1027, 1971.

15. Reeves, J.P. and Sutko, J.L. Sodium-calcium ion exchange in cardiac membrane vesicles. Proc. Natl. Acad. Sci. USA. 76: 590-594, 1979.

16. Heyliger, C.E., Takeo, S. and Dhalla, N.S. Alterations in sarcolemmal Na^+-Ca^{2+} exchange and ATP-dependent Ca^{2+} binding in hypertrophied heart. Can. J. Cardiol. 1: 328-339, 1985.

17. Frank, J.S., Philipson, K.D. and Beydler, S. Ultrastructure of isolated sarcolemma from dog and rabbit myocardium. Circ. Res. 54: 414-423, 1984.

18. Panagia, V., Lamers, J.M.J., Singal, P.K. and Dhalla, N.S. Ca^{2+}- and Mg^{2+}-dependent ATPase activities in the deoxycholate-treated rat heart sarcolemma. Int. J. Biochem. 14: 387-397, 1982.

19. Panagia, V., Pierce, G.N., Dhalla, K.S., Ganguly, P.K., Beamish, R.E. and Dhalla, N.S. Adaptive changes in subcellular calcium transport during catecholamine-induced cardiomyopathy. J. Mol. Cell. Cardiol. 17: 411-419, 1985.

20. Ganguly, P.K., Rice, K.M., Panagia, V. and Dhalla, N.S. Sarcolemmal phosphatidylethanolamine N-methylation in diabetic cardiomyopathy. Circ. Res. 55: 504-512, 1984.

21. Akesson, B. Structural requirements of the phospholipid substrate for phospholipid N-methylation in rat liver. Biochim. Biophys. Acta 752: 460-466, 1983.

22. Crews, F.T. Phospholipid methylation and membrane function. In: Phospholipids and Cellular Regulation, Vol. 1 (edited by J.F. Kuo), CRC Press, Boca Raton, 1985, pp. 131-158.

23. Panagia, V., Ganguly, P.K. and Dhalla, N.S. Characterization of heart sarcolemmal phospholipid methylation. Biochim. Biophys. Acta 792: 245-253, 1984.

24. Sastry, B.V.R., Statham, C.N., Meeks, R.G. and Axelrod, J. Changes in phospholipid methyltransferases and membrane microvisconity during induction of rat liver microsomal cytochrome P-450 by phenobarbital and 3-methylcholanthrene. Pharmacology 23: 211-222, 1981.

25. Panagia, V., Ganguly, P.K., Elimban, V. and Dhalla, N.S. Ca^{2+} binding and Ca^{2+}-ATPase activities in heart sarcolemma upon phospholipid methylation. J. Mol. Cell. Cardiol. 15 Suppl. 4, 35, 1983.

26. Takeo, S., Elimban, V. and Dhalla, N.S. Modification of cardiac sarcolemmal Na^{+}-Ca^{2+} exchange by diltiazem and verapamil. Can. J. Cardiol. 1: 131-138, 1985.

27. Trosper, T.L. and Philipson, K.D. Effects of divalent and trivalent cations on Na^{+}-Ca^{2+} exchange in cardiac sarcolemmal vesicles. Biochim. Biophys. Acta 731: 63-68, 1983.

28. Boelsterli, V.A., Rakhit, G. and Balasz, T. Modulation by S-adenosyl-L-methionine of hepatic Na^{+}, K^{+}-ATPase, membrane fluidity and bile flow in rats with ethinyl estradiol-induced cholestasis. Hepatology 3: 12-17, 1983.

29. Hattori, H. and Kanfer, J.N. Inhibition of rat brain microsomal Na^{+}, K^{+}-ATPase by S-adenosylmethionine. J. Neurochem. 42: 204-208, 1984.

30. Okumura, K., Ogawa, K. and Satake, T. Phospholipid methylation in canine cardiac membranes. Relations to beta-adrenergic receptors and digitalis receptors. Jpn. Heart J. 24: 215-225, 1983.

31. Panagia, V., Okumura, K., Makino, N. and Dhalla, N.S. Stimulation of Ca^{2+}-pump in rat sarcolemma by phosphatidylethanolamine N-methylation. Biochim. Biophys. Acta 856: 383-387, 1986.

32. Ganguly, P.K., Panagia, V., Okumura, K. and Dhalla, N.S. Activation of Ca^{2+}-stimulated ATPase by phospholipid N-methylation in cardiac sarcoplasmic reticulum. Biochem. Biophys. Res. Commun. 130: 472-478, 1985.

10

Na$^+$-Ca^{2+} EXCHANGE IN CARDIAC SARCOLEMMAL VESICLES

K.D. PHILIPSON

Departments of Medicine and Physiology and the American Heart Association
Greater Los Angeles Affiliate Cardiovascular Research Laboratories, UCLA
School of Medicine, Los Angeles, California 90024

INTRODUCTION

Like all muscle, cardiac muscle contracts in response to a rise in
the intracellular Ca^{2+} concentration. Much attention has focused on regulation of the Ca^{2+} transport involved in myocardial
excitation-contraction coupling. Myocardial cells contain multiple Ca^{2+}
transport mechanisms, however, and it has not been possible to define the
importance of each pathway in excitation-contraction coupling.
Mitochondria and sarcoplasmic reticulum both have Ca^{2+} influx and efflux
mechanisms. In addition, the sarcolemmal membrane has three Ca^{2+} transport pathways: 1) a voltage-sensitive Ca^{2+} channel which transports
Ca^{2+} into the myocardial cell; 2) an ATP-dependent Ca^{2+} pump which extrudes cellular Ca^{2+}; 3) a Na$^+$-Ca^{2+} exchanger which can move Ca^{2+} in either direction depending on the Na$^+$ and Ca^{2+} gradients and membrane potential. Unlike skeletal muscle, in which Ca^{2+} movements are primarily
intracellular, it has become clear that both intra- and extracellular
sources of Ca^{2+} are important in regulating myocardial contraction.

In 1968, Reuter and Seitz (1) identified Na$^+$-Ca^{2+} exchange in guinea
pig atria. Extensive efforts since then have implicated an importance
for myocardial Na$^+$-Ca^{2+} exchange. For example, the positive inotropic
effect of digitalis is likely to involve altered Na$^+$-Ca^{2+} exchange activity. Nevertheless, the exact role of Na$^+$-Ca^{2+} exchange remains a controversial issue.

Due to the complexities of the myocardium, it is difficult to investigate Na$^+$-Ca^{2+} exchange in intact cardiac tissue. Recently, the ability
to measure Na$^+$-Ca^{2+} exchange in isolated sarcolemmal vesicles (2, 3, 4)
has greatly aided study of this transport mechanism. Using vesicles,
Na$^+$-Ca^{2+} exchange is most easily measured as Na$_i^+$-dependent Ca^{2+} uptake.
Initial rates of up to 30 nmol Ca^{2+}/mg protein/sec can be achieved.

GENERAL PROPERTIES OF VESICULAR Na^+-Ca^{2+} EXCHANGE

Na^+-Ca^{2+} exchange is an electrogenic process in sarcolemmal vesicles: exchange activity can be modulated by membrane potential (5, 6) and, in addition, the exchanger can generate a membrane current (7). These observations suggest that the stoichiometry of exchange is 3 or more Na^+ ions for each Ca^{2+} ion. Initial observations indicate a stoichiometry of 3 Na^+/Ca^{2+} (8, 9) but further confirmation would be desirable. Apparent $K_M(Ca^{2+})$ values from 2 to 40 μM have been reported. Many factors can modulate the $K_M(Ca^{2+})$ as described below. The apparent $K_M(Na^+)$ is about 20-30 mM.

SYMMETRY OF Na^+-Ca^{2+} EXCHANGE

To measure Na^+-Ca^{2+} exchange, vesicles are usually first loaded with Na^+ by passive diffusion. Sarcolemmal preparations contain both inside-out and right-side-out vesicles, and both types of vesicles will passively take up Na^+. When Na_i^+-dependent Ca^{2+} uptake is initiated both types of vesicles take up Ca^{2+} by Na^+-Ca^{2+} exchange. If the inside-out and right-side-out vesicles have different Na^+-Ca^{2+} exchange properties, this could complicate the data and lead to misinterpretations. To circumvent this problem, we have developed a technique which takes advantage of the fact that the ATP-dependent Na^+ pump and Na^+-Ca^{2+} exchange proteins are present in the same vesicles. Na^+ will be actively transported only into inside-out sarcolemmal vesicles due to the asymmetric orientation of the Na^+ pump. Thus, by initiating active Na^+ transport we are able to selectively Na^+ load inside-out sarcolemmal vesicles in preparation for Na^+-Ca^{2+} exchange. Using this approach, we find the exchanger to be largely symmetric. The Ca^{2+} binding sites on the two surfaces of the exchanger appear similar, as do the Na^+ binding sites (10, 11).

MODULATION OF Na^+-Ca^{2+} EXCHANGE ACTIVITY

Many factors can stimulate the Na^+-Ca^{2+} exchange activity of cardiac sarcolemmal vesicles. These factors include the following: membrane potential (5-7), high pH (12), mild proteinase treatment (13), EGTA (14), intravesicular Ca^{2+} (15), redox modification (16), and a variety of anionic amphiphiles (discussed in more detail below). The major effect of each of these perturbations (except membrane potential) is to increase the apparent affinity of the exchanger for Ca^{2+}. Physiological significance of most of these effects is uncertain. No highly specific inhibitors of Na^+–Ca^{2+} have been described.

INTERACTIONS OF CHARGED AMPHIPHILES WITH THE Na^+–Ca^{2+} EXCHANGER

In a series of investigations (17–22), we found sensitive interactions between the Na^+–Ca^{2+} exchanger and charged lipid components. Anionic phospholipids, fatty acids, and other anionic amphiphiles all stimulate Na^+–Ca^{2+} exchange. In contrast, cationic amphiphiles inhibit exchange activity. The exchanger is more sensitive to membrane perturbation than other sarcolemmal transporters such as the Na^+,K^+–ATPase or the ATP–dependent Ca^{2+} pump.

Unsaturated fatty acids stimulated Na^+–Ca^{2+} exchange more potently than saturated fatty acids (21), and we speculated that the unsaturation increased stimulation by disordering the lipid bilayer in the exchanger microenvironment. Methyl esters of fatty acids have no effect on Na^+–Ca^{2+} exchange indicating the requirement for negative charge at the membrane surface. We also did experiments using stearic acid labelled at different positions with a doxyl group to modulate Na^+–Ca^{2+} exchange activity (22). We were able to map the locations within the bilayer where perturbation most sensitively affected Na^+–Ca^{2+} exchange. We modeled our findings as follows: For a fatty acid to stimulate Na^+–Ca^{2+} exchange, a negative charge is necessary to interact with the exchanger at the membrane surface. Stimulation is enhanced by perturbation within the lipid bilayer. A perturbation is most effective at a location near the center of the bilayer.

PHYSIOLOGICAL SIGNIFICANCE

The cardiac Na^+–Ca^{2+} exchange mechanism could be important for either myocardial Ca^{2+} influx or efflux. Under normal conditions it is probable that a majority of the excitation–dependent Ca^{2+} influx is through the Ca^{2+} channel. This is indicated by the potency of a variety of organic Ca^{2+} channel blockers to uncouple excitation from contraction.

The high activity of Na^+–Ca^{2+} exchange in cardiac sarcolemmal vesicles has suggested an important role for Na^+–Ca^{2+} exchange in cellular Ca^{2+} efflux. Vesicular Na^+–Ca^{2+} exchange, however, is usually measured under conditions which are far from physiologic. Using sarcolemmal vesicles, we have estimated the possible significance of Ca^{2+} efflux mediated by Na^+–Ca^{2+} exchange under approximate in vivo ionic conditions (23). Under these conditions, vesicular Na^+–Ca^{2+} exchange is relatively low. We estimate that the capacity of the Na^+–Ca^{2+} exchange system to extrude intracellular Ca^{2+} is about 1.2 μmol Ca^{2+}/kg wet weight/s, which approximately equals the capacity of the sarcolemmal ATP-dependent Ca^{2+} pump (23). Thus, the relative importance of Na^+–Ca^{2+} exchange versus ATP-dependent Ca^{2+} pumping in mediating myocardial Ca^{2+} efflux is an unresolved issue.

REFERENCES

1. Reuter, H., and Seitz, N. J. Physiol. 195:451–450, 1968.
2. Reeves, J.P., and Sutko, J.L. Proc. Natl. Acad. Sci. USA 76: 590–594, 1979.
3. Philipson, K.D. Ann. Rev. Physiol. 47:561–571, 1985.
4. Reeves, J.P. Curr. Top. Memb. Transp. 25:77–127, 1985.
5. Philipson, K.D., and Nishimoto, A.Y. J. Biol. Chem. 255: 6880–6882, 1980.
6. Caroni, P., Reinlib, L., and Carafoli, E. Proc. Natl. Acad. Sci. USA 77:6354–6358, 1980.
7. Reeves, J.P., and Sutko, J.L. Science 208:1461–1464, 1980.
8. Pitts, B.J.R, J. Biol. Chem. 254:6232–6235, 1979.
9. Reeves, J.P., and Hale, C.C. J. .Biol. Chem. 259:7733–7739, 1984.
10. Philipson, K.D., and Nishimoto, A.Y. J. Biol. Chem. 257: 5111–5117, 1982.
11. Philipson, K.D. Biochem. Biophys. Acta 821:367–376, 1985.
12. Philipson, K.D., Bersohn, M.M., and Nishimoto, A.Y. Circ. Res. 50:287–293, 1982.
13. Philipson, K.D., and Nishimoto, A.Y. Am. J. Physiol. 243: C191–C195, 1982.
14. Trosper, T.L., and Philipson, K.D. Cell Calcium 5:211–222, 1984.
15. Reeves, J.P., and Poronnik, P. Submitted.
16. Reeves, J.P., Bailey, C.A., and Hale, C.C. J. Biol. Chem. 261: 4948–4955, 1986.
17. Philipson, K.D., Frank, J.S., and Nishimoto, A.Y. J. Biol. Chem. 258:5905–5910, 1983.
18. Philipson, K.D., and Nishimoto, A.Y. J. Biol. Chem. 259:16–19, 1984.
19. Philipson, K.D. J. Biol. Chem. 259:13999–14002, 1984.
20. Philipson, K.D., Langer, G.A., and Rich, T.L. Am. J. Physiol. 248: H147–H150, 1985.
21. Philipson, K.D., and Ward, R. J. Biol. Chem. 260:9666–9671, 1985.
22. Philipson, K.D., and Ward, R. Submitted.
23. Philipson, K.D., and Ward, R. J. Mol. Cell. Cardiol. In press.

11

NA/K PUMP FUNCTION IN CULTURED EMBRYONIC CHICK HEART CELLS

L. ANDERSON LOBAUGH, S. LIU & M. LIEBERMAN

Department of Physiology, Duke University Medical Center,
Durham, North Carolina, 27710, USA

INTRODUCTION

The goal of research in our laboratory is to characterize the mechanisms responsible for ion transport across the cardiac sarcolemma using a multidisciplinary approach that combines biochemical and biophysical techniques. Cultured chick embryo heart cells are an ideal preparation for these studies because cells can be grown in one of several physiologically stable configurations ideally suited for a particular experimental technique (1): confluent mass cultures for biochemical measurements; small ($\sim$ 100 μm diameter) aggregates for voltage-clamp analysis; polystrands for isotope flux and ion-selective microelectrodes (ISME). In addition, cultured myocyte preparations are free from the physical (diffusional barriers) and biological (altered metabolic state) limitations associated with dissected cardiac muscle preparations and isolated heart cells, respectively.

The activity of the majority of sarcolemmal transport mechanisms heretofore described in cardiac cells is dependent either directly or indirectly on energy derived from the transmembrane Na gradient. Na-linked transport processes are involved in most aspects of cardiac cell physiology, including excitation and contraction (Na/Ca exchange (2,3)), pH regulation (Na/H exchange (4,5)) and possibly cell volume regulation (Na+K+2Cl cotransport (6,7)). Thus, complete characterization of the ATP-driven Na/K pump, the mechanism responsible for maintaining the Na gradient, is central to understanding ion transport across the cardiac cell. The following studies address the substrate-dependence and activity of the cardiac cell Na/K pump using both biochemical and ISME techniques. Typically, Na/K pump function is studied using protocols that evaluate the consequences of Na/K pump inhibition. An additional advantage of cultured myocytes is that Na/K pump capacity can be increased by growing cells under conditions of partial Na/K pump inhibition thereby producing a preparation with an increased density of Na/K pump sites (8,9,10). These pump-induced preparations (PIPs) can be used to study the physiologic consequences of increasing maximal Na/K pump capacity. A brief electrophysiological characterization of PIPs is also presented.

RESULTS AND DISCUSSION

Substrate-dependence and electrogenicity of the Na/K pump

$Effect$ of K_O on Na/K $pump$ $activity$. K_O activation of the Na/K pump was studied using Na-loaded (20 min $0K_O$) muscle cell-enriched mass cultures exposed for 30 s - 1.5 min to buffer containing 0.2 - 8.0 mM $^{42}K \pm 0.1$ mM ouabain. As expected for a multiple-site interaction between K_O and the Na/K pump, the relationship between the initial rate of ouabain-sensitive ^{42}K uptake and K_O was sigmoidal with a Hill coefficient = 1.95 ± 0.27 and $V_{max} = 151 \pm 40$ nmol/mg protein/min (n=4-8). Ouabain-sensitive ^{42}K uptake was half-maximal in 2.7 mM K_O, consistent with half-maximal activation by 2.6 - 10 mM K_O in sheep Purkinje fibers (11,12), and somewhat higher than half-maximal activation by 0.9 - 1.2 mM in canine Purkinje fibers (13) and 1.5 mM in guinea-pig atria (14).

Fig. 1 shows the effect of incubating muscle cell-enriched mass cultures in decreased K_O on cell Na and K content as determined by atomic absorption spectrophotometry (closed circles). A significant increase in Na_i and decrease in K_O occurred only in $K_O \leq 2$ mM, implying (in contrast to the above data) that Na/K pump activity is saturated by $K_O > 2$ mM. Several possible explanations for this discrepancy exist: First, ^{42}K uptake was measured in cells containing a high $\lfloor Na_i \rfloor$, which may cause a decrease in the affinity of the Na/K pump for K_O (15). Secondly, a rise in $\lfloor Na_i \rfloor$ may stimulate Na/K pump activity to offset the inhibition caused by a decrease in K_O. Data in Fig. 1 (open circles) support the latter suggestion: the rise in Na_i in low K_O is more severe than the fall in K_i when the decrease in cell water that occurs in low K_O (16) is taken into account[1]. The results suggest that

---

[1]The decrease in total cell cation content $((Na+K)_i)$ in $K_O < 2$ mM is indicative of a decrease in cell water (16,18) and serves to accentuate the increase in $\lfloor Na_i \rfloor$ and blunt the decrease in $\lfloor K_i \rfloor$.

cardiac myocytes have a large reserve Na/K pump capacity (17) capable of buffering $[K_i]$ in response to acute changes in K_o by increasing Na_i-activation of the Na/K pump.

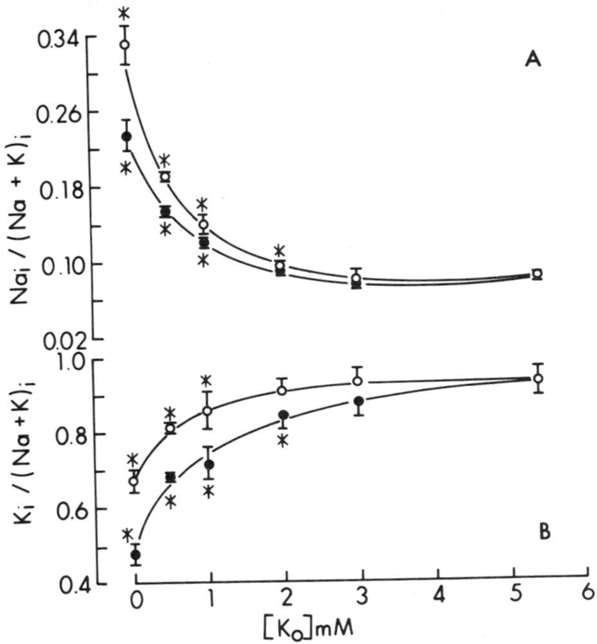

Figure 1: Effect of 20 min incubation in low K_o on intracellular Na and K concentrations. Open circles represent cell Na and K content normalized to $(Na+K)_i$ measured in the indicated K_o to "correct" the data for cell shrinkage in low K_o. These data are indicative of cation concentration in low K_o. In contrast, closed circles represent content data normalized to a constant $((Na+K)_i$ in $5.4K_o)$. Mean $\pm$ SEM (n=6-9).

Effect of Na_i on Na/K pump activity. The relationship between a_{Na}^i and Na/K pump activity was examined directly by Na-loading polystrand preparations for various periods of time in $0.5K_o$ and following the time course of changes in a_{Na}^i during reactivation in $5.4K_o$ with a Na-selective microelectrode (Fig. 2B; 19). A representative record of Na efflux accompanied by membrane hyperpolarization during Na/K pump reactivation is shown in Fig. 2A. The initial change in a_{Na}^i (< 60 s) is linear on a semi-logarithmic plot with an apparent rate coefficient = 0.021 s^{-1} (τ = 47 s) regardless of the initial Na load. Calculated net Na efflux is linearly related to $[Na_i]$ over the range of 14 - 25 **mM** in agreement with previous data obtained from Purkinje fibers (12,20).

A double reciprocal plot of active Na efflux versus $\lfloor Na_i \rfloor 3$ is linear with K_M = 20 mM and V_{max} = 47 pmol/cm^2/s (19). These data are consistent with half-maximal activation of Na/K pump current in internally-perfused isolated guinea pig ventricular myocytes by 10-20 mM Na_i (21) and saturation of Na/K pump activity only at Na_i > 50 mM (22). V_{max} obtained from this analysis is consistent with V_{max} = 37 $\pm$ 10 pmol/cm^2/s calculated from the initial rate of ouabain-sensitive ^{42}K uptake reported above[2] (net active K influx should be 2/3 net active Na efflux for a coupling ratio of 2K:3Na).

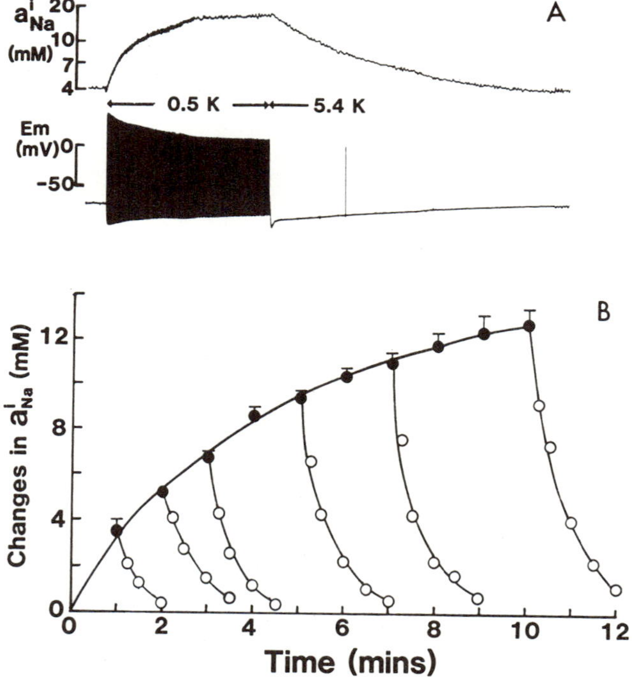

Figure 2: (A) The upper panel is a representative trace of Na efflux during Na/K pump reactivation from 0.5 to 5.4K_0, and the lower panel shows the accompanying changes in E_m. (B) Change in a$^i_{Na}$ during exposure to 0.5K_0 (●) and return to 5.4K_0 (O). Mean $\pm$ SEM.

These data demonstrate that Na/K pump activity in cardiac myocytes is very sensitive to changes in Na_i in the physiologic range, and suggest that this cation is likely to be involved in the regulation of Na/K pump activity <u>in vivo</u>.

---

[2]V_{max} was calculated assuming V/A = 10^{-4} cm (25) and cell volume = 6.8 ul/mg protein (as measured following a 60 min incubation in 0K_0 (16)).

<u>Effect of cell ATP content on Na/K pump activity</u>. Previous studies in this laboratory (23) have shown that cell ATP content decreases by 50 % during a 10 min exposure of muscle cell-enriched mass cultures to 0.1 mM rotenone (inhibitor of oxidative phosphorylation). Exposure of polystrands to rotenone for 5 min results in a 10 mM decrease in a_K^i, along with delayed after-depolarizations and slow depolarization to ~ - 45 mV. These arrhythmic oscillations are similar to those induced by K-free and ouabain-containing solutions (19,24), suggesting that rotenone causes a decrease in Na/K pump activity secondary to a fall in cell ATP content.

<u>Electrogenicity of the Na/K pump</u>. The Na/K pump is believed to be electrogenic with a coupling ratio of 3 Na:2 K (17,24). Earlier attempts to demonstrate electrogenicity of the Na/K pump in cardiac preparations were confounded by hyperpolarization due to depletion of K_O (Rb_O) in the narrow extracellular clefts of dissected preparations during reactivation (26). When a_K^i in polystrands is monitored continuously with ISME, the transient hyperpolarization that accompanies reactivation of the Na/K pump (Fig. 3A) is beyond the most negative known ionic equilibrium potential, E_K, suggestive of an outward Na/K pump current.

As expected for an Na/K pump current dependent on Na_i, the magnitude of the hyperpolarization following reactivation is related to the magnitude of the Na-load during Na/K pump inhibition (Fig. 3B). Passive Na influx following Na/K pump inhibition (9.6 $pmol/cm^2/s$) reflects steady-state Na/K pump activity that is equivalent to a current of 0.31 $\mu A/cm^2$. This finding is consistent with previous reports of 0.15 - 0.32 $\mu A/cm^2$ for sheep Purkinje fibers (20,27) and 0.81 $\mu A/cm^2$ for guinea pig atrial cells (28). Net Na efflux from polystrands during reactivation with Na_i = 25 mM (12.7 $pmol/cm^2/s$) is equivalent to an Na/K pump current of 1.2 $\mu A/cm^2$, a value similar to maximal ouabain-sensitive current (3 $\mu A/cm^2$) reported for isolated guinea pig myocytes clamped at 0 mV and internally perfused with 34 mM Na_i (29). The results demonstrate that the Na/K pump makes a direct contribution to the electrical activity of both resting and stimulated cardiac cells.

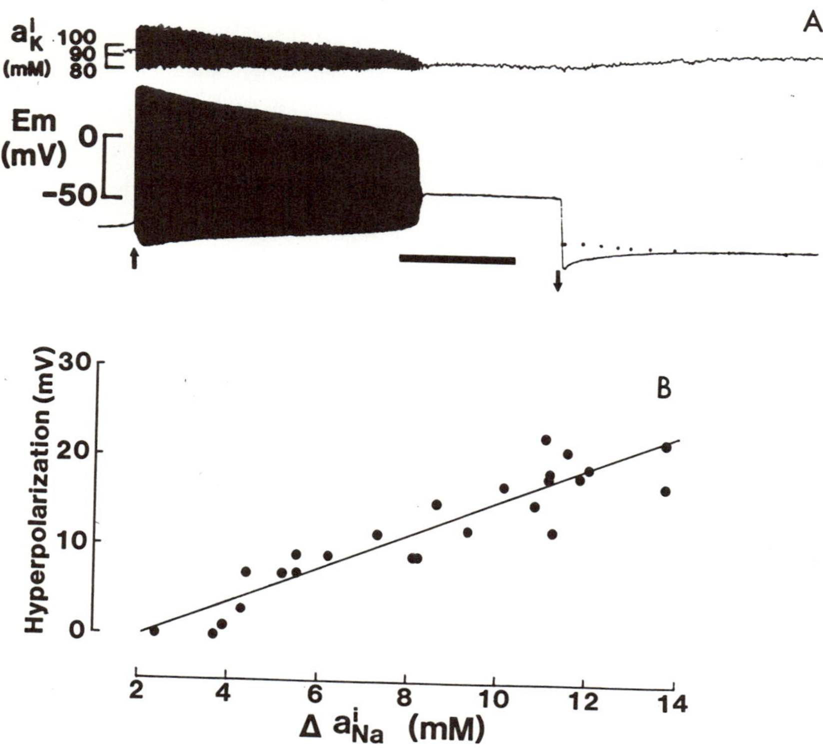

Figure 3: (A) Demonstration of Na/K pump electrogenicity. a_K^i and E_m were measured during Na/K pump inhibition in OK_0 (first arrow) and following restoration of $5.4K_0$ (second arrow). E_m hyperpolarized rapidly beyond E_K (dotted line) during reactivation of the Na/K pump, whereas a_K^i recovered slowly. The horizontal bar represents 1 min. (B) Relationship between Na/K pump reactivation-induced hyperpolarization and Na_i-load.

Na/K pump activity in pump-induced preparations (PIPs).

Induction of Na/K pump sites. Incubation of cultured human fibroblasts under conditions of partial Na/K pump inhibition (ouabain-containing or low K_0 medium) causes an initial rise in Na_i and fall in K_i followed by an increase in Na/K pump site density and partial recovery of cell cation content (30). Recent studies in this laboratory (8) and others (9,10) have demonstrated that cultured heart cells incubated in low K (0.5 - 1 mM) medium undergo a similar induction of Na/K pump sites. Fig. 4 shows the time course of increase in ^{3}H-ouabain binding sites in muscle cell-enriched cultures incubated in 0.5 mM K medium (LK). The number of ^{3}H-ouabain binding sites is increased by 71 $\pm$ 7 % above control after 24 h in LK (n=12). Secondary chick embryo heart fibroblast cultures do not show an increase in 3_H-ouabain binding sites after 24 h incubation in LK (p>.05), implying that induction of Na/K pumps in muscle cell-enriched preparations is myocyte-specific. The functionality of induced Na/K pumps is documented by the partial recovery of cell Na and K content towards control values after 12 h in LK following an initial 3-fold increase in Na_i and 30 % decrease in K_i (8).

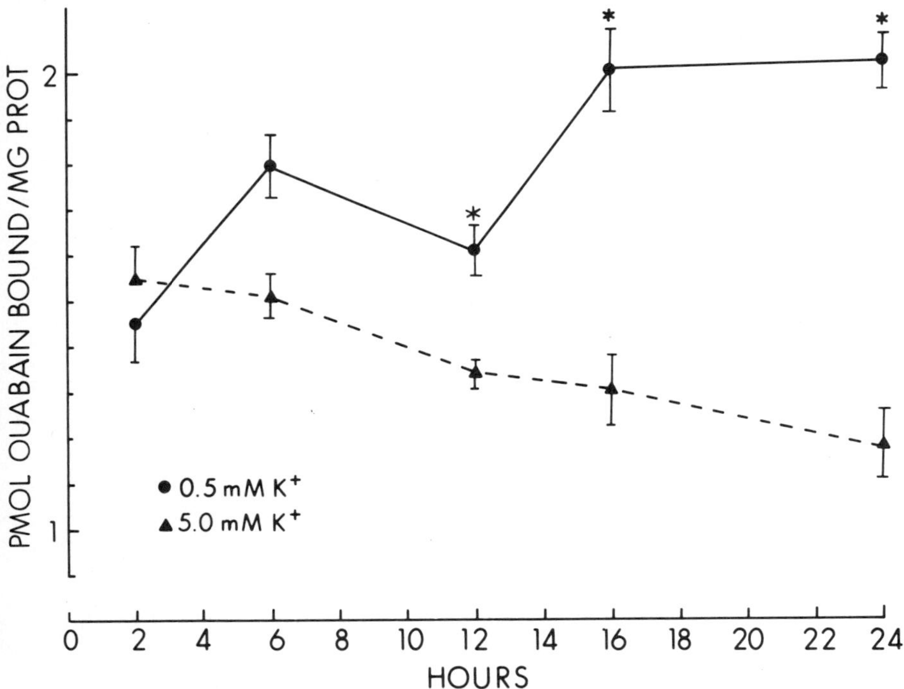

Figure 4: Effect of incubation in 0.5 mM K medium (circles) or 5 mM K medium (triangles) on specific binding of 0.1 uM ^{3}H-ouabain to muscle cell-enriched cultures. Mean ± SEM (n=3-12). (*): Differs from control (5 mM K) cells at this time point (p<.05).

<u>Electrophysiology of PIPs</u>. When PIPs are returned to 5 mM K medium, Na/K pump site density slowly returns to control over an 8 h period (31). Therefore, PIPs can be studied in control solution for several hours while retaining an increased Na/K pump capacity. A comparison of the spontaneous action potentials of PIPs and control polystrands in $5.4K_o$ is shown in Fig. 5A. Although currents underlying the action potential are complex, several changes in PIPs action potential configuration are suggestive of increased hyperpolarizing Na/K pump current: maximal diastolic potential is increased and action potential

duration is shortened. Fig. 5B shows the hyperpolarization produced by Na/K pump reactivation in $5.4K_O$ following 5 min incubation in $0.5K_O$ + 1 mM ouabain to Na-load the preparations (increase in a_{Na}^i (~13 mM) is similar in PIPs and control preparations). The magnitude of membrane hyperpolarization in PIPs is increased compared to control, consistent with an increased Na/K pump current. However, the magnitude of membrane hyperpolarization during Na/K pump reactivation following 5 min in $0.5K_O$ is also greater in PIPs than control (19), despite greater Na_i-activation in control preparations (increase in a_{Na}^i during $0.5K_O$ incubation ~3 mM and ~10 mM in PIPs and control preparations, respectively). These data suggest a possible increase in specific membrane resistance in PIPs. Further studies are required to determine if the electrophysiological behavior of PIPs can be explained solely by an increased Na/K pump capacity.

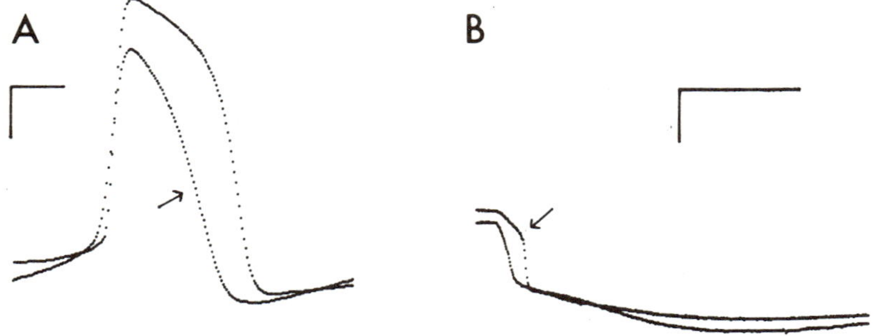

Figure 5: (A) Spontaneous action potentials recorded from PIPs (arrow) and control preparations in $5.4K_O$. (B) E_m during Na/K pump reactivation in $5.4K_O$ following 5 min incubation in $0.5K_O$ + 1 mM ouabain. E_m prior to reactivation = –45 mV in PIPs (arrow) and –50 mV in control preparations. Horizontal bars ((A) 50 msec; (B) 1 min) are set at 0 mV; vertical bars represent 20 mV.

SUMMARY

Cultured heart cells are a convenient preparation with which to study myocyte Na/K pump activity because they can be grown in several physiologically stable configurations conducive to either biochemical or electrophysiological measurements. Myocyte Na/K pump activity can be acutely altered by changes in substrate concentration (Na, K, ATP).

Under physiologic conditions, Na/K pump activity is virtually saturated
by $[K_o]$ but is extremely sensitive to changes in $[Na_i]$. The Na/K pump
is electrogenic and Na/K pump current may directly affect both the
resting potential and action potential of cardiac cells. Myocytes with
enhanced Na/K pump capacity (PIPs) can be produced by long-term
exposure of cultured cells to 0.5 mM K medium. The direct contribution
of Na/K pump current to cardiac cell electrophysiology, as well as the
secondary effects of Na/K pump activity on Na-linked transport
processes, can then be studied by comparing PIPs and control
preparations.

ACKNOWLEDGEMENTS

We would like to acknowledge the excellent technical assistance of
Ms. Dora Lyons, Ms. Connie Ganong & Mr. S. Charles Henry. Special
thanks to Dr. J. Stimers for assisting with data analysis. Supported
in part by NIH grants HL27105, HL17670, HL07101 and an NSF predoctoral
fellowship to LAL.

REFERENCES

1. Lieberman, M., Horres, C.R., Shigeto, N., Aiton, J.F. and Johnson,
    E.A. In: Excitable Cells in Tissue Culture (Eds. P.G. Nelson and
    M. Lieberman), Plenum Press, New York, 1981, pp. 379-408.
2. Chapman, R.A. Am. J. Physiol. 245: H535-H552, 1983.
3. Mullins, L.J. Ion Transport in the Heart. Raven Press, New York,
    1981.
4. Piwnica-Worms, D., Jacob, R., Horres, C.R. and Lieberman, M. J.
    Gen. Physiol. 85: 43-64, 1985.
5. Lazdunski, M., Frelin, C. and Vigne, P. J. Mol. Cell. Cardiol.
    17: 1029-1042, 1985.
6. Liu, S., Jacob, R., Piwnica-Worms, D. and Lieberman, M. Fed.
    Proc. 45: 653a, 1986. (Abstract).
7. Frelin, C., Chassande, O. and Lazdunski, M. Biochem. Biophys.
    Res. Commun. 134: 326-331, 1986.
8. Anderson, L.D., Henry, S.C. and Lieberman, M. J. Gen. Physiol.
    82: 18a, 1983. (Abstract).
9. Werdan, K., Schneider, G., Krawietz, W. and Erdmann, E. Biochem.
    Pharmacol. 33: 1161-1164, 1984.
10. Kim, D., Marsh, J.D., Barry, W.H. and Smith, T.W. Circ. Res. 55:
    39-48, 1984.
11. Eisner, D.A. and Lederer, W.J. J. Physiol. 303: 441-474, 1980.
12. Eisner, D.A., Lederer, W.J. and Vaughan-Jones, R.D. J. Physiol.
    317: 189-205, 1981.
13. Gadsby, D. Proc. Natl. Acad. Sci. 76: 1783-1787, 1980.
14. Glitsch, H.G., Grabowski, W. and Thielen, J. J. Physiol. 276:
    515-524, 1978.
15. Sachs, J.R. J. Physiol. 273: 489-514, 1977.

16. Gaynes, S., Lobaugh, L. and Lieberman, M. Circulation 72: III-326, 1985. (Abstract).
17. Akera, T. and T.M. Brody. Ann. Rev. Physiol. 44: 375-388, 1982.
18. Lee, P., Kirk, R.G. and Hoffman, J.F. J. Membrane Biol. 79: 119-126, 1984.
19. Liu, S. Electrophysiological Studies of Transmembrane Coupled Ion Movements in Cultured Chicken Embryo Heart Cells. Ph.D. Dissertation, Duke University, 1986.
20. Eisner, D.A., Lederer, W.J. and Vaughan-Jones, R.D. J. Physiol. 317: 163-187, 1981.
21. Nakao, M. and Gadsby, D.C. J. Gen. Physiol. 86: 30a, 1985. (Abstract).
22. Gadsby, D.C. and Nakao, M. J. Physiol. 369: 247P, 1985. (Abstract).
23. Murphy, E., Aiton, J.F., Horres, C.R. and Lieberman, M. Am. J. Physiol. 303: C316-C321, 1983.
24. Horres, C.R., Aiton, J.F., Lieberman, M. and Johnson, E.A. J. Mol. Cell. Cardiol. 11: 1201-1205, 1979.
25. Horres, C.R. and Lieberman, M. J. Membrane Biol. 34: 331-350, 1977.
26. Eisner, D.A., Lederer, W.J. and Vaughan-Jones, R.D. In: Electrogenic Transport: Fundamental Principles and Physiological Implications (Eds. M.P. Blaustein and M. Lieberman), Raven Press, New York, 1984, pp. 193-213.
27. Isenberg, G. and Trautwein, W. Pflugers Arch. 350: 41-54, 1974.
28. Daut, J. and Rudel, R. J. Physiol. 330: 243-264, 1982.
29. Gadsby, D., Kimura, J. and Noma, A. Nature 315: 63-65, 1985.
30. Cook, J.S., Karin, N.J., Fishman, J.B., Tate, E.H., Pollack, L.R. and Hayden, T.L. In: Regulation and Development of Membrane Transport Processes (Ed. J.S. Graves), John Wiley and Sons, New York, 1985, pp. 3-20.
31. Lobaugh, L.A. and Lieberman, M. J. Gen. Physiol. 86: 31-32a, 1985. (Abstract).

12

CHARACTERISTICS OF Ca^{2+}/Mg^{2+} ATPASE IN HEART SARCOLEMMA TREATED WITH TRYPSIN

M.B. ANAND-SRIVASTAVA, N.S. DHALLA

Experimental Cardiology Section, Department of Physiology, University of
Manitoba, Faculty of Medicine, Winnipeg, Canada R3E 0W3.

INTRODUCTION

Both biochemical and histochemical techniques have demonstrated the
presence of an ATP-hydrolyzing enzyme in heart sarcolemma, which is
activated by millimolar concentrations of various divalent cations including
Ca^{2+} or Mg^{2+} (1-5). Earlier studies have revealed that the activity of this
sarcolemmal Ca^{2+}/Mg^{2+} ATPase was decreased by different agents, which have
been shown to exert cardiodepressant effects (6-8). Furthermore,
interventions, which are known to increase cardiac contractile force, were
shown to increase the sarcolemmal Ca^{2+}/Mg^{2+} ATPase activity (9,10). The
activation of this enzyme system was found to exhibit a closed relationship
with the increase in cardiac contractile force at different concentrations
of Ca^{2+} (11). The activities of sarcolemmal Ca^{2+}/Mg^{2+} ATPase have been
shown to increased under pathological situations which favour the occurrence
of intracellular Ca^{2+} overload (13,14) but were depressed in other types of
failing hearts (15,16). These observations support the view that Ca^{2+}/Mg^{2+}
ATPase may be involved in Ca^{2+}-gating mechanisms and thus may play an
important role in regulating the contractile force development in the
cardiac muscle (11,16).

Treatment of heart sarcolemma with detergents such as deoxycholate and
lubrol was found to decrease Ca^{2+} ATPase activity to a greater extent than
Mg^{2+} ATPase activity (17). On the other hand, treatment of heart sarcolemma
with trypsin was shown to release Ca^{2+} dependent ATPase, which exhibited
negligible Mg^{2+} ATPase activity (18,19). Since a large proportion of $Ca^{2+}/$
Mg^{2+} ATPase activity in heart sarcolemma remained associated with the
membrane after trypsin treatment (18), it is the purpose of this study to
investigate the properties of this trypsin-resistant component of the $Ca^{2+}/$
Mg^{2+} ATPase in order to gain further information regarding the structure-
function relationship of this enzyme system.

MATERIALS AND METHODS

Rat heart sarcolemmal membrane was isolated by the hypotonic-shock
LiBr treatment according to the procedure described elsewhere (18). The
sarcolemmal membrane (2 mg/ml) was digested with various concentrations of
trypsin at room temperature for different time intervals in a medium
containing 50 mM Tris-HCl, pH 7.5, and 20 mM KCl. The reaction was stopped
by the addition of 2 - 3 fold of soybean trypsin inhibitor. The tubes were
centrifuged at 1,000 x g for 10 min. The residue was washed twice with 1 mM
Tris-HCl, pH 7.0, suspended in the same buffer and aliquots were used for
ATPase activity and morphological studies. Ca^{2+} ATPase or Mg^{2+} ATPase
activities were measured in the presence of Ca^{2+} or Mg^{2+} in a medium
containing 50 mM Tris-HCl, pH 7.5 (18) and the concentrations of Pi and
proteins were determined by the methods of Taussky and Shorr (20) and Lowry
et al (21), respectively. For morphological studies, the pellets were fixed
in 1% glutaraldehyde in a 0.1 M phosphate buffer pH 7.4 for 16 hr. These
specimens were further fixed with 1% osmium tetraoxide, dehydrated in a
graded ethanol series and embedded in Epon 812. Sections of these specimens
were cut with a Porter - Blum MT-11 ultramicrotome using glass knives,
stained with uranyl acetate and lead citrate, and examined with a Zeiss
electron microscope (EM 9S). The results were analyzed statistically by
using the Student's t test.

RESULTS

The effectiveness of trypsin treatment on heart sarcolemma was tested
by examining the trypsin-treated membrane electron microscopically after
fixing and embedding (Fig. 1). These studies indicated dramatic
morphological alterations in the membrane appearance due to trypsin
treatment. For obtaining trypsin-treated preparations with maximal specific
enzyme activity, the conditions for trypsin treatment were thoroughly worked
out. The results shown in Table 1 indicate that the presence of different
ligands such as Ca^{2+}, Mg^{2+} or ATP at high concentrations in the medium
during incubation of heart sarcolemma with trypsin increased the Ca^{2+}/Mg^{2+}
activities to a lesser extent in comparison to that seen in their absence.
By changing different experimental conditions including changes in pH and
cation concentrations of the incubation medium, it was found that the Ca^{2+}
ATPase and Mg^{2+} ATPase activities of the trypsin-treated membrane were
maximal when the trypsin treatment was carried out in a medium containing

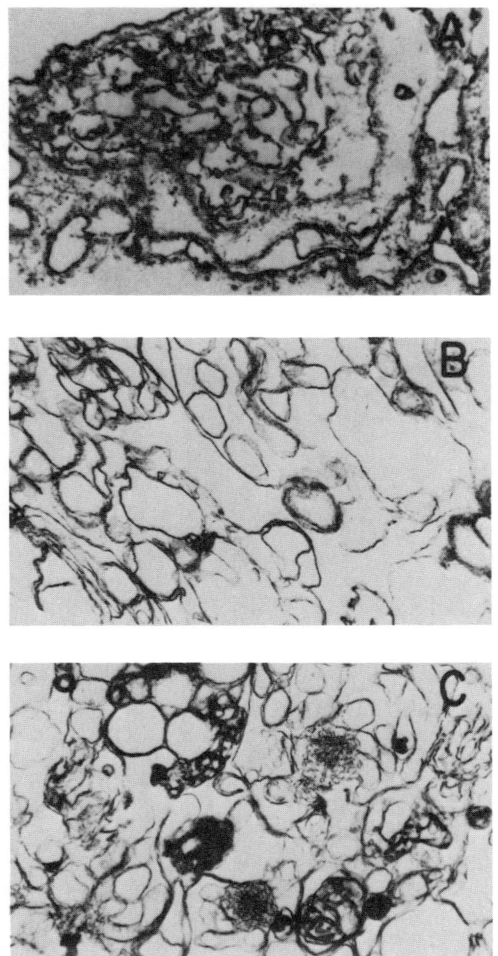

Figure 1. Electron micrographs of heart sarcolemma with or without trypsin treatment. A, Control; B, Trypsin (100 μg/mg membrane protein) treatment for 10 min; and C, Trypsin (100 μg/mg membrane protein) treatment for 30 min. (X26,730).

50 mM Tris-HCl, pH 7.5, and 20 mM KCl.

The Ca^{2+}/Mg^{2+} ATPase activities were also measured after digestion of heart sarcolemma with different concentrations of trypsin for 10 min or for different intervals of time by employing 100 μg trypsin/mg membrane protein.

Table 1. Effect of trypsin digestion in the presence or absence of various ligands on Ca^{2+}/Mg^{2+} ATPase activities of heart sarcolemma.

| | ATPase activities (μmole Pi released/mg protein/hr) | | | |
| | Control | | Treated | |
Additions	1.25 mM Ca^{2+}	1.25 mM Mg^{2+}	1.25 mM Ca^{2+}	1.25 mM Mg^{2+}
None	30.1 ± 2.2	23.9 ± 1.7	63.9 ± 2.8	63.5 ± 2.7
4 mM Ca^{2+}	32.1 ± 1.8	25.1 ± 1.3	51.3 ± 2.2*	49.9 ± 2.1*
4 mM Mg^{2+}	28.0 ± 1.9	23.2 ± 1.2	52.0 ± 2.4*	50.8 ± 1.8*
4 mM ATP	30.7 ± 2.3	23.6 ± 1.4	51.2 ± 2.3*	51.3 ± 2.1*

* Significantly different from values obtained in the absence of ligands ($P < 0.05$). Sarcolemma was treated with trypsin at a concentration of 100 μg/mg of membrane protein for 10 min in the presence or absence of divalent cations of ATP. The concentration of ATP for ATPase determination was 1.25 mM. Each value is a mean ± S.E. of 4 experiments.

The data in Fig. 2 shows that the protein content of the membrane decreased by about 60% after 100 μg trypsin/mg membrane protein and further increase in trypsin concentration did not produce a further decrease in protein content. On the other hand, maximal specific activity of the Ca^{2+} ATPase was achieved at 100 – 150 μg trypsin/mg membrane protein whereas that for the Mg^{2+} ATPase was seen at about 200 μg trypsin/mg membrane protein concentration. Varying the time of digestion indicated that the maximum decrease in membrane proteins was obtained in 10 min whereas the maximal Ca^{2+} ATPase and Mg^{2+} ATPase activities were apparent at 10 and 40 min of digestion with trypsin (Fig. 3).

In another series of experiments, the Ca^{2+}/Mg^{2+} ATPase activities of the trypsin-treated preparations were measured by using different concentrations of Ca^{2+} or Mg^{2+}. When micromolar concentrations of Ca^{2+} or Mg^{2+} were employed, increases in Ca^{2+} ATPase or Mg^{2+} ATPase activities of the trypsin treated sarcolemma were evident at each concentration (Fig. 4). It was interesting to note that the activation pattern of the Mg^{2+} ATPase, unlike that of the Ca^{2+} ATPase, in the trypsin treated preparation gave the

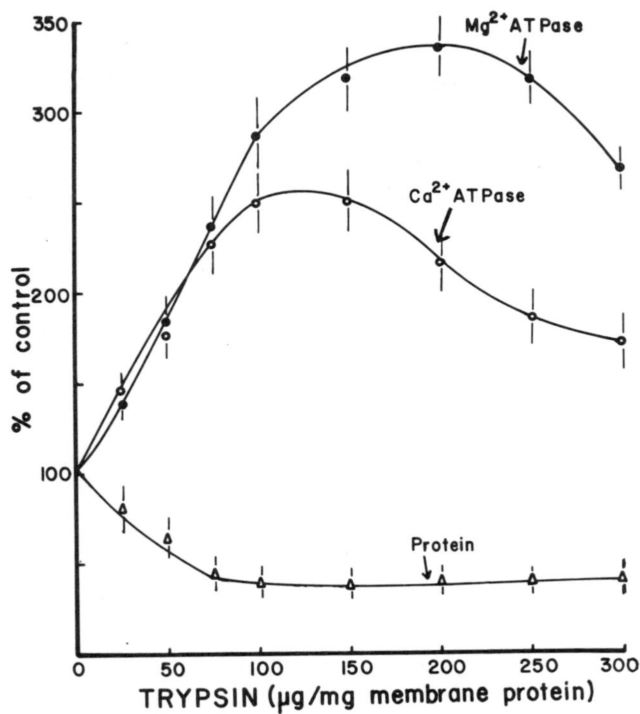

Figure 2. Effect of different concentrations of trypsin treatment on Ca^{2+} ATPase, Mg^{2+} ATPase activities and protein content of heart sarcolemma. The time of incubation with trypsin was 10 min. The concentrations of Ca^{2+} or Mg^{2+} and ATP were 1.25 mM. Each value is a mean ± S.E. of 4 experiments.

appearance like that for an allosteric enzyme. However, no further effort was made to characterize this enzyme system for the present study. Both Ca^{2+} ATPase and Mg^{2+} ATPaes activities were also determined by employing high concentrations (in the millimolar range) of Ca^{2+} and Mg^{2+}, respectively. The data in Fig. 5 indicate no changes in the Ka value (58 µM) for Ca^{2+} ATPase in trypsin treated preparations whereas Vmax value was markedly increased. Likewise, an increase in the specific activity of Mg^{2+} ATPase in trypsin-treated membranes was also associated with an increase in the Vmax value without any changes in the Ka value (72 µM) (Fig. 6).

Since Ca^{2+}/Mg^{2+} ATPase system in heart sarcolemma has been shown to possess low and high affinity sites for ATP (4), the specific activities of

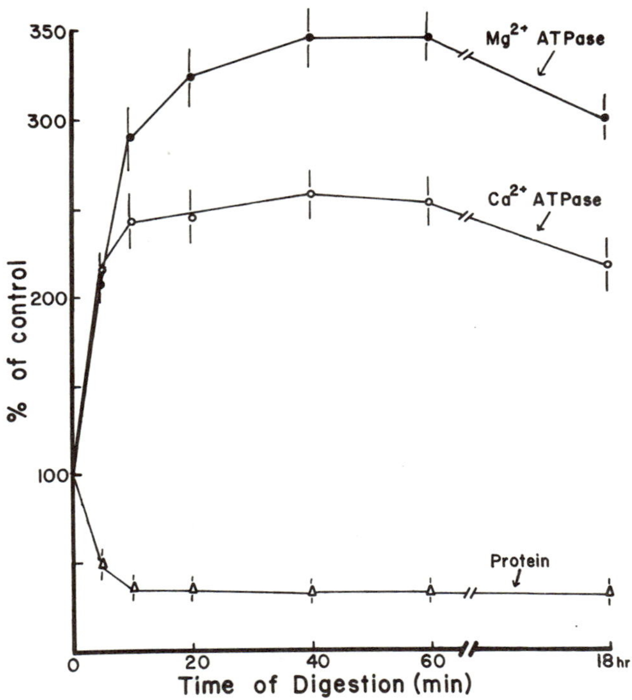

Figure 3. Effect of time of digestion of sarcolemma with trypsin at a concentration of 100 μg/mg membrane protein on Ca^{2+} ATPase, Mg^{2+} ATPase activity and protein content. The concentrations of Ca^{2+} or Mg^{2+} and ATP were 1.25 mM. Each value is a mean ± S.E. of 4 experiments.

both Ca^{2+} ATPase and Mg^{2+} ATPase in trypsin treated membranes were determined by using micromolar concentrations (high affinity site) and millimolar concentrations (low affinity site) of ATP. The data shown in Fig. 7 indicates that Km values for the high affinity sites of Ca^{2+} ATPase (68 μM) and Mg^{2+} ATPase (86 μM) of the trypsin-treated membranes were not different from the control. On the other hand, Vmax values for the high affinity sites of Ca^{2+} ATPase increased from 13 to 50 μmoles Pi/mg/hr and those for Mg^{2+} ATPase increased from 16 to 50 μmoles Pi/mg/hr upon trypsin treatment. When ATP hydrolysis was also carried out by employing millimolar concentrations of ATP, the results shown in Fig. 8 indicate that Km value (333 μM) for the low affinity sites for Ca^{2+} ATPase or Mg^{2+} ATPase in

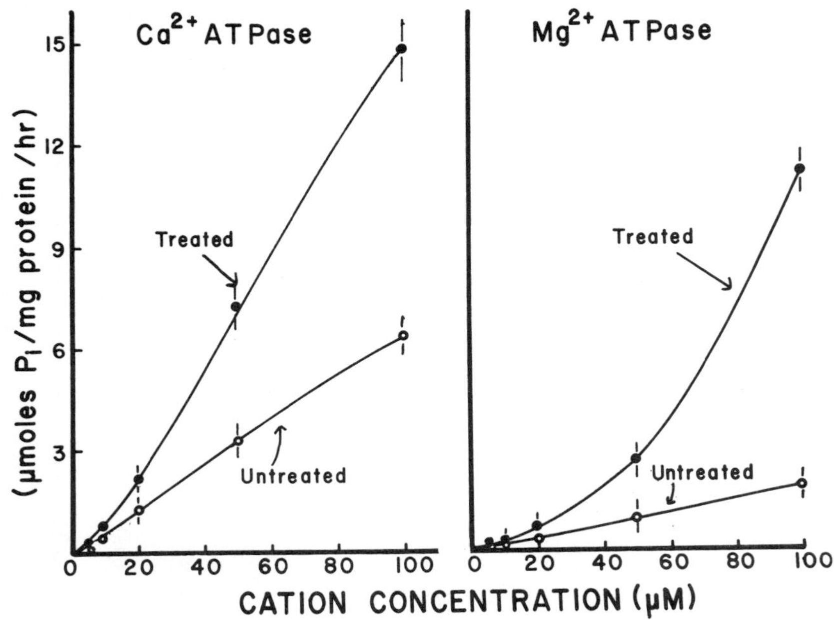

Figure 4. Effect of low (μM) concentrations of Ca^{2+} or Mg^{2+} on ATP hydrolysis by heart sarcolemma pre-treated with trypsin at a concentration of 100 μg/mg of protein for 10 min. ATP concentration was 4 mM. The results are the mean ± S.E. of 4 experiments.

trypsin-treated preparation was not different from the control whereas the Vmax value for Ca^{2+} ATPase increased from 43 to 99 μmoles Pi/mg/hr and that for Mg^{2+} ATPase increased from 30 to 80 μmoles Pi/mg/hr.

The interaction of Ca^{2+} and Mg^{2+} was examined in control and trypsin treated preparations to determine if any changes are produced by one cation when the enzyme is fully activated by the other cation. For this experiment, either Ca^{2+} (4 mM) concentration was kept constant and an increasing amount of Mg^{2+} was added or Mg^{2+} (4 mM) concentration was kept constant and an increasing amount of Ca^{2+} was added. The results shown in Table 2 indicate that Ca^{2+} ATPase activity of the trypsin-treated preparation decreased to a lesser extent by the addition of Mg^{2+} in comparison to the control preparation whereas an equal degree of depression

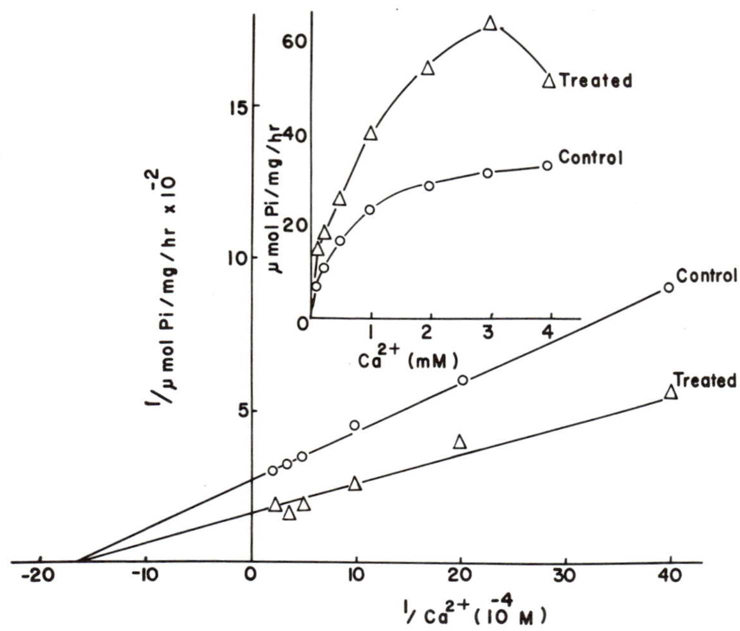

Figure 5. Effect of high (mM) concentrations of Ca^{2+} on ATP hydrolysis by heart sarcolemma pretreated with trypsin at a concentration of 100 μg/mg of protein for 10 min. ATP concentration was 4 mM. The results are typical of 4 experiments.

was noted in control and trypsin-treated membrane Mg^{2+} ATPase upon the addition of Ca^{2+}. It should be pointed out that the pH optima (7.5 to 8.0) for the Ca^{2+} ATPase or Mg^{2+} ATPase activities in the trypsin-treated preparations were similar to those of the control membranes.

DISCUSSION

The experiments described in this study reveal that the specific activities of the Ca^{2+} and Mg^{2+} ATPases in trypsin-treated preparations were increased by 2.5 and 3 fold respectively. This change was associated with alterations in morphological appearance of heart sarcolemma and can be explained mainly on the basis of a decrease in membrane proteins. However, it should be noted that the maximal Ca^{2+} ATPase and Mg^{2+} ATPase activities

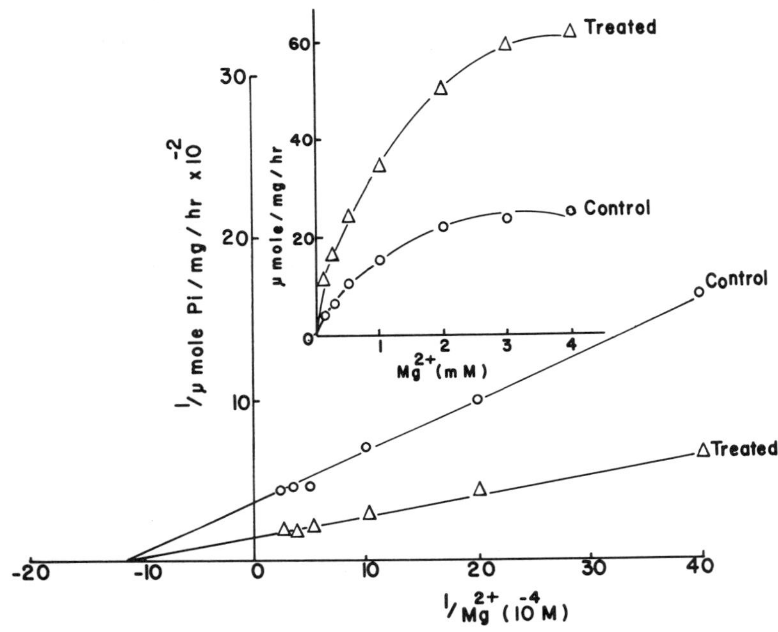

Figure 6. Effect of high (mM) concentrations of Mg^{2+} on ATP hydrolysis by heart sarcolemma pretreated with trypsin at a concentration of 100 μg/mg of protein for 10 min. ATP concentration was 4 mM. The results are typical of 4 experiments.

were seen when 100 - 150 μg and about 200 μg/mg membrane protein concentrations of trypsin were employed, respectively, whereas trypsin concentrations greater than 100 μg/ mg membrane protein did not produce any further loss of membrane proteins. Likewise, the maximal Ca^{2+} ATPase and Mg^{2+} ATPase activities were observed in 10 and 40 min of incubating heart sarcolemma with 100 μg trypsin/mg protein, respectively. Thus trypsin can be seen to produce some different types of direct effects on the Ca^{2+} ATPase and Mg^{2+} ATPase systems of heart sarcolemma. Alternatively, there appears to be some degree of difference for Ca^{2+} ATPase and Mg^{2+} ATPase activities with respect to the protein- protein interaction in the heart sarcolemmal membrane.

The observed increase in the specific activities of Ca^{2+} ATPase and

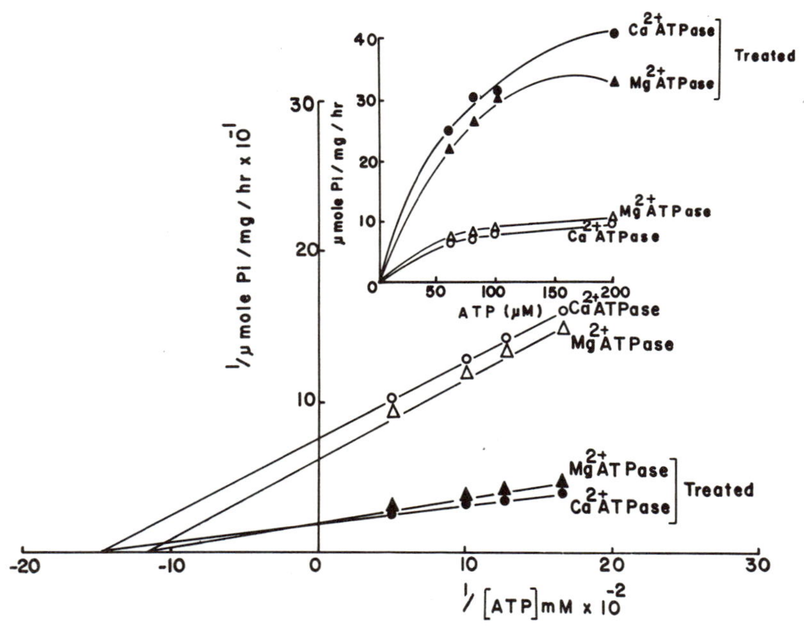

Figure 7. Effect of low (μM) concentrations of ATP on ATP hydrolysis by control and trypsin-treated (at a concentration of 100 μg/mg membrane protein for 10 min) heart sarcolemma in the presence of 4 mM Ca^{2+} or Mg^{2+}. The results are typical of 4 experiments.

Mg^{2+} ATPase in trypsin-treated sarcolemma was found to be associated with an increase in their Vmax values without any changes in their Ka values. Likewise, no changes in the Km values for both the low and high affinity sites were apparent whereas their Vmax values were increased in trypsin-treated preparations. Furthermore, these changes in the enzyme activities in trypsin-treated preparations were not due to any alterations in their pH optima. The inhibitory response of Ca^{2+} ATPase in trypsin-treated preparations to Mg^{2+} was also similar to that of Mg^{2+} ATPase to Ca^{2+}. In spite of these similarities between Ca^{2+} ATPase and Mg^{2+} ATPase systems of trypsin-treated heart sarcolemma, some differences in these enzyme were evident. For example, the Km value for the high affinity sites of Ca^{2+} ATPase was lower than that for the Mg^{2+} ATPase. The activation pattern of the Mg^{2+} ATPase in trypsin-treated preparations at low concentrations of

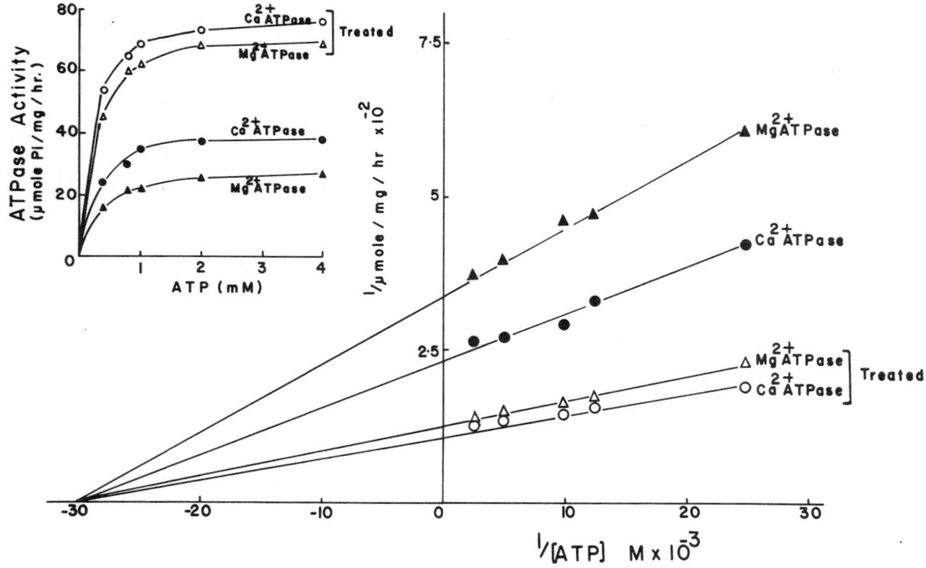

Figure 8. Effect of high (mM) concentrations of ATP on ATP hydrolysis by control and trypsin-treated (at a concentration of 100 μg/mg membrane protein for 10 min) heart sarcolemma in the presence of 4 mM Ca^{2+} of Mg^{2+}. The results are typical of 4 experiments.

Mg^{2+}, unlike that for the Ca^{2+} ATPase, was readily identifiable for its allosteric nature since the curve was sigmoidal in shape. These rather minor differences in results can, however, be explained on the basis of some differences in the accessibility of Ca-ATP and Mg-ATP for the active enzyme sites in the membrane preparation. Alternatively, some trypsin-sensitive Ca^{2+} ATPase, which was released in the supernatant during trypsin digestion (18), may still be present in the trypsin-treated preparations employed in this study. Thus it appears that Ca^{2+} ATPase and Mg^{2+} ATPase activities in heart sarcolemma treated with trypsin may be due to the presence of a single enzyme component.

SUMMARY

Digestion of sarcolemma with trypsin produced dramatic changes in the membrane structure. The specific activities of Ca^{2+} ATPase and Mg^{2+} ATPase in the trypsin-treated preparations increased by 2.5 and 3 fold respectively

Table 2. Effect of Ca^{2+} or Mg^{2+} on Ca^{2+}/Mg^{2+} ATPase activities from control and trypsin treated sarcolemma

Additions Ca^{2+} or Mg^{2+}	ATPase activity (% of control)			
	Ca^{2+} ATPase		Mg^{2+} ATPase	
	Control	Treated	Control	Treated
50 µM	86.5 ± 6.2	104.4 ± 5.9	100.7 ± 3.7	98.3 ± 3.2
100 µM	77.2 ± 6.7	101.5 ± 4.7	96.4 ± 2.9	94.3 ± 3.4
0.5 mM	62.8 ± 8.0	104.1 ± 4.8	93.5 ± 2.8	96.5 ± 3.5
1.0 mM	63.7 ± 8.7	98.7 ± 3.2	91.5 ± 2.8	92.7 ± 2.6
2.0 mM	61.4 ± 7.5	95.2 ± 5.1	88.8 ± 3.0	88.9 ± 2.8
3.0 mM	59.2 ± 6.2	93.3 ± 5.6	85.9 ± 3.1	81.1 ± 2.5
4.0 mM	57.3 ± 6.0	87.4 ± 6.9	81.9 ± 3.6	81.5 ± 2.6

ATP concentration in the incubation medium was 4 mM. Ca^{2+} ATPase and Mg^{2+} ATPase activities were monitored in the presence of 4 mM Ca^{2+} or Mg^{2+}. Different concentrations of Mg^{2+} were added to the assay medium for Ca^{+} ATPase activity whereas different concentrations of Ca^{2+} were added to the assay medium for Mg^{2+} ATPase activity. Each value is a mean ± S.E. of 4 experiments.

whereas the membrane protein decreased by about 60%. Although increases in both Ca^{2+} ATPase and Mg^{2+} ATPase activities in trypsin-treated preparations with millimolar concentrations of cations were associated with increases in their Vmax values without any changes in their Ka values, the activation of Mg^{2+} ATPase, unlike Ca^{2+} ATPase, in micromolar cationic concentrations appeared to be allosteric in nature. The Vmax values, but not the Km values, for low and high affinity sites for ATP in trypsin-treated membranes for both Ca^{2+} ATPase and Mg^{2+} ATPase were higher than the control; however, the Km value for the high affinity sites for Ca^{2+} ATPase was lower than that for the Mg^{2+} ATPase. Although pH optima for Ca^{2+} ATPase and Mg^{2+} ATPase in trypsin-treated membranes were similar to the control values, Ca^{2+} ATPase in the trypsin-treated preparations was inhibited to a lesser extent by Mg^{2+} in comparison to the control whereas the magnitudes of inhibition in Mg^{2+} ATPase activities by Ca^{2+} in both preparations was similar. These results indicate only minor differences with respect to the properties of Ca^{2+} ATPase and Mg^{2+} ATPase in trypsin-treated heart sarcolemma.

203

ACKNOWLEDGEMENTS

The work reported here was supported by a grant from the Medical Research Council of Canada.

REFERENCES

1. McNamara, D.B., Singh, J.N. and Dhalla, N.S. J. Biochem. 76: 603-609, 1974.
2. Dhalla, N.S., Anand, M.B. and Harrow, J.A.C. J. Biochem. 79: 1345-1350, 1976.
3. Anand, M.B., Chauhan, M.S. and Dhalla, N.S. J. Biochem. 82: 1731-1739, 1977.
4. Anand-Srivastava, M.B., Panagia, V. and Dhalla, N.S. Advances in Myocardiol. 3: 359-371, 1982.
5. Malouf, N.N. and Meissner, G. J. Histochem. Cytochem. 28: 1286-1294, 1980.
6. Dhalla, N.S., Lee, S.L., Anand, M.B., Chauhan, M.S. Biochem. Pharmacol. 26: 2055-2060, 1977.
7. Dhalla, N.S., Harrow, J.A.C. and Anand, M.B. Biochem. Pharmacol. 27: 1281-1283, 1978.
8. Harrow, J.A.C., Das, P.K. and Dhalla, N.S. Biochem. Pharmacol. 27: 2605-2609, 1978.
9. Ziegelhoffer, A., Anand-Srivastava, M.B., Khandelwal, R.L. and Dhalla, N.S. Biochem. Biophys. Res. Commun. 89: 1073-1081, 1979.
10. Dhalla, N.S., Ziegelhoffer, A. and Makino, N. In: Pathobiology of Cardiovascular Injury (Eds. H.L. Stone and W.B. Weglicki), Martinus Nijhoff Publishing, Boston, 1985, pp. 222-231.
11. Dhalla, N.S., Pierce, G.N., Panagia, V., Singal, P.K. and Beamish, R.E. Basic Res. Cardiol. 77: 117-139, 1982.
12. Moffat, M.P. and Dhalla, N.S. Can. J. Cardiol. 1: 194-200, 1985.
13. Dhalla, N.S., Smith, C.I., Pierce, G.N., Elimban, V., Makino, N. and Khatter, J.C. In: The Regulation of Heart Function (Ed. H. Rupp), Thieme, New York, 1986, pp. 121-136.
14. Tomlinson, C.W., Lee, S.L. and Dhalla, N.S. Circ. Res. 39: 82-92, 1976.
15. Panagia, V., Singh, J.N., Anand-Srivastava, M.B., Pierce, G.N., Jasmin, G. and Dhalla, N.S. Cardiovasc. Res. 18: 567-572, 1984.
16. Dhalla, N.S., Ziegelhoffer, A. and Harrow, J.A.C. Can. J. Physiol. Pharmacol. 55: 1211-1234, 1977.
17. Panagia, V., Lamers, J.M.J., Singal, P.K. and Dhalla, N.S. Int. J. Biochem. 14: 387-397, 1982.
18. Dhalla, N.S., Anand-Srivastava, M.B., Tuana, B.S. and Khandelwal, R.L. J. Mol. Cell. Cardiol. 13: 413-423, 1981.
19. Tuana, B.S. and Dhalla, N.S. J. Biol. Chem. 257: 14440-14445, 1982.
20. Taussky, H.H. and Shorr, E. J. Biol. Chem. 202: 675-685, 1983.
21. Lowry, O.H., Rosebrough, N.Y., Farr, A.L. and Randall, R.J. J. Biol. Chem. 193: 265-275, 1951.

D. SARCOPLASMIC RETICULUM FUNCTION

13

DEPRESSION OF CANINE VENTRICULAR SARCOPLASMIC RETICULUM BY THE CALCIUM CHANNEL AGONIST, BAY K 8644

Deepak Bose, Takakazu Kobayashi, Larry V. Hryshko & Teresa Chau

Departments of Pharmacology & Therapeutics & Internal Medicine, Faculty of Medicine, University of Manitoba, Winnipeg, Man, Canada, R3E 0W3

INTRODUCTION

Ca channel agonists are novel compounds which increase cardiac contractile force by increasing slow inward Ca current through the sarcolemma (1,2,3). The presently available compounds are dihydropyridine analogs with structural similarities with agents such as nifedipine, which are Ca channel antagonists. The present study resulted from some chance observation which were made with BAY K 8644, a prototype Ca channel agonist first discovered by Schramm et al (4). This compound was being used by us to evaluate an experimental model designed to test the effects of cardioactive agents on the contribution of transsarcolemmal and transsarcoplasmic reticular Ca movement to inotropy. We observed that BAY K 8644, impaired Ca release from the sarcoplasmic reticulum in addition to its well known effect of increasing transsarcolemmal Ca influx.

MATERIALS AND METHODS

Experimental Preparation:

Isolated trabecula were obtained from the right ventricle of dogs (5-12 kg of either sex) anesthetized with pentobarbital (30 mg/kg IV). The muscle was bathed in Krebs Henseleit solution having a composition (in mM) of (NaCl 118, KCl 4.7, KH_2PO_4 1.2, $MgSO_4$ 1.1, $CaCl_2$ 2.5, $NaHCO_3$ 25 and dextrose 11). Isometric contractions, transmembrane potential changes and laser light scattering were studied. These methods will be described later. The ambient solution was kept at 37° and bubbled with 95% O_2 - 5% CO_2 to maintain a pH of 7.4.

Tension Measurement:

For most experiments thin segments of trabecula (<= 1 mm diameter and 10-15 mm long) were attached to field electrodes and stimulated with square pulses, (1-5 msec in duration, having a voltage that was 20% higher than threshold. The stimulus pulse was obtained from a custom designed computerized pulse sequencer (5) driving a constant current stimulator (Pulsar 6I; F. Haer). The stimulus protocol consisted of regular pulses at 1000 - 2000 msec interval. The pulse train was interrupted from 5 - 480 sec to study the effect on the post-rest beat. Isometric mechanograms were recorded on a Grass Polygraph with the help of a Grass FT03 C force transducer.

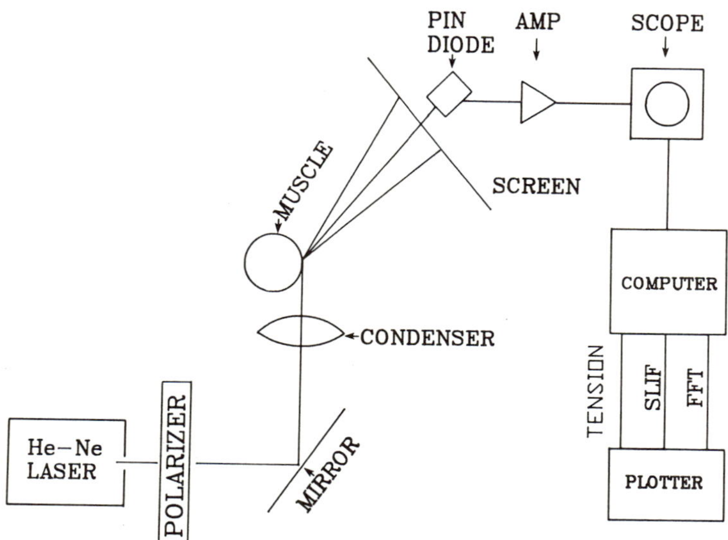

Fig. 1. Experimental setup for measuring scattered intensity light fluctuation (SLIF) in canine ventricular trabecular muscle. Isometric tension, SLIF and magnitude spectrum of SLIF (FFT) were recorded.

The experimental setup is shown in the above figure. Thin bundles (~300 um) were used and tension was measured in these experiments with a solid state transducer (Aksjeselskapet AME-801) connected to a bridge preamplifier and a Nicolet Model 3091 digital oscilloscope. Incident laser beam of approximately 200 um diameter from a 7 milliwatt He-Ne laser (632.8 nm wave length; Spectraphysics) was directed towards the edge of the bundle of dog ventricular trabecula. This was made possible with an optical system consisting of a pinhole and the objective lens of an Olympus IMT-2 inverted phase contrast microscope. The scattered light was collected at an angle of 30° with a PIN photodiode (S 1188; Hamamatsu Photonics). Signal was analyzed during a 30 second period when the muscle was not stimulated. The electrical transform of the light signal was amplified and recorded on a digital storage oscilloscope (Nicolet Model 3091). The data was transferred serially from the oscilloscope to a Mind microcomputer running the MS DOS 3.1 operating system. A data acquisition software package which utilizes the ASYST (MacMillan Software Co., Rochester, N.Y., USA) programming environment was developed by us to analyse the raw light and tension signals. The light data was analysed for its spectral content using an FFT routine in ASYST. The areas under the the magnitude spectrum signal were measured for specific frequency bands between 0.3 - 10 hz.

Electrophysiological studies:

Conventional glass microelectrodes (tip resistance 10 - 30 megohms) were used to record transmembrane electrical potential from ventricular muscle cells. The preparation was similar to the one previously described for mechanical measurements. The electrode was attached to a high input impedence preamplifier (A & M Systems, Model 1600). Electrical signals were stored on magnetic tape (Vetter Model D Instrumentation Tape Recorder) and paper (Gould Model 280 or 440 Recorder). Data were analyzed with a Waveform Analyzer (Data Precision - Model Data 6000). Hard copies were obtained on a digital X-Y recorder (Hewlett Packard Model 7470 or 7475).

Drugs and Chemicals:

BAY K 8644 and ryanodine were kind gifts from Drs. A. Scriabine (Miles Lab., USA) and R. Rogers (Merck, Sharp and Dohme, USA) respectively. All other chemicals were obtained from Sigma Chemicals (USA) or Fisher Scientific (Canada).

RESULTS

In the studies carried out by us, three general experimental approaches were used. They are simple, non-biochemical and are able to examine different aspects of cardiac cellular function.

Biphasic contractions: This is an experimental model in which the ventricular twitch is converted from a contraction with a single peak to one with two peaks. The interesting feature is that each peak reveals, semiquantitatively, the contribution of Ca from transsarcoplasmic reticular or transsarcolemmal pathways for the contraction. When ~ 90% of normal Ca in the Krebs-Henseleit bathing medium was replaced by Sr, the canine right ventricular trabecula showed 2 peaks of isometric contraction, in response to a single electrical stimulation and in the presence of a single action potential. The first peak (P1) had a normal latency and time to peak tension and the second slower one (P2), had a longer latency and time to peak tension and also a slower relaxation.

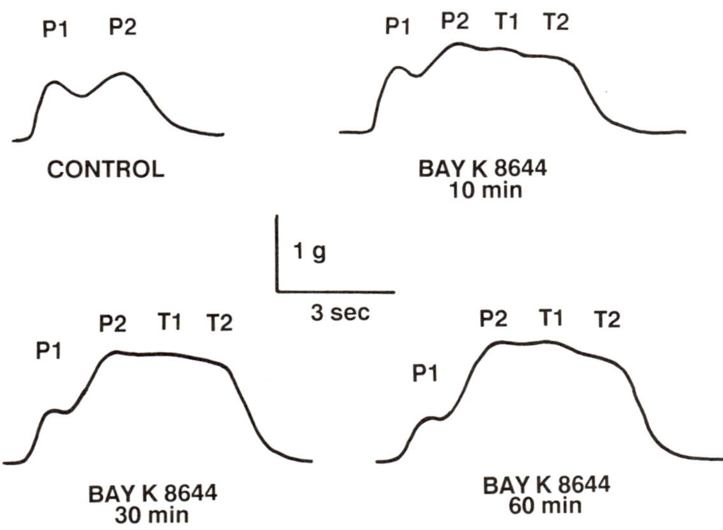

Fig. 2. Biphasic contractions of trabecular muscle obtained in the presence of 2.5 mM Sr and 0.15 mM Ca. Recordings taken before and various times after treatment with BAY K 8644 (1 uM). Note increase in P2 and appearance of tonic phases (T1 and T2) after BAY K 8644. However, P1 after a transient increase became smaller.

P1 represents Ca released from the sarcoplasmic reticulum while P2 depended on Sr entry across the sarcolemma through channels similar to those permitting Ca influx and also possibly through Na-Ca exchange as previously described by us in details (6). P1 was blocked by ryanodine, which impairs Ca release by the sarcoplasmic reticulum (7) and P2 was preferentially blocked by the inorganic Ca channel blocker, Mn (8).

Fig. 2 shows that 10 min after exposing the canine right ventricular trabecula to BAY K 8644 (1 uM), there was a large increase in P2 as well as a modest increase in P1. With time P2 increased further and was prolonged into a tonic phase which usually had 2 components (T1-T2). Sixty minutes after BAY K 8644, P1 decreased in amplitude to about 80% of the control.

were surprising because previous studies failed to show any effect of BAY K 8644 on the sarcoplasmic reticulum or on the contractile apparatus using skinned fibers (9). Our own work (Kim and Bose, unpublished) on isolated sarcoplasmic reticulum vesicles obtained from the canine ventricle revealed no effect of BAY K 8644 on ^{45}Ca influx or efflux. We therefore made use of another interesting experimental tool which is a good indicator of sarcoplasmic reticulum activity. This is the phenomenon of post-rest potentiation.

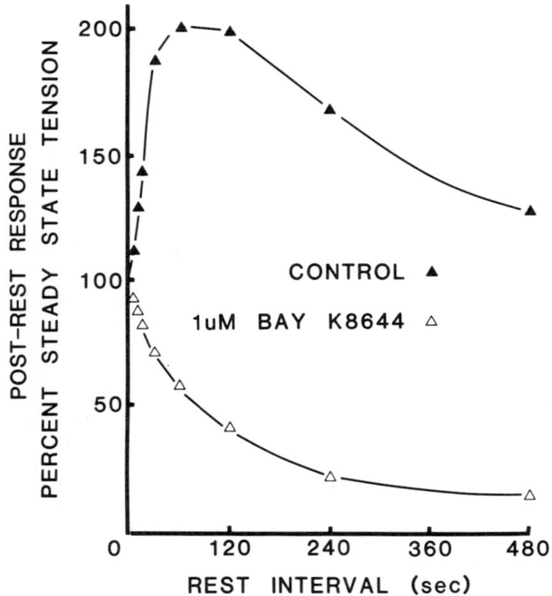

Fig. 3. Effect of varying rest intervals on post-rest contraction in the presence and absence of BAY K 8644 (1 uM).

Rest-potentiation: When variable periods of rest were interposed within a train of regularly spaced stimuli, 2000 msec apart, the first post-rest beat showed a characteristic response. The amplitude of this contraction increases at first and reaches a maximum after 60 to 120 sec and decreases thereafter (Fig. 3). With rest periods longer than those shown in the figure (i.e. about 20 - 30 minutes), the first beat is markedly diminished and resembles the P2 or slow phase of the biphasic response obtained in the presence of Sr and a minimal amount of Ca. The potentiated 1st post-rest beat was much more dependent on Ca released from the sarcoplasmic reticulum than a normal steady state beat. Post-rest contraction was depressed by ryanodine, a drug which is believed to block Ca release from the sarcoplasmic reticulum (7) or according to some others increase loss of Ca from the sarcoplasmic reticulum (10). After the normal post-rest potentiation there was a phase of tension undershoot. The magnitude of this undershoot also increased with the duration of rest. BAY K 8644 showed a very unexpected effect on the post-rest phenomenon. The normal post-rest potentiation in the untreated muscle was converted into a rest-depression by treatment with BAY K 8644 (1 uM). Electrophysiological data suggest that this depression was due to an effect on the sarcoplasmic reticulum and not on the sarcolemma.

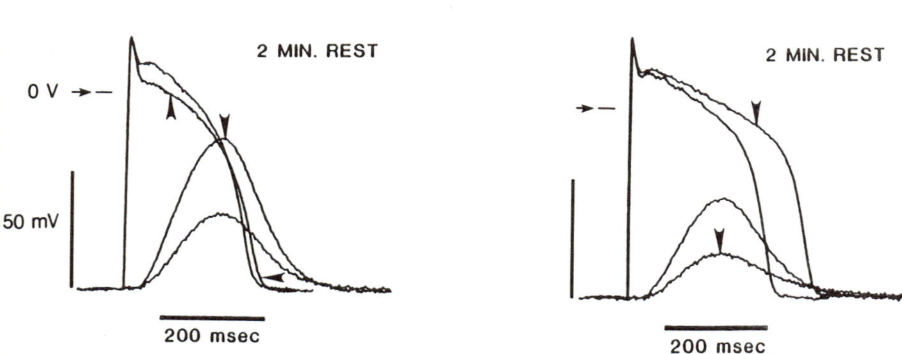

Fig. 4. Superimposed transmembrane action potential and tension recordings in the absence (CONTROL) and presence of BAY K 8644 (1 uM). Post-rest beats have been marked with arrows. Note conversion of post-rest potentiation to depression after BAY K 8644.

BAY K 8644 reduced the size of the post-rest beat inspite of a marked prolongation of the action potential duration and an elevation in the amplitude of the plateau. This is in keeping with the known effect of BAY K 8644 on I_{si} (11). It is interesting that the inhibitory effect of BAY K 8644, a positive inotropic agent, on post-rest beat resembles that of the negative inotrope, ryanodine (12).

These results raised some questions about the mechanism of the depressant effect of BAY K 8644 on the sarcoplasmic reticulum. We initially suspected that BAY K 8644 may be causing Ca overload of the cell, resulting in impaired contractile function due to metabolic impairment (13,14). This idea had to be abandoned as a result of the following experiment (Fig. 5). Post-rest contraction of the control muscle preparations (1 mM Ca) in the top shows potentiation after a 2 min rest period. In the presence of 5 mM external Ca the potentiation is less, possibly because the amplitude of the pre-rest steady-state beat was increased. In the bottom panel similar recordings made in the presence of BAY K 8644 show post-rest depression in the control (lower left) which was reduced in the presence of the higher Ca concentration. This is contrary to what one would expect if BAY K 8644 was causing a state of Ca overload.

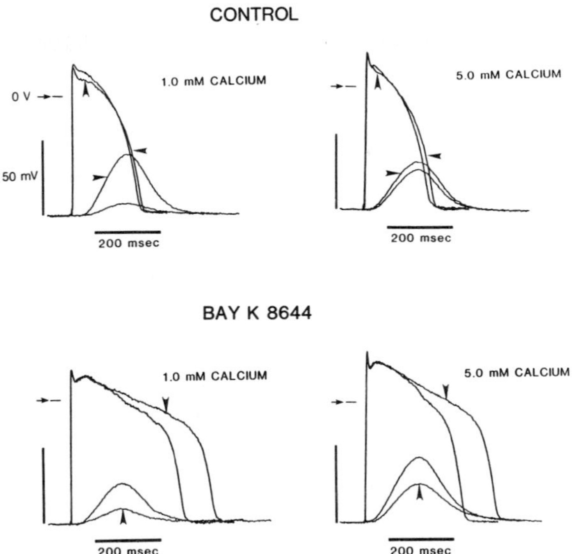

Fig. 5. Transmembrane potential and tension recordings in normal and post-rest (120 sec) beats (marked by arrows) in the absence (CONTROL) and presence of BAY K 8644 (1 uM). The effects were studied in the presence of low (1 mM) and high (5 mM) external Ca.

Intensity Fluctuation Spectroscopy: The second hypothesis tested by us is based on the observation that the size of a stimulated cardiac contraction depends on the amount of Ca released asynchronously during the preceding diastole (15). This is explained on the basis of an increased state of refractoriness of the Ca release process caused by the spontaneous Ca release during the preceding diastole. We investigated the possibility that BAY K 8644 may be releasing Ca from the sarcoplasmic reticulum during diastole, as is seen in the presence of toxic concentrations of cardiac glycosides. There may be no overt indication of such a process in the form of tension oscillations because the release is asynchronous (15). In order to test this possibility we employed the method of *Intensity Fluctuation Spectroscopy* described by Lakatta's group (16, 17,18). Microscopic sarcomere motion, even during diastole but which is undetectable to the tension transducer, perturb the speckle pattern that is characteristic of coherent light scattered by an optically inhomogenous structure. Such fluctuation of scattered light or *SLIF* can be subjected to fluctuation analysis and the spectral content of the fluctuating signal can be measured in terms of frequency and/or magnitude of the frequency components. Some agents which cause increased Ca loading of the cell, e.g. digitalis, low Na_{ext}, low external K and high external Ca, increase SLIF (16). Fig 6 is a record of isometric tension and SLIF.

Fluctuation analysis of the 30 sec segment of light recording during diastole was done. Note that after addition of BAY K 8644, there was a marked increase in tension amplitude but the magnitude of SLIF decreased by 40% (Fig. 6).

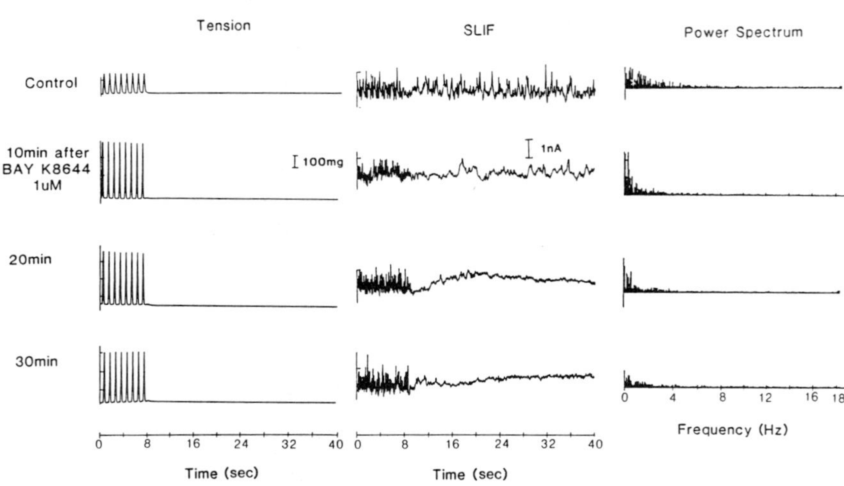

Fig. 6. Recording of isometric tension (left panel), SLIF (middle panel) and power spectrum (right panel) in control and various times after BAY K 8644.

In contrast to the above, after addition of the digitalis-like agent, ouabagenin, tension increased along with a slight increase in SLIF but subequently there is a marked increase in SLIF as toxicity supervened (Fig. 7). It should be mentioned that the post-rest beat is either not decreased or only slightly reduced after inotropic or toxic concentrations of ouabagenin (not shown).

The following results show that both the normal decrease in post-rest tension with long rest as well as the depression of the post-rest beat with BAY K 8644 may depend on the Na-Ca exchange process. Inhibition of the Na-Ca exchange process by reducing Na_{ext} by 75% markedly reduced the inhibition of post-rest contraction by BAY K 8644 (Fig 8).

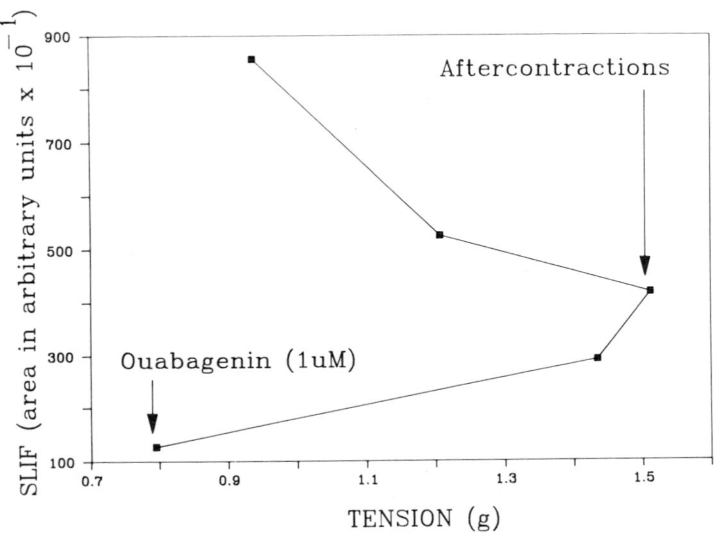

Fig. 7. Plot of isometric tension vs power spectrum of SLIF after ouabagenin. Note that as tension increase, there is a small increase in SLIF but when toxicity develops in the form of aftercontractions, contractions decrease while SLIF continues to increase.

Similar results were obtained by inhibiting the Na pump with ouabain thereby dissipating the transmembrane Na gradient or by exposing the muscle to low Na only during the rest period.

DISCUSSION

BAY K 8644 is a novel inotropic agent acting by increasing the open time of the Ca channel (19, 20). Inspite of this its clinical utility in heart failure is diminished by its non-selective effect on vascular Ca channels. This leads to unacceptable vasoconstriction in coronary and other vascular beds. The present experiments revealed that the action of BAY K 8644 is more complex than previously thought. A second effect in the form of contractile depression was seen, especially if the muscle was allowed to rest. This depression was shown by two methods: a) biphasic contractions in the presence of Sr and Ca in the external medium have been shown to indicate the relative contributions of transarcolemmal and transsarcoplasmic reticular Ca flux to

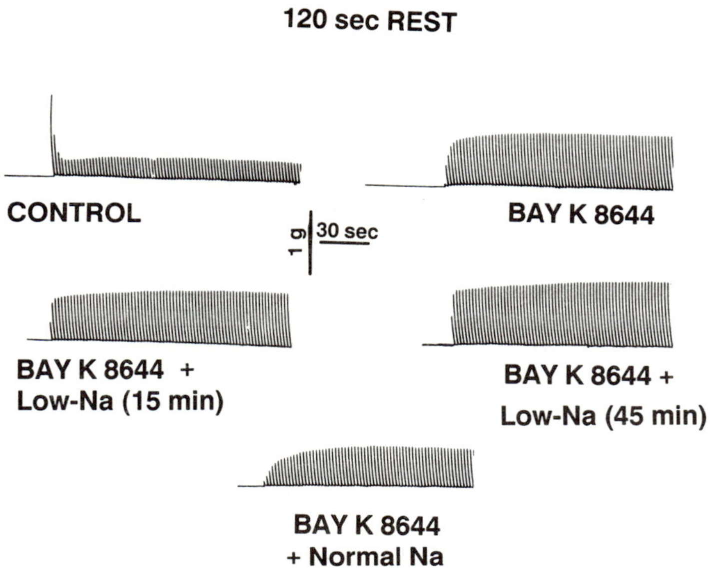

120 sec REST

Fig. 8. Contractions after 120 rest periods in the absence (control) and presence of BAY K 8644 (1 uM). Reduction of external Na to 30% of normal (low-Na) decreased post rest depression by BAY K 8644.

contraction (6). Increase in the size of P2 phase and the prolongation of the contraction into tonic phases is consistent with increase in the duration of opening of the divalent cation channel. In addition the early increase in the size of P1 indicates increase in Ca release from the sarcoplasmic reticulum. It has been proposed that the slow Ca channels contribute to the filling of sarcoplasmic reticular Ca stores (21) which may lead secondarily to increased Ca release from this pool during stimulation. However it was surprising to note that with time the contribution of Ca from the sarcoplasmic reticulum decreased, as seen by a decrease in the amplitude of P1. This occured inspite of a progressive increase in the size of P2. Thus the decrease in the P1 phase of contraction is unlikely to be due to a generalized depression in energy production during Ca overload of the cardiac cell (13). A more dramatic impairment of Ca availability from the sarcoplasmic reticulum is seen in the form of a conversion of post-rest potentiation into post-rest depression. Post-rest potentiation has been shown to be due to increased availability of Ca from the sarcoplasmic reticulum as a result of an increase in the releasable pool, probably due to recycling within the sarcoplasmic reticulum (12, 22), although other explanations are possible such as recovery from refractoriness of the Ca release process (23). Prolonged rest of the dog ventricle causes a decrease in the post-rest potentiation process, eventually leading also to post-rest depression (12). It has been suggested that during rest a 'leak' process may lead to gradual depletion of Ca from the sarcoplasmic reticulum (12, 24, 25). It has also been recently proposed (24) that Na-Ca exchange mediates this Ca loss from the cell. In view of these findings it would be reasonable to assume that the post-rest depression of contraction induced by BAY K 8644 indicates a faster and perhaps greater loss of Ca from the sarcoplasmic reticulum. This conclusion could not be arrived at from studies done on skinned muscle (9) or on isolated sarcoplasmic reticular vesicles (Kim & Bose, unpublished). Hence it appears that the intact cell is necessary to reveal the depressant effect of BAY K 8644 on the sarcoplasmic reticulum. Whether it indicates a need for an intact t-tubule-sarcoplasmic reticulum junction or the presence of an intact cell membrane to allow the Na-Ca exchange process to have full effect is not clear. Qualitatively, BAY K 8644 had an effect on the post-rest beat which was similar to that of ryanodine, a negative inotropic agent and a well known depressant of Ca release from the sarcoplasmic reticulum (7). Increase in extracellular Ca decreased the post-rest depression in the presence of BAY K 8644. This finding rules out the possible role of Ca overload due to BAY K 8644 in the post-rest depression. It is also unlikely that during the post-rest beat inward Ca current is decreased compared to the normal steady-state contraction because the action potential plateau was higher in amplitude after rest and the duration of the plateau as well as the total action potential was longer. Taking all these into consideration it is reasonable to conclude that the post-rest beat is determined largely by Ca release from the sarcoplasmic reticulum. When this is decreased by BAY K 8644, increase in the transmembrane Ca influx is unable to compensate.

Recently, asynchronous Ca release has been shown to occur from the cardiac sarcoplasmic reticulum during diastole (12,13,13a). Such release does not often lead to detectable increases in externally manifested tension but lead to optical changes in the contratile apparatus revealed as fluctuation in the intensity of coherent light scattered by the muscle (SLIF) and seen as a *speckle pattern*. The amount of such diastolic Ca release can also seen with the help of aequorin injected into the cardiac cell (15). It has been proposed that contraction is influenced by the amount and pattern of Ca release from the sarcoplasmic reticulum during the preceding diastolic interval (15). We tested the hypothesis that post-rest depression was due to such a phenomenon. Our results indicate that such a hypothesis is incorrect and indeed the amount of SLIF decreased significantly after BAY K 8644. This is in contrast to other inotropic procedures e.g. ouabagenin, low-Na_{ext} and external cooling (16, 17, 18; unpublished observations). Hence the effect of BAY K 8644 is rather unique among inotropes. It is also interesting that unlike ouabagenin, there was no increase in diastolic tension even with very high concentrations of BAY K 8644 and it was also relatively difficult to obtain oscillatory aftercontractions (unpublished observations). Hence it seems that inotropy due to increased duration of Ca channel opening

218

does not produce the same extent of toxicity due to Ca overload as procedures which increase Ca_i indirectly through inhibition of Na pump and/or directly by affecting Na-Ca exchange.

Lastly, it seems that Na-Ca exchange is likely to control the decay of contraction after rest and also after BAY K 8644. In the presence of low-external Na, BAY K 8644-induced depression of post-rest contraction was reduced. In preliminary experiments, we have also found that this procedure reduces the effect of rest in potentiating the action potential duration prolonging effect of BAY K 8644 (unpublished observations). Hence it would appear that both the mechanical as well as electrophysiological effect of BAY K 8644 after rest depend on the Na-Ca exchange process. It will be interesting to see if part of the plateau prolonged by rest in the presence of BAY K 8644 is due to an electrogenic Na-Ca exchange process causing a net inward current due to an excess of Na entering the cell in exchange for Ca leaving the cell. As an alternative the effect of low Na_{ext} in shortening the action potential duration and in preserving the post-rest beat amplitude may be due to an increase in Ca_i. This may protect Ca stores in the sarcoplasmic reticulum from depletion by BAY K 8644 and also cause a more rapid inactivation of the Ca current (26, 27, 28).

We have shown three experimental models to test the involvement of sarcolemma and sarcoplasmic reticulum in inotropy. We have also shown a rather unique and yet unreported action of BAY K 8644 which results in impaired Ca delivery from the sarcoplasmic reticulum. This action is seen only in the intact tissue. Whether this is in anyway connected with increased Ca entry is not clear. Such an explanation is unlikely because it is not seen with other inotropes which increase Ca influx. Finally, it will be interesting to see if our predictions of lower incidence of toxic arrhythmias with BAY K 8644 compared to digitalis will be confirmed by whole animal experiments and if so it will be of even greater interest to search for more specific Ca channel agonists which will be relatively cardioselective. One will also need to examine whether the effectiveness of BAY K 8644 in pathological states such as ischemia, is different from those of other inotropes.

SUMMARY

The mechanical and electrical effects of the Ca channel agonist, BAY K 8644 were studied in the dog ventricular trabecula. In addition to the expected positive inotropic effected seen during stimulation of the preparation at a steady rate, the drug showed indication of impairment of Ca availability from the sarcoplasmic reticulum. These were detected by 3 techniques: i) there was a decrease in the amplitude of the early phase (P1) of biphasic contractions seen when approximately 90% of external Ca was replaced by Sr, ii) conversion of post-rest potentiation to post-rest depression and iii) decrease in intensity fluctuation of He-Ne laser light scattered by the muscle (SLIF). Reduction in post-rest potentiation was inhibited by reducing extracellular Na concentration, suggesting a possible role of the Na-Ca exchange in mediating this phenomenon. In contrast to the effects of BAY K 8644 on SLIF another positive inotrope, ouabagenin increases the magnitude of SLIF. Positive inotropic effects of BAY K 8644 were associated with fewer arrhythmic effects than that due to ouabagenin. These results show that Ca channel agonists with selectivity towards the heart may possess some advantages over digitalis-like inotropic agents due to their ability to impair availability of Ca from the sarcoplasmic reticulum.

ACKNOWLEDGEMENTS: This work was supported by grants from the Manitoba Heart Foundation.

REFERENCES

1. Fleckenstein, A. Annu. Rev. Pharmacol. Toxicol. 17: 149-166, 1977.
2. Sanguinetti, M.C. and Kass, R.S. J. Molec. and Cell. Cardiol. 16: 667-670, 1984.
3. Lee, K.S. and Tsien, R.W. Nature (London) 302: 790-794, 1983.
4. Schramm, M., Thomas, G., Towart, R. and Franckowiak, G. Nature (London) 303: 535-537, 1983.
5. Boyechko, G. and Bose, D. J. Pharmacol. Methods 12: 45-52, 1984.
6. King, B.W. and Bose, D. Circ. Res. 52: 65-75, 1983.
7. Sutko, J.L., Willerson, J.T., Templeton, G.H., Jones, L.R. and Besch, H.R. jr. J. Pharm. exp. Ther. 209: 37-47, 1979.
8. King, B.W. Ph.D. Thesis, University of Manitoba, 1982.
9. Thomas, G., Grob, R., Pfitzer, G. and Ruegg, J.C. Naunyn Schmiedeberg's Arch. Pharmakol. 328: 378-381, 1985.
10. Hilgeman, D.W., Delay, M.J., Langer, G.A. Circ. Res. 53: 779-793, 1983.
11. Thomas, G., Chung, M. and Cohen, C.J. Circ. Res. 56: 87-96, 1985.
12. Bose, D., King, B.W. and Chau, T. Fed. Proc. 43: 3132Abs., 1984.
13. Gerstenblith, G., Hoerter, J.A., Jacobus, W.E., Lakatta, E.G., Miceli, M.V., and Renlund, D.G. J. Physiol (Lond) 334: 105P, 1986.
14. Vassalle, M. and Lin, C.I. Am. J. Physiol 236: H689-H697, 1979.
15. Allen, D.G., Eisner, D.A., Pirolo, J.S. and Smith, G.L. J. Physiol (Lond) 364: 169-182, 1985.
16. Lappe, D.L. and Lakatta, E.G. Science 207: 1369-1371, 1980.
17. Lakatta, E.G. and Lappe, D.L. J. Physiol (Lond) 315: 369-394, 1981.
18. Kort, A.A. and Lakatta, E.G. Circ. Res 54: 396-404, 1984.
19. Kokubun, S. and Reuter, H. Proc. Natl. Acad. Sci. 81:4824-4827, 1984.
20. Nilius, B., Hess, P., Lansman, J.B. and Tsien, R.W. Nature 316: 443-446, 1985.
21. Bean, B.P. J. Gen. Physiol. 86: 1-30, 1985
22. Bers, D.M. Am. J. Physiol. 248: H366-H381, 1985.
23. Fabiato, A. J. Gen. Physiol. 85: 247-289, 1985.

24. Sutko, J.L., Bers, D.M. and Reeves, J.P. Am. J. Physiol. 250: H654-H661, 1985.
25. Bers, D.M. and Macleod, K.T. Circ. Res. 58: 769-782, 1986.
26. Mitchell, M.R., Powell, T., Terrar, D.A. and Twist, V.W. Proceedings of the Royal Society B 219: 447-469, 1983.
27. Josephson, I.R., Sanchez-Chapula, J. and Brown, A. Circ. Res. 54: 157-162, 1984.
28. Kass, R.S. and Sanguinetti, M.C. J. Gen. Physiol. 84: 705-726, 1984.

14

BIOPHYSICAL ASPECTS OF Ca^{2+}-TRANSPORT SITES IN SKELETAL AND CARDIAC SARCOPLASMIC RETICULUM $(Ca^{2+} + Mg^{2+})$-ATPase

Adil E. Shamoo[*], Tom R. Herrmann[†], Preeti Gangola[*] and Nanda B. Joshi[*]

[*]Membrane Biochemistry Research Laboratory, Department of Biological Chemistry, University of Maryland School of Medicine, Baltimore, Maryland 21201, USA, and [†]Physics Department, Eastern Oregon State College, Le Grande, Oregon, USA

INTRODUCTION

Calcium is involved in a variety of cell functions, such as controlling cell division and growth, muscle contraction, hormone secretion, and in the excitation-contraction coupling mechanism (1). Intracellular calcium is regulated by the plasma membrane and the subcellular organelles. The plasma membrane extrudes calcium via the Ca^{2+}-pump $((Ca^{2+} + Mg^{2+})$-ATPase) and via the $Ca^{2+} : Na^{2+}$ countertransport system (1). The subcellular organelles that contribute to Ca^{2+}-regulation are mainly the sarcoplasmic reticulum, via the Ca^{2+}-pump, and the mitochondria via the Ca^{2+} uniport system (2,3). Sarcoplasmic reticulum plays primary role in the regulation of cytoplasmic calcium in skeletal muscle and thus in the contraction-relaxation cycle. In cardiac muscle the important role of sarcoplasmic reticulum in regulating the contraction-relaxation cycle, is more complex since the organelles function is regulated by Catecholamines (4).

In both cardiac and skeletal systems, the $(Ca^{2+} + Mg^{2+})$-ATPase has been identified as the site of both $(Ca^{2+} + Mg^{2+})$-activated ATP hydrolysis and active Ca^{2+}-transport (5-7). This enzyme has a reported molecular weight of 110,000 daltons (8-10). In skeletal muscle, the $(Ca^{2+} + Mg^{2+})$-ATPase transports two Ca^{2+} ions for each ATP hydrolyzed (11). However, in cardiac muscle saroplasmic reticulum, the Ca^{2+}/ATP hydrolyzed ratio has been reported to be from one to two (for details see the discussion in Shamoo et al (7)).

RESULTS AND DISCUSSION

Skeletal Muscle

The $(Ca^{2+} + Mg^{2+})$-ATPase of skeletal muscle sarcoplasmic reticulum (SR) is the sole protein responsible for the active transport of calcium into the SR (6,12). The entire machinery for active transport of calcium resides in the 110,000 dalton, single polypeptide constituting the $(Ca^{2+} + Mg^{2+})$-ATPase (9). The molecule contains two high-affinity Ca^{2+} binding sites, an ATP binding site, an energy transduction unit, and it must contain a transmembrane proteinaceous channel which allows the movement of Ca^{2+} across the lipid bilayer (13-15). During the pumping cycle, an acid-stable phosphorylated intermediate of the enzyme is formed. In intact SR vesicles there is a tight coupling between Ca^{2+}-uptake and $(Ca^{2+} + Mg^{2+})$-ATPase activity with a stoichiometry of 2 Ca^{2+} transported per ATP hydrolyzed in the presence of oxalate, precipitating anion (16). However, even in the absence of oxalate the coupling ratio is strictly 2 in the initial phase of the reaction (17).

Regulation of Cardiac $(Ca^{2+} + Mg^{2+})$-ATPase

Cyclic AMP is known to be a regulator of myocardial contractility (18). This regulation is believed to be achieved, at least in part, by regulating calcium transport into the sarcoplasmic reticulum (18). Several groups (19-21); and Kirchberger _et al_. (22,23) have shown that calcium transport into the sarcoplasmic reticulum is stimulated by the presence of cyclic AMP and cyclic AMP-dependent protein kinase. A 22,000 dalton protein from cardiac sarcoplasmic reticulum has been shown to be specifically phosphorylated by a cyclic AMP-dependent protein kinase (24).

Cyclic AMP-dependent protein kinase also stimulates the phosphorylation of a smaller molecular weight protein (6000-9000 daltons) (25,27,82). The physiological role of this protein is not yet elucidated. Several workers have suggested that the 6000 dalton protein is a monomer of phospholamban (28-30). From amino acid analysis of the isolated protein, the minimal molecular weight is about 5,500 (26-29). The molecular weight of phospholamban appears to be 27,000 daltons in SDS-gels and thus consistant with a pentamer of 5,500 daltons subunits. Our laboratory has published data indicating that phospholamban and the 5,500 dalton proteins are chemically distinct (26,27).

Our laboratory was the first to report the purification of native phospholamban (27). Deoxycholate (DOC) at 5×10^{-6} M rendered most of phospholamban soluble. Further treatment of the cardiac SR with DOC resulted in the solubilization of the $(Ca^{2+} + Mg^{2+})$-ATPase and its subsequent purification.

Treatment of cardiac SR vesicles with DOC to solubilize phospholamban results in a drastic decrease in Ca^{2+}-uptake (basal levels), accompanied by an increase in Ca^{2+} permeability, with no change in $(Ca^{2+} + Mg^{2+})$-ATPase activity (31-38). If the vesicles are first phosphorylated and then DOC treated, phospholamban is not solubilized and none of the aformentioned alterations in SR functions results (33,37,38). Therefore, it appears that phospholamban acts like a subunit required for the basal normal levels of Ca^{2+}-uptake (37,38).

The purified $(Ca^{2+} + Mg^{2+})$-ATPase has been reconstituted into azolectin vesicles in the presence and absence of phosphate as a calcium precipitating anion to enhance trapped calcium (37). Such reconstituted $(Ca^{2+} + Mg^{2+})$-ATPase vesicles clearly show an ATP dependent Ca^{2+} uptake. The co-reconstitution of phosphorylated phospholabman with the ATPase had no effect on ATP-dependent Ca^{2+}-uptake in these experiments. However, the reconstitution of phosphorylated phospholamban alone into vesicles resulted in an increase in Ca^{2+} permeability (37). The lack of any effects of phosphorylated phospholamban on ATP-dependent Ca^{2+}-uptake by such reconstituted ATPase could merely reflect that the proper conditions for reconstitution in order to observe regulation have not been found.

Calmodulin has been shown to stimulate numerous "pumping" systems in various tissues (39). Katz's group (40,41) have shown that calmodulin increases calcium transport in "crude" cardiac sarcoplasmic reticulum. It is postulated that the calmodulin-Ca^{2+} system is involved in the regulation of transient Ca^{2+} fluxes that occur from beat to beat in contractile activity, whereas the c-AMP dependent system induces an activation of the Ca^{2+}-uptake. The molecular mechanisms involved in the interaction of phospholamban with the $(Ca^{2+} + Mg^{2+})$-ATPase and the mechanisms of phosphorylation at either (or both sites) remain to be characterized.

Dissection of Skeletal $(Ca^{2+} + Mg^{2+})$-ATPase

Our laboratory, in collaboration with Dr. MacLennan's group in Toronto, has produced evidence that the $(Ca^{2+} + Mg^{2+})$-ATPase contains a calcium ionophorous site distinct from the site of phosphorylation of the enzyme. We utilized tryptic digestion (13-15) to probe the interaction between the ATP hydrolytic site and calcium transport site of the $(Ca^{2+} + Mg^{2+})$-ATPase. The initial cleavage, which we have designated TD1, results in two peptides: A (55k dalton) and B (45k dalton). Currently, the accepted molecular weight of the B fragment (formerly called 45k) is about 54K dalton. The TD1 cleavage has no effect on the functional integrity of the enzyme: hydrolytic and transport activities remain at the levels of undigested control. However, concomitantly with the second cleavage (TD2) of the A peptide to A_2 (22k dalton) and A_1 (33k dalton) fragments, calcium transport is abolished. The inhibition of calcium transport is parallel to the rate of disappearance of the A fragment.

We have also shown that the intact parent enzyme $((Ca^{2+} + Mg^{2+}$-ATPase)) , the 55k dalton fragment; and the 25k dalton fragment all exhibit the same Ca^{2+}-ionophorous activity in black lipid membranes (13,42-44). We have subsequently further traced the location of the ionophorous site within the primary structure of the enzyme to the 22k dalton fragment and possibly to the 13k dalton fragment (14,15,44,45). We have also shown that the A_1 (33k) dalton fragment contains the site of phosphorylation (14). The tryptic digestion pattern, the ionophoric activity, and the selectivity of each fragment reported by us have been confirmed recently by an independent study (46). Reports from our laboratory have demonstrated that the two high affinity sites for Ca^{2+} are heterogeneous and that they differ in their sensitivity to temperature and tryptic digestion (14,15).

Monomeric Nature of $(Ca^{2+} + Mg^{2+})$-ATPase

In 1974, we (47) showed that purified, solubilized $(Ca^{2+} + Mg^{2+})$-ATPase endows black lipid membranes with Ca^{2+}-selective ionophoric activity. Primarily from this data on $(Ca^{2+} + Mg^{2+})$-ATPase (13), we proposed that the three elements of the active transport enzyme are: "channel", a selective gate (ionophore or ion binding) and an energy transducer. In this same paper we clearly concluded that the functional $(Ca^{2+} + Mg^{2+})$-ATPase is a monomer and stated: "For the case of Ca^{2+} transport in the $(Ca^{2+} + Mg^{2+})$-ATPase, the energy transducer represents the site of ATP hydrolysis (30,000 dalton fragment), the gate represents the Ca^{2+}-ionophore (20,000 dalton fragment) and the nonselective channel represents the 45,000 dalton fragment". In the same review, we further stated "The model provides energy coupling without the need for a membrane in contrast to the chemiosmotic hypothesis. The membrane in the proposed model provides the translocation of the ion. The transport of an ion occurs each time the ATPase cleaves an ATP molecule regardless of the membrane. Transport in a homogeneous medium cannot be measured unless the transport elements are all lined up in a certain direction".

The SR $(Ca^{2+} + Mg^{2+})$-ATPase has been solubilized in several non-ionic detergents with the retention of full hydrolytic activity (48-53). However, retention of hydrolytic activity alone is by itself not sufficient to show active transport of Ca^{2+}. Using variety of methods, indirect evidence of interaction among the ATPase molecules as a contributor to Ca^{2+}-uptake was also suggested (52,54-59). Hymel et al (60) using radiation inactivation suggested that the functional enzyme is a dimer. In 1980 (61) we were first to show unequivically that purified $(Ca^{2+} + Mg^{2+})$-ATPase solubilized in 2% $C_{12}E_8$ was capable of ATP synthesis due to a sudden change in pH. Furthermore, we showed that if the enzyme is in the TD2 form, the ATP synthesis is abolished. From these data, our conclusions then and now are the same. In the 1980 paper we stated "The obvious conclusion drawn from our experiment is that the enzyme alone is responsible for the synthesis of ATP. This is because synthesis is measured with the solubilized enzyme and with solubilized tryptically digested enzyme."

We further showed (14,15) that the loss of Ca^{2+}-uptake and the loss of the 55,000 dalton fragment of the ATPase are parallel in time, further indicating the monomeric nature of the functional enzyme. We have provided a theoretical analysis of the data supporting that the loss of Ca^{2+}-uptake is due to the cleavage of a monomer and not a dimer(62). Subsequently, we also showed that there are two high affinity Ca^{2+} binding sites per single polypeptide as have others (15,63-65). Martin et al. (66) and Vilsen and Anderson (67) showed that solubilized and monomeric $(Ca^{2+} + Mg^{2+})$-ATPase in $C_{12}E_8$ is capable of ATP synthesis and Ca^{2+} occlusion. These authors came to the same conclusion that the single polypeptide is inherently capable of Ca^{2+}-pumping. It appears that these authors had no access to our publications.

Lanthanide Spectroscopy

Spectroscopically useful lanthanide ions are known as Ca^{2+} analogues in a variety of biological systems (68). We have utilized laser-excited Eu^{3+} luminescence techniques (69,70) to characterize the Ca^{2+} binding sites in $(Ca^{2+} + Mg^{2+})$-ATPAse of SR. The method involves direct excitation of the $^7F_0$ to $^5D_0$ transition in Eu^{3+} ions by means of an intense pulsed laser light source. The excitation profiles and fluorescence decay constants are highly sensitive to the environment of the Eu^{3+} ions and therefore used to characterize the distinct Eu^{3+} binding sites in the system. This particular excitation pathway is non-degenerate, thereby eliminating ligand field splitting and simplifying the interpretation of excitation spectra. Fluorescence lifetime measurements in H_2O and D_2O allow the determination of number of the water molecules in the first coordination sphere of the Eu^{3+} ion. Number of water molecules in the first coordination sphere of Eu^{3+} bound to protein are determined as described by Horrocks et al., (71). The lifetime (τ) is measured in H_2O-D_2O buffer mixtures with different mole fractions of H_2O. Decay constants k $(= \tau^{-1})$ are plotted as a function of χ, the mole fraction of H_2O, and the decay constant in 100% D_2O is then estimated by extrapolation. The following equation is used to estimate q, the number of water molecules:

$$q = -(1.05 \text{ ms}) (k_{D_2O} - k_{H_2O})$$

We have characterized Eu^{3+} as a biochemical analog of Ca^{2+}, to correlate the data from Eu^{3+} luminescence measurements with biochemical processes. We studied the effects of Eu^{3+} on Ca^{2+} binding, phosphoenzyme formation, ATPase activity and Ca^{2+} uptake in native SR vesicles. In cardiac SR, it was gratifying to observe that Eu^{3+} does not interfer with c-AMP dependent phosphorylation of phospholamban. Eu^{3+} inhibits all four components, a) Ca^{2+} binding, b) Ca^{2+}-uptake, c) ATPase activity and, d) E-P formation, of the catalytic cycle in parallel (72-76). Table 1

TABLE 1

K_I of Eu^{3+} to $(Ca^{2+} + Mg^{2+})$-ATPase

	K_I (M)	
Preparation	Skeletal	Cardiac
SR	$\sim 1 \times 10^{-5}(*)$	5×10^{-8}
DOPC-ATPase	1.2×10^{-8}	-

* This is $K_{0.5}$.

summarizes the data on Eu^{3+} inhibition of the ATPase function for both skeletal and cardiac SR. It is noteworthy that Eu^{3+} was three orders of magnitude less effective in competing with Ca^{2+} in skeletal SR-ATPase than in cardiac SR-ATPase. This difference maybe due to other Eu^{3+} binding proteins and/or charged phospholipids that are more abundant in skeletal than cardiac SR. We have conducted a detailed study of Eu^{3+} binding to various phospholipids (77). To enhance the signal for Eu^{3+} bound at the Ca^{2+} site for the skeletal ATPase, we were compelled to purify the ATPase and exchange its lipids with phospholipid-dioleoyl phosphatidylcholine (DOPC) a neutral phospholipid which binds Eu^{3+} only weakly (73,74). The DOPC exchanged ATPase then showed k_I for Eu^{3+} similar to that observed with cardiac SR-ATPase. These two preparations are suitable for further studies.

Luminescence Studies of Eu^{3+} Binding to $(Ca^{2+} + Mg^{2+})$-ATPase

In K-MOPS buffer at pH 6.8, Eu^{3+} exhibits a single symmetrical excitation peak at 578.8 nm, similar to that of free aquo ion. Upon binding of Eu^{3+} to $(Ca^{2+} + Mg^{2+})$-ATPase the peak shifts to 579.3 nm and is not symmetrical. Further, the fluorescence intensity increases 5 fold due to the increase in quantum yield upon removal of waters of hydration (Table 2) (74,75).

TABLE 2

Effect of ATP on the Fluorescence Characteristics of Eu^{3+} Bound to SR $(Ca^{2+} + Mg^{2+})$-ATPase

Medium	Peak Position nm	τ μsec	No. of H_2O's	Estimated No. of Ligands	Estimated No. of H_2O's for Ca^{2+}
Mops	578.8	114 ± 5	9	0	8
ATP	579.05	165 ± 2	6.0	3	5
Skeletal					
DOPC-(Ca^{2+} + Mg^{2+})- ATPase	579.3	236 ± 4 580 ± 10	4.0 1.5	5 7.5	3 0.5
DOPC-(Ca^{2+} + Mg^{2+})- ATPase + ATP	579.3	310 ± 10 700 ± 15	0.0 0.6	9 8.4	0 0
Cardiac					
SR	579.3	302 ± 5 847 ± 15	2.8 1.0	6.2 8	1.8 0
SR + ATP	579.3	502 ± 16 1193 ± 48	1.3 0.5	7.7 8.5	0.3 0

The excitation peak at 579.3 nm is attributed to Eu^{3+} bound to the high affinity Ca^{2+} binding sites. The non-Lorentzian nature of the excitation spectrum indicates the presence of more than one emitting species which may be due to Eu^{3+} bound to low affinity Ca^{2+}

binding sites or to other non-specific sites. The experiments described here were performed at a Eu^{3+}-to-protein ratio of 2:1 (mole:mole). We expect that under such conditions Eu^{3+} preferably will bind to high affinity sites and the concentration of Eu^{3+} bound to low affinity will be negligibly small. The two high affinity sites are indistinguishable in terms of the excitation peak position. The shift in peak position indicate that two positive charges on Eu^{3+} have been neutralized by the ligand.

The fluorescence decay of Eu^{3+} in $(Ca^{2+} + Mg^{2+})$-ATPase is multi-exponential, indicating the presence of more than one emitting species in the system. Decay curves were analyzed by a nonlinear least squares fit method assuming two fluorescence lifetimes. Table 2 gives the data on lifetimes and number of water molecules in the first coordination sphere of Eu^{3+} for both skeletal and cardiac ATPase. As the fluorescence decay of Eu^{3+} is sensitive to ligand binding, the two decay components observed in ATPase represent two distinct Eu^{3+} binding sites in the protein. In MOPS buffer, in the absence of ATPase, the decay was single exponential with a lifetime of 114 µsec. All the lifetime data described here are for 579.3 nm excitation.

Number of Water Molecules Coordinated to Eu^{3+} Sites

The number of water molecules are determined to be 4 and 1.5 for skeletal ATPase and 2.8 and 1.0 for cardiac ATPase (Table 2), with an uncertainty of ± .5 (78). Addition of the ATP to Eu^{3+}-ATPase complex, under the conditions of hydrolysis, caused a diminution of fluorescence intensity with the excitation peak remaining at 579.3 nm. The decay curve was multi-exponential, but both components decay with longer lifetimes as compared to those in the absence of ATP. The number of water molecules in the presence of ATP are 0 and 0.6 for skeletal ATPase and 1.3 and 0.5 for cardiac ATPase. In the presence of nonhydrolyzing ATP analogs, AMP-PNP and AMP-PCP, neither the lifetimes nor the number of H_2O molecules change.

These data indicate that the two calcium ions in the binding sites of $(Ca^{2+} + Mg^{2+})$-ATPase are highly coordinated by the protein and they are even further occluded, down to near zero or one water molecule of solvation, "during" the transport process. Table 2 also gives the estimated number of ligands provided for Eu^{3+} by, for example, the peptidic region of the ATPase that binds the ion. The estimation is simply based on the assumption that Eu^{3+} ion need nine coordination ligands (9 H_2O's) and thus whatever H_2O's are missing from 9 must be provided by the peptide region of binding. The last column of Table 2 gives the estimated number of H_2O's surrounding Ca^{2+}, based on the knowledge that Ca^{2+} needs 8 coordination ligands.

Estimation of Inter-Binding-Site Distances in Skeletal (Ca^{2+} + Mg^{2+})-ATPase

Horrocks et al (79) have documented that energy transfer measurements between certain lanthanide donor and acceptor ions can give a reliable estimate of inter-ion distance in proteins.

Both Eu^{3+} and Tb^{3+} bound to the ATPase exhibited multi-exponential decay rates of luminescence. The association constants of lanthanides to Ca^{2+}-binding ligands are usually much higher than Ca^{2+} due to their higher charge in about the same ionic radius as Ca^{2+}. Since the K_A for Ca^{2+} at the high-affinity sites of the ATPase is between 1 and 4 µM (15), we expect lanthanides to bind at these sites with a K_A of less than 1 µM. Our data indicate the K_I for Eu^{3+} is near 1 nM (74). Scott (80) has reported that Ca^{2+} protects the ATPase from inhibition of hydrolytic activity by Tb^{2+}, obtaining a K_I' value on the order of 1 µM.

TABLE 3

Intersite Distance in Angstroms (A°) for skeletal ATPase

Acceptor	Tb^{3+} as Donor	Eu^{3+} as Donor
Ho^{3+}	9.0	-
Er^{3+}	8.2	-
Nd^{3+}	8.6	7.8 - 8.2
Pr^{3+}	-	8.6

Table 3 gives the intersite distances in angstroms based on

averages for lifetimes with Tb^{3+} and Eu^{3+} as donors and other lanthanides as acceptor. We have chosen to use primarily the short lifetime component for calculation of inter-site distance since it is dominant and can be determined by the curve-fitting algorithm with the least statistical uncertainty (See reference 81 for details). The calculated inter-ionic site distances are in the 8 to 9 Å range.

<u>Prediction, Synthesis and Characterization of one of the Calcium Transport Sites for Skeletal and Cardiac $(Ca^{2+} + Mg^{2+})$-ATPase</u>

We have discussed earlier the role of tryptic digestion in identifying the partial function associated with each polypeptide, consistant with the total function of the intact enzyme. The peptide region that is affected by TD_2 must be associated with one of the high affinity Ca^{2+}-binding sites that is involved in transport. Moreover, the site must be the site mandatory to be occupied for energy transduction accompanied by Ca^{2+}-transport. This is born out from our data showing clearly that lowering the temperature to 4°C reduces the ratio of transported Ca^{2+}/ATP molecules hydrolyzed to one and is associated with the loss of one of the two high affinity sites. Tryptic digestion causes a similar reduction in the number of high affinity sites but with total loss of Ca^{2+}-transport (14,15).

Recently, MacLennan's and coworkers in collaboration with Green and coworkers (9,10) published the complete sequence of the skeletal and cardiac $(Ca^{2+} + Mg^{2+})$-ATPase. Close inspection of the sequence reveals that the eight amino acids adjacent to TD_2 are unique in that they contain three prolines each seperated from the other by one amino acid. The eight amino acids could form a torus (i.e. nearly circular). Furthermore, there are two asparatic acid for cardiac ATPase where there is one aspartic acid and one glutamic acid for skeletal ATPase out of the other five. The two carboxyl acid side chains could form in part the ligands for calcium binding. The two peptides were synthesized by solid phase peptide synthesis and purified by high pressure liquid chromatography (73). The synthesized peptide (skeletal or cardiac) bind 1.0 Eu^{3+}/peptide and strips off two water molecules (Table 4). The decay rate of Eu^{3+} bound to the peptide is monoexponential consistant with one Eu^{3+} binding to one peptide. The shift in the Eu^{3+} excitation peak upon

TABLE 4

Characteristics of the Ca^{2+}-site Peptide

	Skeletal	Cardiac
No. of Ligands	2	2
Eu^{3+}/peptide stoichiometry	1	1
No. of charges neutralized	1	1

binding to the peptide indicates that the peptide neutralizes one charge; in contrast, the intact enzyme neutralizes two charges. These data are consistant with the hypothesis that this peptide region is the high affinity Ca^{2+}-transport site involved in energy transduction.

<u>Development of the Model for the Regulation of Ca^{2+}-Transport in Cardiac Muscle</u>

In our review paper (35), we proposed a model with a detailed figure for the mechanism of phospholamban regulation of cardiac SR ATPase. In that review we were the first to state: that "When non-phosphorylated, the phospholamban-phosphorylation sites are exposed, the Ca^{2+} and ATP domains of the ATPase are uncoupled and there is no transport" (35). We then went on to say that phosphorylation of the Ca-calmodulin site couples the two systems and that the normal Ca^{2+}-transport is achieved. In the presence of cAMP-dependent protein kinase, Ca^{2+}-transport is further stimulated. These conclusions were based on our previous published work (26,27,32,82). In 1982 we presented a paper at the Symposium on Structure and Function of Sarcoplasmic Reticulum but the conference proceedings appeared in 1985 (36). In this paper we stated: "It can be concluded that in cardiac sarcoplasmic reticulum, the $(Ca^{2+} + Mg^{2+})$-ATPase requires the presence of phosphorylated phospholamban in order to express its calcium transport function." Further data in support of the model was reported in 1984 (33). These data were based not only on the effect of DOC on intact cardiac SR but also on the reconstitution data for the purified $(Ca^{2+} + Mg^{2+})$-ATPase and purified phospholamban originally reported in 1979 (82) and more recently (37). In our latest publications (37) we stated: "After P_1 is occupied then the enzyme is coupled we observe the normal basal "pumping" levels of calcium. However, when P_2 is occupied then the "extra" stimulation of calcium transport takes place. This kind of regulation, therefore, is unique in terms of down-regulation and up-regulation through the regulatory protein. This is the first time that such a hypothesis has been put forward and obviously it requires further testing". More recently (38), we have amplified this concept and presented data showing that phospholamban per se is required for the normal basal levels of Ca^{2+}-transport where upon DOC solubilization, phospholamban is removed but when phospholamban is phosphorylated DOC fails to remove it and thus failed to reduce Ca^{2+}-uptake. These data are consistant with our reconstitution of purified $(Ca^{2+} + Mg^{2+})$-ATPase, where ATP-dependent Ca^{2+}-uptake is demonstrated without phospholamban (37,82). In February 1986, Inui et al. (83) published data confirming our previous finding without the use of purified enzyme, but rather with Triton solubilization of cardiac SR followed by the removal of the detergent. The reconstituted SR contains proteins similar to those in the original SR and it showed an ATP dependent Ca^{2+}-uptake without any effect of phosphorylated phospholamban on Ca^{2+}-transport. These workers came to a similar conclusion, as they state in their summary: "These results suggest that in normal cardiac SR, phospholamban in the dephosphorylated state acts as a suppressor of the Ca^{2+}-pump and that phosphorylation of phospholamban serves to reverse the suppression." It is unfortunate that our publications (just cited) were not available to these authors. Figure 1 is an update of our model reported earlier (35). The figure shows that in an in-vitro preparation when SR vesicles are treated with DOC removing phospholamban and resulting in an uncoupled Ca^{2+}-transport system (38). Thus, phospholamban can be assumed to be either a subunit of the transport system or a coupling protein. The mere presence of phospholamban (in proper configu-

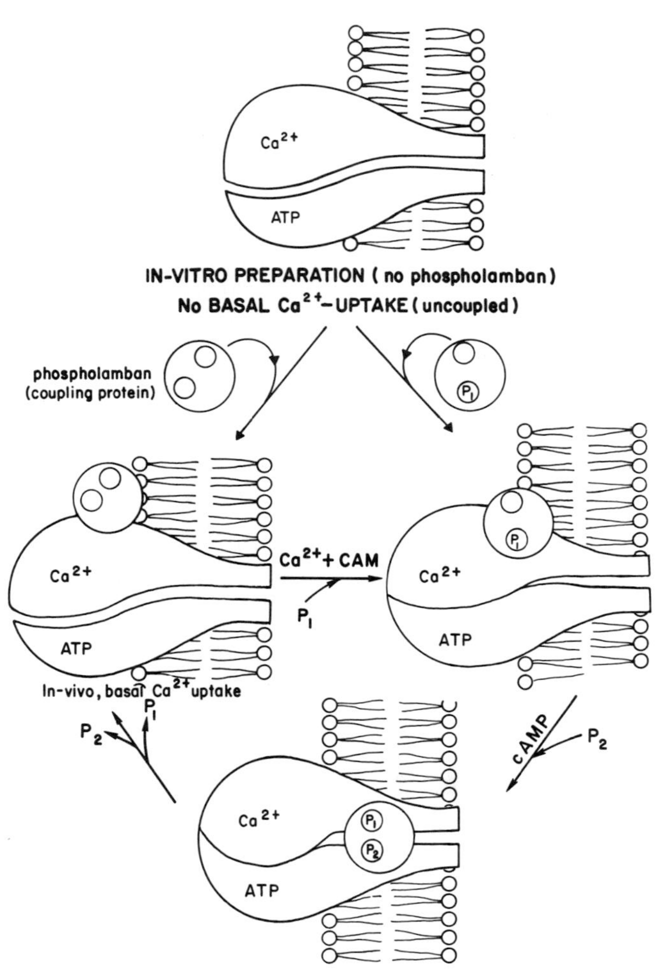

Figure 1

ration) causes coupling which restores the basal, normal levels of Ca^{2+}-transport (38). When phospholamban is then phosphorylated by Ca^{2+}-calmodulin and the cAMP-dependent protein kinase system, Ca^{2+}-uptake is further stimulated as we and others have suggested earlier (36). The figure also shows that when phospholamban is phosphorylated before reconstitution, it can then reconstitute in a configuration which induces coupling directly (38). Further detailed reconstitution experiments will shed light on the mechanism of how phospholamban causes coupling and further stimulation of Ca^{2+}-uptake.

Historical Development of the Model for Ca^{2+}-transport in Skeletal Muscle
----

    In 1975 (84), we suggested that "pump" enzymes involved in ion translocation must have (1) an ATP hydrolytic site, (2) ion binding and translocating site and, (3) a non-selective channel spanning the membrane. This concept was primarily developed and based on our data on the Ca^{2+}-pump from the skeletal muscle SR. In our review in 1977 (13), we elaborated on this concept and generalized it to accomodate the additional data on Ca^{2+}-transport and other known transport systems. Berman has used and amplified this concept and terminology in his elegant review on Ca^{2+}-transport (12). Figure 2 gives a

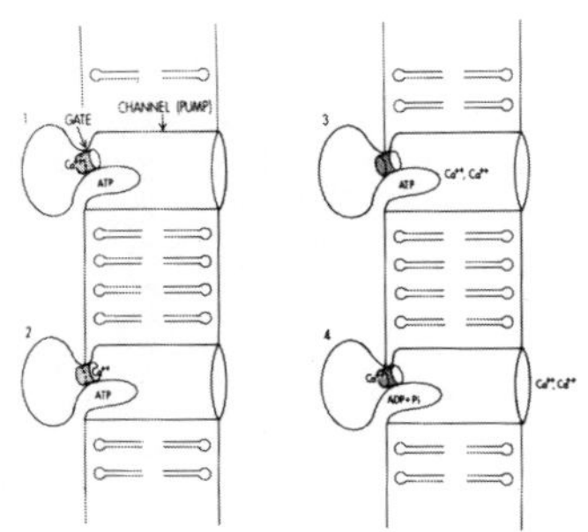

Shamoo and Ryan, 1975

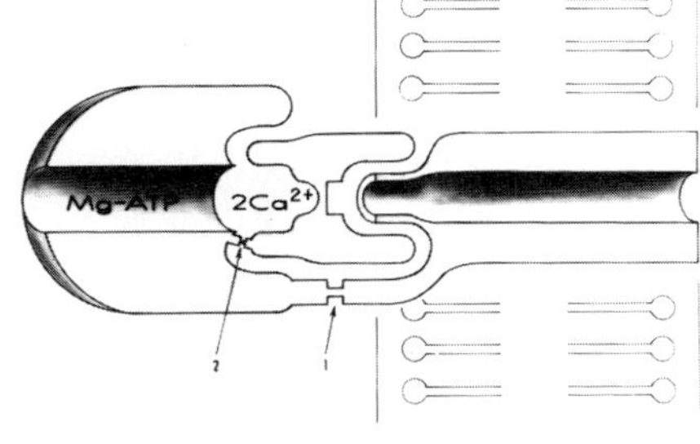

Shamoo and Goldstein, 1977

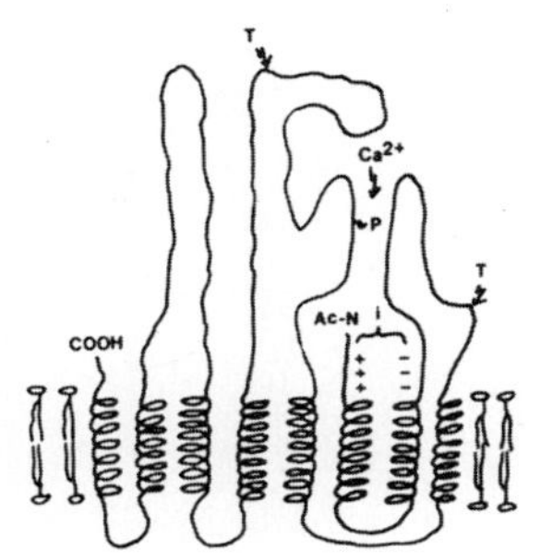

MacLennan et al. and Shamoo, 1980

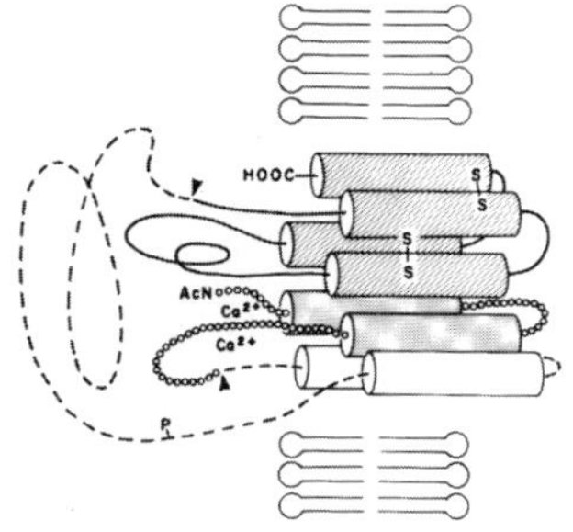

Herrmann and Shamoo, 1982

Figure 2

summary of the historical development of the models. It is clear that our proposed model and the conceptual framework is consistent with the overall known sequence of the enzyme (9,10). However, a major difference is that in our original models and data as well as in our most recent data (73), we show that the site of TD2 is near one of the two high-affinity Ca^{2+}-binding sites, in contrast to the suggestion of MacLennan's et al. (9,10) that the stalk region is where the Ca^{2+} binding sites reside. Furthermore, our recent data (73,81) clearly indicate that the two high affinity calcium binding sites are very close (within 9 A°) and therefore both sites in the three dimensional structure must be at or near the TD2 site.

Prediction of the peptidic region of the two high affinity calcium sites

As we have mentioned earlier, there is one-high affinity site for Ca^{2+} at the TD2 region of the enzyme that is responsible for energy transduction. The other high affinity site for Ca^{2+} appears not to be required for Ca^{2+} transport. Earlier, we predicted and synthesized the peptidic backbone for the Ca^{2+} transport site at TD2. However, the two carboxylic acid side chains are not sufficient to provide calcium with 6-8 coordination ligands (85,86). It has been anticipated that at least four Carboxylic side chains are needed for each calcium site, especially for the skeletal SR (Ca^{2+} + Mg^{2+})-ATPase (87). Thus, with the present knowledge and the following two additional assumptions, one can make the following "working" predictions regarding the two high affinity sites for Ca^{2+}:

1) The two calcium sites reside near the TD2 and the 25,000 dalton fragment shown by us to be a Ca^{2+}-ionophore. This will make the two high affinity sites for Ca^{2+} residue between the N-terminal and the TD2, site excluding the transmembranous region.

2) The "missing" coordination ligand will probably occur in region which two carboxylic acid side chains are separated by no more than 2-4 amino acids and one of these amino acids preferably would be a proline. This one proline will provide the least needed curvature in the peptide. The "one proline" assumption is

Figure 3

SKELETAL
CARDIAC
Ca2+
Val 194
Pro 193
Pro 195
Glu 192
Asp 196
Thr 191
Pro 197
Asp 157
Lys 158
Ile 163
Val 159
Asp 162
Pro 160
Ala 161
Val 146
Ile 145
Pro 147
Asp 144
Gly 148
Arg 143
Asp 149
Glu 40
Leu 41
Gly 46
Pro 42
Glu 45
Ala 43
Glu 44
Asp 192
Thr 191
Lys 143

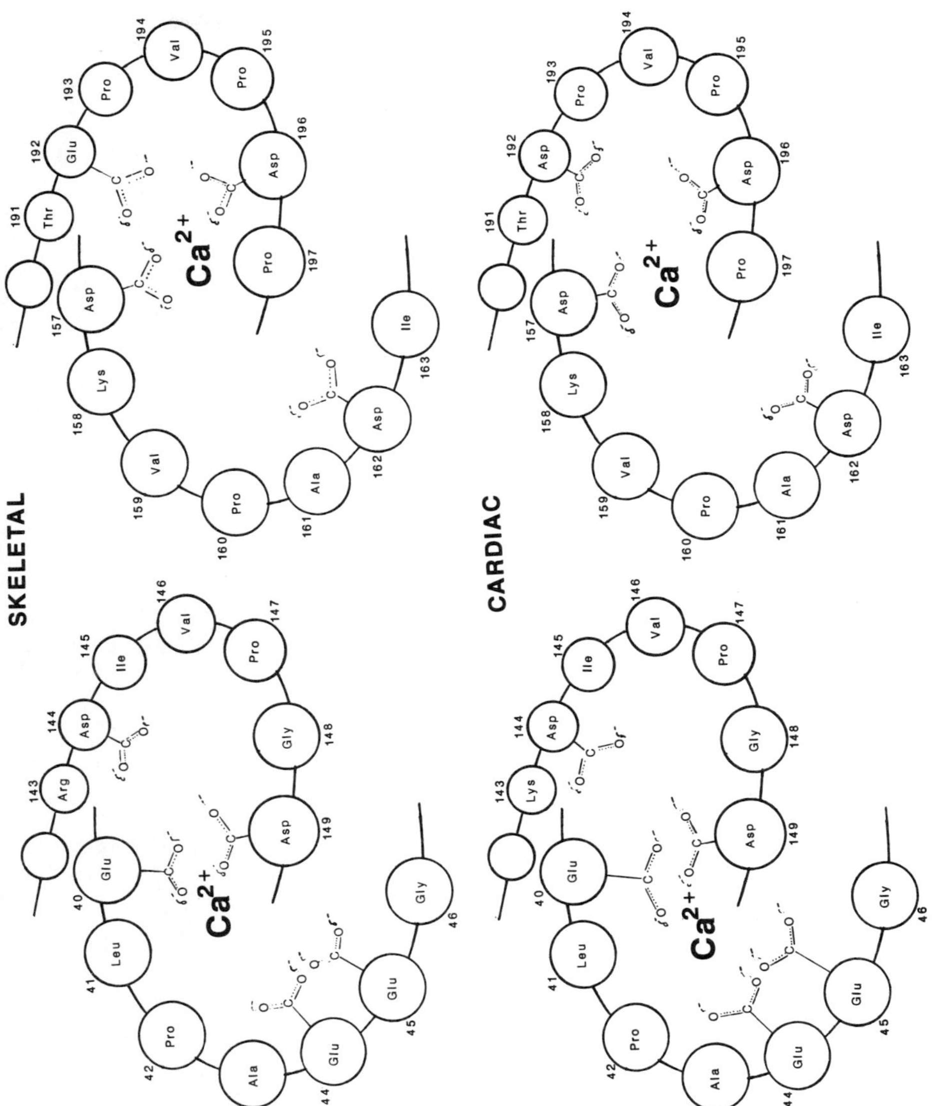

made since no regions with two or three prolines separated by 1-3 amino acids is seen in the sequence of interest except at the TD2 site.

Upon inspection of the amino acid sequence, one finds only three peptide regions satisfying these assumptions. One of these regions must accompany the TD2 site to form the Ca^{2+} transport site and the other two peptide regions may form the other Ca^{2+}-site. Figure 3 present the two predicted calcium sites for the cardiac and skeletal $(Ca^{2+} + Mg^{2+})$-ATPase (88).

ACKNOWLEDGEMENT

This work was supported in part by the National Institutes of Health grant number RO1 HL30677.

<u>REFERENCES</u>

1. Carafoli, E. and Cromption, M. (1978). Curr. Top. Memb. Transp. 10: 151-216.
2. Bygrave, F.L. (1977). Current Topics in Bioenergetics, 6: 259-318.
3. Bygrave, F.E. (1978). Biological Review, 53: 43-79.
4. Katz, A.M., Tada, M. and Kirchberger, M.A. (1975). Advan. Cyclic. Nucleotide Res., 5: 453-472.
5. MacLennan, D.H. (1970). J. Biol. Chem. 245: 4508-4518.
6. Racker, E. (1972). J. Biol. Chem., 247: 8198.
7. Shamoo, A.E. (1985). Overall regulations of calcium transport in muscle. In Current Topics in Membranes and Transport, Vol. 25: 1-7. Edited by A.E. Shamoo, Academic Press, New York, NY.
8. Meissner, G. (1975). Biochim. Biophys. Acta, 389: 51-68.
9. MacLennan, D.H., Brandl, C.J., Korczak, B., Green, N.M. (1985). Nature, 316: 696-700.
10. Brandl, C.J., Green, N.M., Korczak, B. and MacLennan, D.H. (1986). Cell, 44:597-607.
11. Weber, A. (1966). In: "Current Topics in Bioenergetics", Sanadi, D.R. (ed.), Vol. 1, 203-254, Academic Press, New York.
12. Berman, M.C. (1982). Biochim. Biophys. Acta. 694:95-121.
13. Shamoo, A.E. and Goldstein, D.A. (1977). Isolation of ionophores from ion transport systems and their role in energy transduction. Biochim. Biophys. Acta, 472:13-53, 1977.
14. Scott, T.L. and Shamoo, A.E. (1982). J. Membrane Biol. 64:137-144.
15. Scott, T.L. and Shamoo, A.E. (1984). Eur. J. Biochem., 143:427-436.
16. Hasselbach, W. and Makinose, M. (1961). Biochem. Z., 333:518-528.

17. Kurzmack, M., Verjovski-Almeida, S. and Inesi, G. (1977). Biochem. Biophys. Res. Commun., 78:772-776.
18. Fabiato, A. and Fabiato, F. (1975). Nature, 253:556-558.
19. Tada, M., Kirchberg, M.A., Repke, D.I. and Katz, A.M. (1974). J. Biol. Chem., 249:6174-6180.
20. Tada, M., Ohmori, F., Yamada, M. and Abe, H. (1979). J. Biol. Chem., 254:319-326.
21. Tada, M., Yamada, F.O., Kuzuya, T., Inu, M. and Abe, H. (1980). J. Biol. Chem., 255:1985-1992.
22. Kirchberger, M.A., Tada, M., Repke, D.I. and Katz, A.M. (1972). J. Mol. Cell. Cardiol., 4: 673-680.
23. Kirchberger, M.A., Tada, M. and Katz, A.M. (1974). J. Biol. Chem., 249: 6166-6173.
24. Tada, M. and Kirchberger, M.A. (1975). Acta Cardiologia, 30: 231-237.
25. Jones, L.R., Besch, H.R. Jr., Fleming, J.W., McConnaughey, M.M. and Watanabe, A.M. (1979). J. Biol. Chem., 254:530-539.
26. Bidlack, J.M. and Shamoo, A.E. (1980). Biochim. Biophys. Acta., 632:310-325.
27. Bidlack, J.M., Ambudkar, I.S. and Shamoo, A.E. (1982). J. Biol. Chem., 257:4501-4506.
28. Le Peuch, C.J., Le Peuch, D.A.M. and Demaille, J.G. (1980). Biochemistry, 19:3368-3373.
29. Kirchberger, M.A. and Antonetz, T. (1982). J. Biol. Chem., 257:5685-5691.
30. Lamers, J.M. and Stinis, J.T. (1980). Phosphorylation of low molecular weight protein in purified rat heart sarcolemma reticulum. Biochim. Biophys. Acta 624:443-459.
31. Ambudkar, I.S. and Shamoo, A.E. (1982). Biophys. J., 37: 187a.
32. Ambudkar, I.S. and Shamoo, A.E. (1982). In second European Bioenergetics Conference IUB-IU PAB Bioenergetic Groups. University Claude Bernard-Lyon, France July 4-10, EBEC Reports, Vol. 2, 39-40.
33. Ambudkar, I.S. and Shamoo, A.E. (1984). Membrane Biochemistry, 5: 119-130.
34. Shamoo, A.E. and Ambudkar, I.S. (1982). A concerted role for calmodulin and phospholamban in Ca^{2+}-transport. In the Second European Bioenergetics Conference IUB-IUPAB Bioenergetics Groups. University Claude Bernard-Lyon, France. July 4-10, EBEC Reports Vol. 2: pp. 43-44.
35. Shamoo, A.E. and Ambudkar, I.S. (1984). Canadian J. of Physiology and Pharmacology, 62: 9-22.
36. Shamoo, A.E. and Ambudkar, I.S. (1985). Resolution of the regulatory systems of the cardiac sarcoplasmic reticulum Ca^{2+} + Mg^{2+}-ATPase. In "Structure and Function of Sarcoplasmic Reticulum" conference proceedings of a meeting in Kobe, Japan, July 4-10, 1982, pp. 577-590, Editors: Fleischer and Tonomura, Academic Press, New York.
37. Shamoo, A.E., Ambudkar, I.S., Jacobson, M.S. and Bidlack, J. (1985). Regulation of calcium transport in cardiac sarcoplasmic reticulum. In Current Topics in Membranes and Transport, Vol. 25: 131-145. Edited by A.E. Shamoo, Academic Press, New York, NY.
38. Ambudkar, I.S., Fanfarillo, D. and Shamoo, A.E. (1986). Membrane Biochemistry, In press.
39. Cheung, W.Y. (1982). Fed. Proc., 41: 2253-2257.

40. Katz, S. (1980). Mechanism of stimulation of calcium transport in cardiac sarcoplasmic reticulum preparations by calmodulin. Ann. N.Y. Acad. Sci. 356: 267-278.

41. Lopaschuk, G., Richter, B. and Katz, S. (1980). Characterization of calmodulin effects on calcium transport in cardiac microsomes enriched in sarcoplasmic reticulum. Biochemistry 19: 5603-5607.

42. Shamoo, A.E., Ryan, T.E., Stewart, P.S. and MacLennan, D.H. (1976). J. Biol. Chem., 251: 4147-4154.

43. Shamoo, A.E. (1978). J. Membrane Biol., 43: 227-242.

44. Herrmann, T.R. and Shamoo, A.E. (1983). Biochim. Biophys. Acta, 732: 647-650.

45. Shamoo, A.E. and Herrmann, T.R. (1981). Conf. Proc. of the mechanism of gated calcium transport across biological membranes, Editors: Ohnishi and Endo, 193-198, Academic Press.

46. Nikolaeva, L.I., Grishin, E.V., Levitsky, D.O., Loginov, V.A., Molokoedov, A.S. (1985). Isolation and characterization of Ca^{2+}-transporting peptides from the Ca^{2+}-ATPase of rabbit skeletal muscle sarcoplasmic reticulum. Biological Membranes (USSR), 2: 871-879.

47. Shamoo, A.E. and MacLennan, D.H. (1974). Proc. Natl. Acad. Sci. (USA), 71: 3522-3526.

48. le Maire, M., Moller, J.V. and Tanford, C. (1976). Biochemistry, 15: 2336-2341.

49. Dean, W.L. and Tanford, C. (1978). Biochemistry, 17: 1683-1690.

50. Moller, J.V., Lind, K.E. and Andersen, J.P. (1980). J. Biol. Chem., 255: 1912-1920.

51. Moller, J.V. Andersen, J.P. and le Maire, M. (1982). Mol. Cell. Biochem., 42: 83-107.

52. Martin, D.W. (1983). Biochemistry, 22: 2276-2282.

53. Kosk-Kosicka, D., Kurzmack, M. and Inesi, G. (1983). Biochemistry 22: 2559-2567.

54. Vanderkooi, J.M., Ierokomas, A., Nakamura, H. and Martonosi, A. (1977). Biochemistry 16: 1262-1267.

55. Anderson, J.P., Moller, J.V. and Jergensen, P.L. (1982). J. Biol. Chem. 257: 8300-8307.

56. Watanabe, T. and Inesi, G. (1982). Biochemistry 21: 3254-3259.

57. Martonosi, A.N. and Beeler, T.J. (1983). In "Handbook of Physiology, Section 10: Skeletal Muscle" (Peachey, L.D. and Adrian, R.H., eds.), pp. 417-482, American Physiological Society, Bethesda.

58. Ikemoto, N. and Nelson, R.W. (1984). J. Biol. Chem. 259: 11790-11797.

59. Yamamoto, T., Yantorno, R.E., and Tonomura, Y. (1984). J. Biochem. Tokyo 95: 1783-1791.

60. Hymel, L., Maurer, A., Berenski, C., Jung, C. and Fleischer, S. (1985). In Structure and Function of Sarcoplasmic Reticulum. pp. 155-162, Academic Press.

61. Ratkje, S.K. and Shamoo, A.E. (1980). Biophys. J. 40: 523-530.

62. Scott, T., Blumenthal, R. and Shamoo, A.E. (1986). Submitted FEBS Letters.

63. Verjovski-Almeida, S. and Silva, J.L. (1983). Biophys. J. 41: 168a.

64. Murphy, A.J., Pepitone, M. and Highsmith, S. (1982). J. Biol. Chem. 257: 3551-3554.

65. Scofano, H., Barrabin, H., Inesi, G. and Cohen, J.A. (1985). Biochim. Biophys. Acta, 819: 93-104.

66. Martin, D.W., Tanford, C. and Reynolds, J. (1984). Proc. Nat. Acad. Sci. (USA), 81: 6623-6626.
67. Vilsen, B., and Andersen, J.P. (1986). Biochim. Biophys. Acta 855: 429-431.
68. Evans, C.H. (1983). Trends in Biochem. Dec. 445-449.
69. Horrocks, W. DeW. and Sudnick, D.R. (1979). J. Am. Chem. Soc., 101: 334-340.
70. Rhee, M.J., Sudnick, D.R., Arkle, V.K. and Horrocks, W. DeW. (1981). Biochemistry, 20: 3328-3334.
71. Horrocks, W. DeW., Schmidt, G.F., Sudnick, D.R., Kittrell, C., Bernheim, R.A. (1977). J. Am. Chem. Soc., 99: 2378-2380.
72. Gangola, P. and Shamoo, A.E. (1985). Biophys. J., 47: 283a.
73. Gangola, P. and Shamoo, A.E. (1986). J. Biol. Chem. (July), In Press.
74. Gangola, P. and Shamoo, A.E. (1986). Submitted to Eur. J. of Biochem.
75. Joshi, N.B. and Shamoo, A.E. (1986). Biophys. J., 49: 560a.
76. Joshi, N.B. and Shamoo, A.E. (1986). Biophys. J. Submitted for publications.
77. Herrmann, T.R., Jayaweera, A.R. and Shamoo, A.E. (1986). Biochemistry, In Press.
78. Sudnick, D.R. (1979). Ph.D. Thesis, The Pennsylvania State University, University Park, PA.
79. Horrocks, W. DeW, Rhee, M.-J., Snyder, A.P. and Sudnick, D.R. (1980). J. Am. Chem. Soc., 102: 3650-3652.
80. Scott, T.L. (1984). J. Biol. Chem., 259: 4035-4037.
81. Herrmann, T.R., Gangola, P., and Shamoo, A.E. (1986). Eur. J. Biochem., In Press.
82. Bidlack, J.M. and Shamoo, A.E. (1979). Biophys. J. 25: 24a.
83. Inui, M., Chamberlain, B.K., Saito, A. and Fleischer, S. (1986). J. Biol. Chem. 261: 1794-1800.
84. Shamoo, A.E. and Ryan, T.E. (1975). Ann. New York Academy of Sciences, 264: 83-97.
85. Matthews, B.W., Weaver, L.H., Kester, W.R. (1974). J. Biol. Chem. 249: 8030-8044.
86. Williams, R.J.P. (1977). In: Calcium Binding Proteins and Calcium Function. pp. 3-11. Wasserman et al editors. North-Holland, New York.
87. Orlov, S.N., Sitozhevsky, A.V., Pokudin, N.I., Karagodina, Z.V. and Ryazhsky, G.G. (1985). Biological Membranes (USSR) 2: 976-984.
88. Shamoo, A.E. (1986). Nature, Submitted.

15

MECHANISMS OF SARCOPLASMIC RETICULUM FUNCTIONS AND CONSEQUENCES FOR MUSCLE ACTIVITY

WILHELM HASSELBACH

Max-Planck-Institute for Medical Research, Dept. of Physiology, Jahnstr. 29, 69 Heidelberg/FRG

The calcium concept of excitation-contraction coupling evolved from four basic findings:

1) The contractile machinery of all kinds of muscles contains calcium sensitive target proteins with similar calcium affinity (1-3).

2) During muscle contraction, the sarcoplasmic calcium level rises transiently from 0.1 µM to 10 µM (4-6).

3) Active calcium pumps guarantee a low resting calcium level, and a fast removal of calcium from the contractile proteins for relaxation (7-9), and

4) specific calcium storing and releasing structures supply the contractile machinery with calcium (10-12).

During the last decade additional evidence has been provided that in skeletal muscle elements of the sarcoplasmic reticulum membranes were the main sinks and wells for calcium (12). In cardiac muscle, however, the role of the sarcoplasmic reticulum was long disputed because the cardiac cell is equipped with additional effective calcium transport systems and releasing mechanisms (13). Yet as it has convincingly been demonstrated by Fabiato (14) also in the cardiac cell the mechanical performance of its contractile apparatus is governed by the activity of the calcium accumulating and releasing systems of the sarcoplasmic reticulum.

In the following, I want to focus on two interrelated gaps in our current calcium concept of excitation-contraction coupling.

1) The first problem concerns the functional state of the sarcoplasmic reticulum calcium pump in the resting muscle, and

2) the second problem concerns the possible involvement of the sarcoplasmic reticulum calcium pump in calcium release.

In the resting muscle, the total calcium concentration in the cisternal enlargements of the sarcoplasmic reticulum has been determined by Somlyo and co-workers (12). The binding state of calcium in the isolated cisternae can be inferred from the internal space of the sarcoplasmic reticulum membranes, their protein composition, and the calcium binding properties of the proteins accessible from the lumen (Tab. 1). It emerges that a considerable fraction of calcium in the lumen exists as free calcium.

Table 1. Internal Calcium Distribution in Sarcotubular Vesicles

Total Calcium	30 mM	150 nmol/mg (12)
Calsequestrin – Ca		100 nmol/mg (15–17)
ATPase – Ca		20 nmol/mg (18)
Phosphate – Ca		?
Free Ca	6–8 mM	30 nmol/mg

Data used for estimate

ATPase: 3 nmol/mg, $K_{Ca}^{Ca} = 2.10^{-3}$ M, n = 60 nmol/mg (17)

Calsequestrin: 4.5 nmol/mg, $K^{Ca} = 2.10^{-3}$ M, n = 400 nmol/mg

Vesicular volume: 5 µl/mg (15–17)

(12) Somlyo et al., (15) MacLennan and Wong, (16) Meissner, (17) Ikemoto et al., (18) Hasselbach and König.

The protein-bound fraction must be assigned to the low affinity – high capacity calcium binding protein calsequestrin (15–17) but also to low affinity calcium binding sites which reside in the luminal section of the calcium transport protein, number and properties of these sites were obtained by comparing low affinity calcium binding to closed sarcoplasmic reticulum membrane vesicles with that of calcium-permeable ATPase preparations (18–19) (Fig. 1).

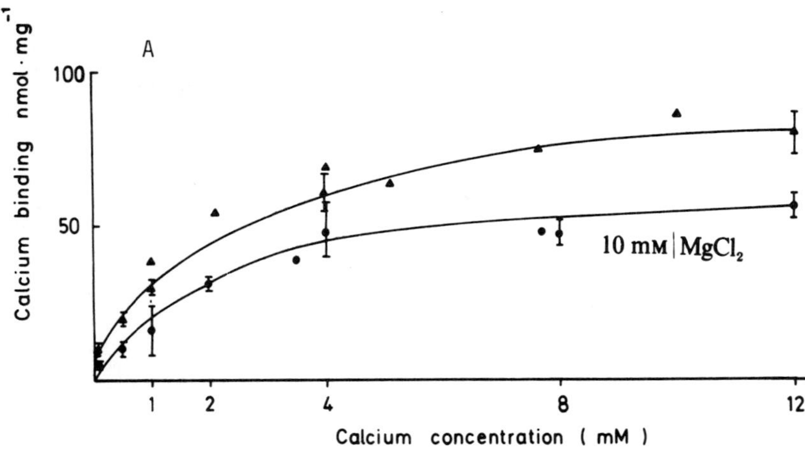

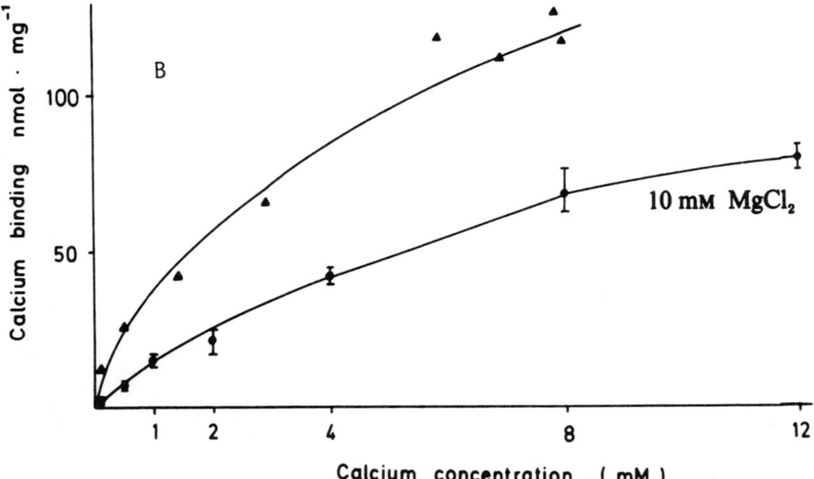

Fig. 1. Low affinity calcium binding to native vesicles and purified calcium transport ATPase.
The membrane preparations were incubated for approximately 1–2 min in 0.1 M KCl, 20 mM imidazole, pH 7.0, 0 mM Mg (▲) or 10 mM Mg (●) and the concentrations of radioactive calcium indicated on the abscissa. The low affinity sites were obtained by subtracting the number of sites titrated at 0.1 mM Ca from the total number of sites. Calcium binding was determined by Millipore filtration technique (18). A) native vesicles, B) purified calcium transport ATPase.

One can estimate that the calcium transport molecule has about six low affinity calcium binding sites. The presence of permanent low affinity calcium binding sites in the transport molecule appears to be in line with its recently proposed molecular structures (19, 20). The question arises whether these sites participate in calcium transport or whether they only serve as additional calcium storage sites. Since we could titrate these sites in the absence of ATP, their direct involvement in calcium transport is not evident.

More interesting than the permanent internal low affinity sites are those which show up only during pump activity. There is general agreement that calcium is moved by an energy-dependent transformation of high into low affinity sites and the enzyme's external high affinity sites disappear and internal low affinity sites appear when the enzyme is phosphorylated either by ATP or by inorganic phosphate (21-25) (Fig. 2).

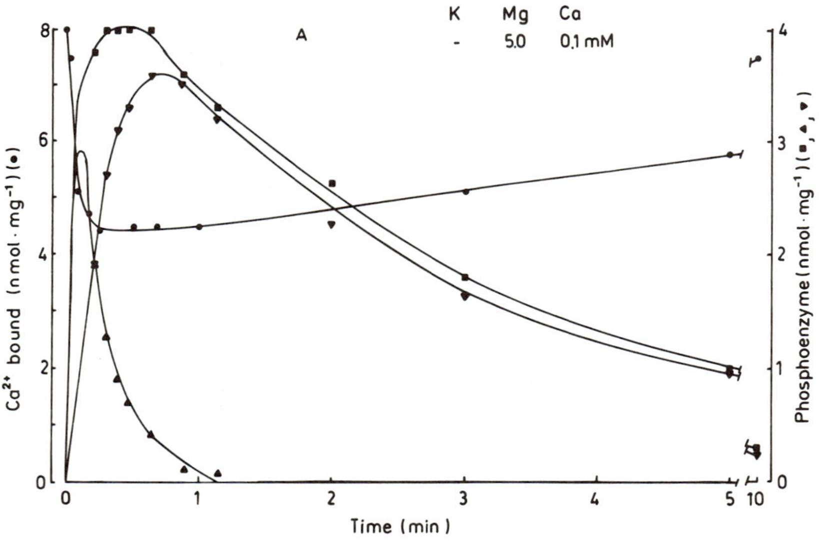

Fig. 2. Calcium and phosphoprotein transient in sarcoplasmic reticulum vesicles at 0° C.
Sarcoplasmic reticulum vesicles made permeable with 10 µM A28137 were phosphorylated with 2 µM γ-labeled P-ATP in the absence of KCl and the presence of 5 mM Mg^{++} and 0.1 mM Ca^{++} at pH 6.1 and 0° C. The formation of total phosphoprotein (■), ADP-sensitive phosphoprotein (▲) and ADP-insensitive phosphoprotein (▼) was monitored. In an identical assay containing no radio-active ATP but 0.1 mM radioactive $CaCl_2$ the time course of calcium binding was measured by Millipore filtration technique (●). Note that the calcium release from the vesicles precedes the formation of ADP-insensitive phosphoprotein and that calcium rebinding occurs more slowly than phosphoprotein decay (23).

This disappearance of high affinity calcium binding sites from the external surface and the concomitant appearance of low affinity sites on the internal surface can most easily be demonstrated by trapping the low affinity state with the phosphate analogue vanadate, which is more slowly handled by the enzyme than phosphate (26, 27). In the resting muscle, the transport system is caught in its low affinity state . The high internal calcium concentration inside the reticulum membrane prevents pump activation even at sufficiently high calcium concentrations in the external medium. Thus, it is difficult to imagine how the calcium transport system should operate as rapidly as required to remove activator calcium from the contractile protein in the living muscle. The only way out of this difficulty is to assume that only those sections of the reticulum can become active from which previously calcium has been released. This leads us to consider some aspects of the mechanism of calcium release.

Recently, studies on calcium release have gained great actuality. Calcium release has been analysed under a great variety of conditions using passively or actively loaded vesicles under physiological or unphysiological conditions (28-31). These experiments have led to the clarification of the conditions under which rapid calcium release can be observed. There exist quite a number of agents or manipulations by which the calcium can be released from the reticulum. We limited ourselves mainly to the calcium release induced by caffeine (10, 30). Caffeine induces calcium release when the conditions listed in Tab. 2 are met (30).

Table 2. Optimal conditions for caffeine-induced calcium release

Medium calcium	0.3-3 μM
Calcium loading	100 nmol/mg
Free ATP	0.4 mM
Ionic strength	0.15
Caffeine concentration	
max. effective	1-2 mM

Similar conditions apply to calcium-induced calcium release. These were recently explored by Meissner (31) for passively loaded preparations in the absence of Mg^{++} ions. The most heavy membrane fraction that can reasonably be separated from myofibrilles and mitochondria exhibits the highest caffeine and calcium sensitivity. This fact suggests that the releasing structures are located in the sarcotubular membrane complex. Yet is does not rule out that the pump itself might be part of the releasing complex (29). The fact that the pump is activated by concentrations of calcium and ATP as they are also required for the activation of calcium release appears to support this notion. In the following some experiments are described that largely exclude an involvement of the active pump in calcium release. We made use of the well-known fact that the pump can irreversibly be inactivated by agents that react with its functional relevant thiol groups. The mercurial salyrgan was used (8). It takes approximately 1 min until the transport ATPase is completely blocked by a large excess of the reagent.

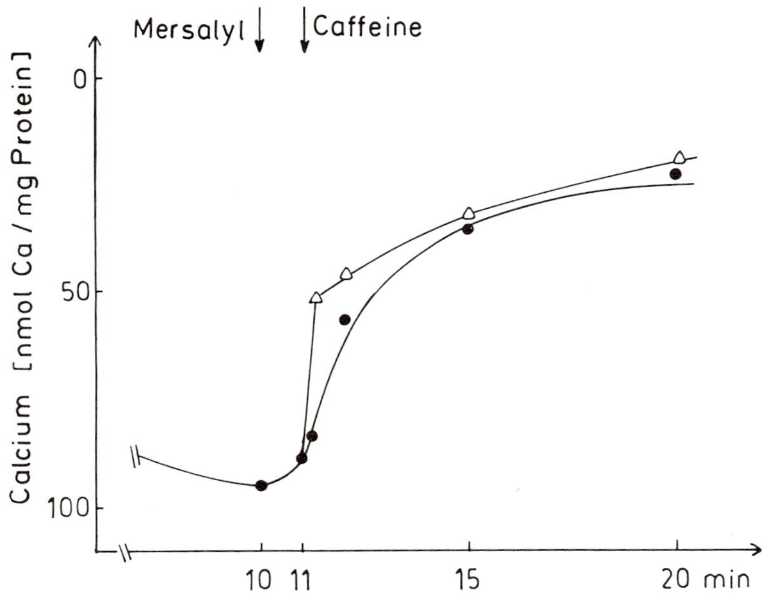

Fig. 3. Caffeine-induced calcium release after blocking the enzyme's thiol residues with mersalyl.
After calcium loading 0.1 mM mersalyl (final concentration) was added (•). 1 min after the addition of mersalyl caffeine was applied (△).

Fig. 3 illustrates that salyrgan by itself induces a slowly starting calcium release. Yet when after complete abolition of pump activity, caffeine or calcium ions are added, a rapid calcium release occurs. Since the pump is inactive, no reuptake of calcium takes place. From this experiment two conclusions can safely be drawn:

1) An intact calcium pump is not required for calcium release and

2) the protein component of the releasing complex does not contain salyrgan-sensitive thiol groups.

How can the finding that the calcium pump is not part of the calcium releasing system be brought together with the truncation of pump activity by high calcium discussed before? An answer might be furnished by observing the activity pattern of the calcium pump during calcium release. Fig. 4 shows the splitting of ATP by the sarcoplasmic reticulum during calcium release and two appropriate controls. The hydrolysis of γ-labelled ATP by calcium loaded vesicles was measured.

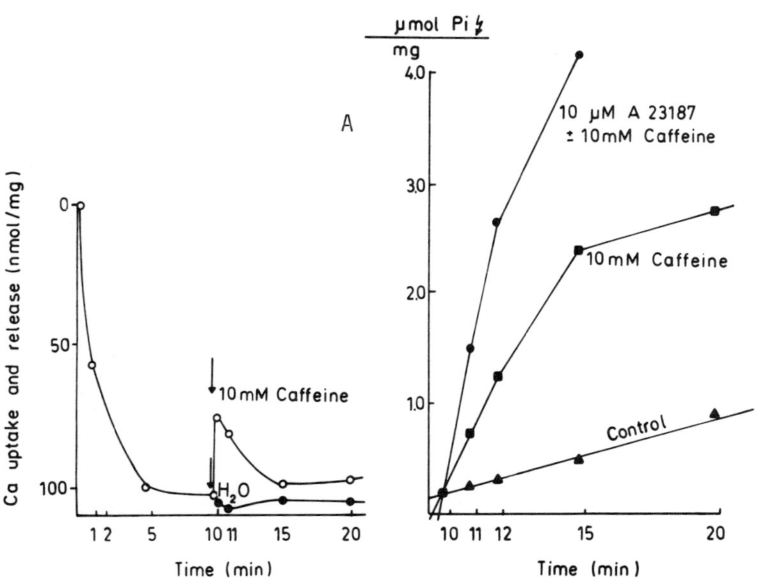

Figure 4. Legend appears on page 250.

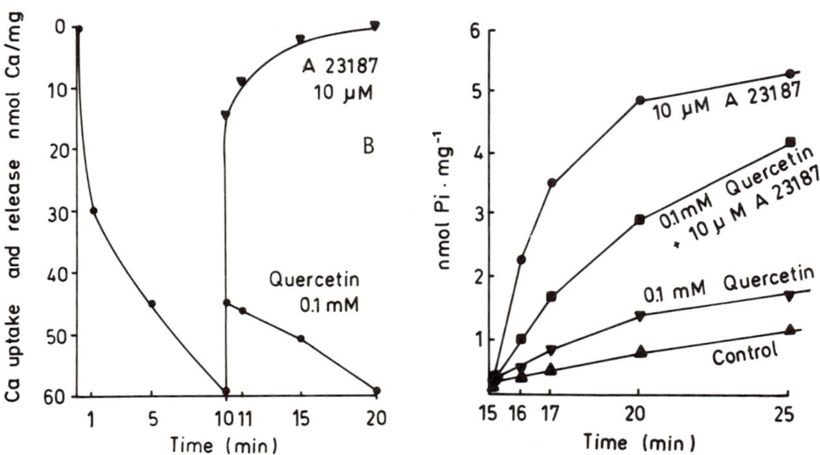

Fig. 4. Calcium release and the concomitant hydrolysis of ATP by the calcium transport ATPase. A) Caffeine-induced calcium release. B) Quercetin-induced calcium release.

Calcium loading of a heavy sarcoplasmic reticulum membrane fraction was energised by ATP plus phosphoenolpyruvate as described by Su and Hasselbach (30). 10 mM caffeine or 0.1 mM quercetin induce a release of 20-30 nmol/mg calcium from an total load of 60-100 nmol calcium/mg resulting in a free calcium concentration of 3 µM in the medium. ATP hydrolysis was monitored using γ-labeled P-ATP which was added after a loading period of 15 min just before caffeine or quercetin addition. Control: no addition of caffeine or quercetin. The measured ATPase activity is composed of the basic activity and the steady-state hydrolysis. The basic activity measured in the presence of 2 mM EGTA amounts to 80% of the total control activity. Maximal activity in the presence of 10 µM A23187 is not affected by caffeine. In contrast quercetin considerably depresses calcium activated ATP hydrolysis. Addition of 10 mM caffeine or 0.1 mM quercetin to the calcium loaded preparation induces a transient hydrolysis of ATP which is considerably smaller than the respective maximal activities although the calcium concentration in the medium should allow maximal activation of the enzyme. During the period of enhanced activity approximately 2 µmol calcium/mg protein are hydrolysed while only 30 nmol calcium/mg are accumulated by the preparation.

The low hydrolytic activity is composed of two components, the so-called basic splitting - measured in the presence of excess EGTA - which is completely unrelated to pump activity, and the steady-state hydrolysis required to maintain the concentration gradient. The low steady-state splitting resulting from the two measured activities is indicative for the enzyme being in its low affinity state discussed above. The uninhibited activity is about 50 times higher and arises when the vesicles were made permeable with a calcium ionophore. Caffeine addition does not at all affect the fully activated ATP hydrolysis, a fact that should be stressed. On addition of 10 mM caffeine to the calcium loaded preparation approximately 30% of the stored calcium are released which rises the calcium concentration sufficiently high to fully activate ATP hydrolysis. Yet, only a partial activation followed by a rapid return to the low steady-state level is observed. The same activity pattern is found when calcium release is induced by quercetin which is a very effective releasing agent. But quercetin, in contrast to caffeine, quite severely interferes with ATPase and transport activity of the preparation. The quercetin-induced release only remains transient when the quercetin concentration does not exceed 0.1 mM. As observed with caffeine the transient activity only reaches approximately 30% of the maximal value possible in the presence of quercetin. In both releasing experiments the amount of ATP hydrolysed far exceeds the amount of calcium which has been released and is pumped back. The observed behaviour is most possibly explained in the following way:

1) The sarcoplasmic reticulum preparation contains release competent and release incompetent structures which both take part in calcium uptake. When calcium uptake has reached steady state, the calcium concentration inside the vesicular membranes is high and in the external medium low.

2) Caffeine or quercetin effect a complete release of calcium from the release competent fraction only.

3) Calcium is slowly reaccumulated by the release incompetent fraction, but not by the release competent fraction.

4) ATP hydrolysis mainly arises from the fraction which has lost its calcium but which is unable to reaccumulate it.

Splitting subsides after calcium has slowly been removed by the release incompetent membrane fraction. Accumulation proceeds slowly because the calcium concentration inside these vesicles is high. When we try to apply these results to the living muscle, the current concept has to be refined in the following details:

1) The reticulum as it exists in the resting muscle is unable to rapidly remove calcium from the cytoplasma because the activity of its pump is suppressed by high internal calcium which forces the

enzyme into its inactive state.

2) Activation of the pump not only requires the occurrence of calcium in the cytoplasma but also its disappearance from the internal space of the reticulum.

3) At every excitation event calcium is released only from a fraction of the sarcotubular complex and it is this membrane population which must accomplish rapid calcium reuptake.

4) The calcium channels in the release competent structure must immediately close to achieve an effective reuptake of calcium.

REFERENCES:

1) Weber, A., Winicur, S., J.Biol.Chem. 236, 3198-3202, 1961.
2) Ebashi, S., Nature 200, 1010, 1963.
3) Potter, J.D. and Gergely, J., Biochemistry 13, 2697-2703, 1974.
4) Portzehl, H., Caldwell, P.C. and Rüegg, J.C., Biochim. Biophys.Acta 79, 581-591, 1964.
5) Blinks, J.R., Eur.J.Cardiol. 1/2, 135-142, 1973.
6) Melzer, W., Schneider, M.F., Simon, B.J. and Szucs, G., J.Physiol. 373, 481-511, 1986.
7) Gilbert, D.L. and Fenn, W.O., J.Gen.Physiol. 40, 393-408, 1957.
8) Hasselbach, W. and Makinose, M., Biochem.Zeitschrift 333, 518-528, 1961.
9) Caroni, P. and Carafoli, E., J.Biol.Chem. 256, 3263-3270, 1981.
10) Weber, A., J.Gen.Phys. 52, 760-772, 1968.
11) Hasselbach, W., Fed.Proc. 23, 909-912, 1964.
12) Somlyo, A.V., McClellan, G.,Gonzales-Serratos, H. and Somlyo, A.P., J.Biol.Chem. 260, 6801-6807, 1985.
13) Langer, G.A., Frank, J.S., Philipson, K.D., Pharmac.Thera. 16, 331-376, 1982.
14) Fabiato, A., Am.Physiol.Soc. 247, C1-C14, 1983.
15) MacLennan, D.H. and Wong, P.T., Proc.Natl.Acad.Sci.USA 68, 1231-1235, 1971.
16) Meissner, G., Biochim.Biophys.Acta 389, 51-68, 1975.
17) Ikemoto, N., Nagy, B., Bhatnagar, G.M. and Gergely, J., J.Biol.Chem. 249, 2357-2365, 1974.
18) Hasselbach, W. and König, V., Z.Naturforsch. 35c, 1012-1018, 1980.
19) Miyamoto, H. and Kasai, M., J.Biochem. 85, 765-773, 1979.
20) MacLennan, D.H., Brandl, Ch.J., Korczak, B. and Green, N.M., Nature 316, 696-700, 1985.
21) Ikemoto, N., J.Biol.Chem. 251, 7275-7277, 1976.
22) De Meis, L. and Inesi, G., Biochemistry 24, 922-925, 1985.
23) Hasselbach, W., Agostini, B., Medda, P. Migala, A. and Waas, W. in Structure and Function of Sarcoplasmic Reticulum. eds. S.Fleischer and Y.Tonomura, Acad.Press 1985, pp. 19-49.
24) Jencks, W.P. in: Advances in Enzymology, John Wiley & Sons, New York, Vol. 51, New York 1980, pp. 75-106.
25) Tanford, Ch., CRC Crit.Rev.Biochem. 17, 123-151, 1984.
26) Medda, P. and Hasselbach, W., Eur.J.Biochem. 137, 7-14, 1983.
27) Hasselbach, W., Medda, P., Migala, A. and Agostini, B., Z.Naturforsch. 38c, 1015-1022, 1983.

28) Miyamoto, H., and Racker, E., FEBS Lett. $\underline{133}$, 235-238, 1981.
29) Mészáros, L. and Ikemoto, N., J.Biol.Chem. $\overline{260}$, 16076-16079, 1985.
30) Su, J.Y. and Hasselbach, W., Pfl.Arch. $\underline{400}$, $\overline{14}$-21, 1984.
31) Meissner, G., Darling, E. and Eveleth, $\overline{J.}$, Biochemistry $\underline{25}$, 236-244, 1986.

16

PROTEIN PHOSPHORYLATION IN CARDIAC SARCOPLASMIC RETICULUM AND ITS
FUNCTIONAL CONSEQUENCES

M. TADA, M. KADOMA AND J. FUJII

Division of Cardiology, Departments of Medicine and Pathophysiology,
Osaka University School of Medicine, Fukushima-ku, Osaka 553, Japan

INTRODUCTION

The β-adrenergic action of catecholamines is known to exhibit
remarkable influence on the excitation-contraction (E-C) coupling of the
myocardium to alter the contractility of heart muscle. Cyclic AMP (cAMP)
serves as a second messenger of such a catecholamine action, activating
cAMP-dependent protein kinase. Protein kinase catalyzes phosphorylation of
at least three kinds of important proteins in the myocardial cells,
phospholamban of sarcoplasmic reticulum (SR), a protein of sarcolemma, and
myofibrillar protein troponin I. It is intriguing to note that all of
these phosphorylation reactions are associated with Ca related events
within the cell, thus serving to link the interplay between cAMP and Ca^{2+}.
Among these, phosphorylation of phospholamban and its functional
consequences are extensively defined, in that phospholamban presumably
serves to modulate Ca pump ATPase of SR by augmenting the key elementary
steps of ATPase (1). The cAMP-mediated cascade of intracellular reactions,
leading to increased turnover of Ca fluxes, may largely contribute to alter
the contraction-relaxation process of the myocardium (2).

ROLE OF PHOSPHOLAMBAN IN REGULATION OF Ca PUMP ATPase

Ca pump of cardiac SR is energized by Ca^{2+}-dependent ATPase of E_1E_2
type. During translocation of Ca across the SR membrane, the ATPase
undergoes a complex series of reactions in which phosphorylated
intermediates (EP) are sequentially formed and degraded. A line of
evidence has indicated that the turnover rate of ATP hydrolysis coupled
with Ca transport is enhanced when phospholamban is phosphorylated by cAMP-
dependent protein kinase. Under these conditions, both the rates of
formation and decomposition of intermediate EP are significantly enhanced.

<u>Steady-state kinetics of Ca pump ATPase</u>.

Table 1 summarizes the effects of phospholamban phosphorylation on enzymatic parameters of Ca^{2+}-dependent ATPase. The Lineweaver–Burk plot indicated that V_{max} of ATPase is markedly enhanced by phosphorylation of phospholamban (3). These results are consistent with the observations that the Ca^{2+}-dependence profiles of ATPase and Ca transport at the steady state are significantly shifted toward low Ca^{2+} concentration, due to phospholamban phosphorylation. When the rates of Pi liberation (v) and EP levels were simultaneously determined as a function of pCa, the value of $v/[EP]$, which was independent of Ca^{2+}, was greatly enhanced by phospholamban phosphorylation, indicating that the rate–determining step of EP decomposition is markedly enhanced (3). These results are consistent with the finding that the rate constant k_d of EP decomposition was enhanced. When the rate of EP formation was determined by a special means (see below), phosphorylation of phospholamban also resulted in a marked increase in this step.

<u>Presteady–state kinetics of Ca pump ATPase</u>.

The step at which EP is formed is an extremely rapid process, taking place within tens of milliseconds (4). Employing a rapid mixing device, the rate of EP formation was determined in reactions initiated at two different states of the ATPase (5). These two states of the enzyme are distinct from each other in terms of their affinities for Ca^{2+}. The state of enzyme having a high affinity for Ca^{2+} is designated as Ca^{2+}-bound

Table 1. Comparison of Enzymatic Parameters of Ca^{2+}-dependent ATPase of Unphosphorylated (Control) and Phosphorylated Cardiac SR

Cardiac SR	Maximal velocity V_{max}	EP decomposition $v/[EP]$	k_d	EP formation $t_{1/2}$
	nmol Pi/mg·min	sec^{-1}	sec^{-1}	msec
Control	26.3	0.54	0.55	42.7
Phosphorylated	54.3	1.14	1.03	21.7

$v/[EP]$: The rate of ATP hydrolysis per unit of EP concentration at steady state.

k_d : Estimated from the rate of decay in EP amount after EP formation is terminated by excess EGTA.

$t_{1/2}$: Time at which a half of maximal EP is attained.

enzyme (E_1 in Equation 1), while the state of the enzyme having low affinity for Ca^{2+} is designated as Ca^{2+}-free enzyme (E_2 in Equation 1). These two enzyme states are interconvertible and operationally defined, when the enzyme is incubated with Ca-EGTA buffer (Ca^{2+}-bound enzyme : E_1) or incubated with EGTA (Ca^{2+}-free enzyme : E_2). In reactions initiated at Ca^{2+}-bound enzyme, the initial rates of EP formation were virtually unaltered by phospholamban phosphorylation, whereas EP levels were slightly augmented (5) (Fig. 1). In reactions initiated at Ca^{2+}-free enzyme, the initial rate of EP formation was much lower than that initiated at Ca^{2+}-bound enzyme, since the EP formation requires the initial conversion of Ca^{2+}-free to Ca^{2+}-bound enzyme (E_2 to E_1 in Equation 1), which is rate-determining. Under these conditions, phosphorylation of phospholamban

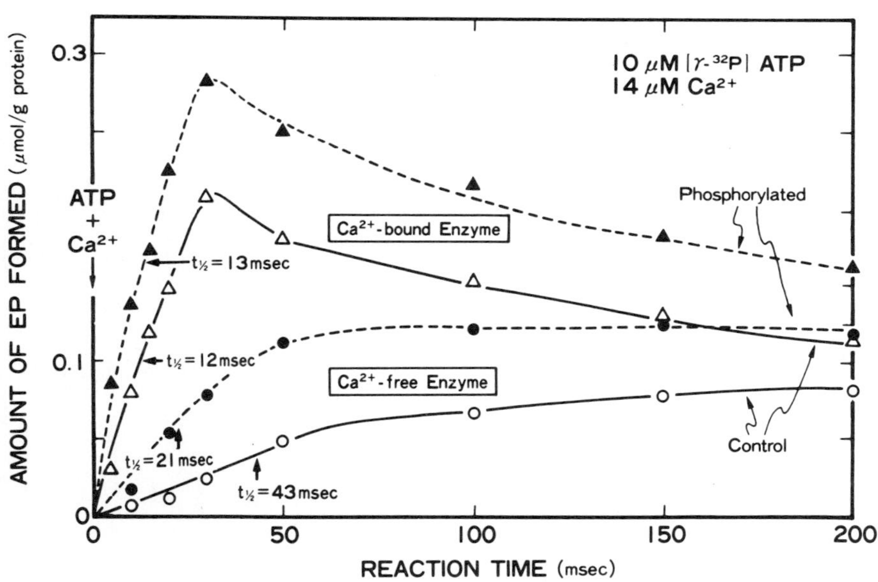

Fig. 1: Effect of treatment with cAMP-dependent protein kinase on the initial rate of Ca^{2+}-dependent formation of EP of ATPase of Ca^{2+}-free and Ca^{2+}-bound cardiac SR. Following pretreatment with protein kinase and anion exchange resin, cardiac SR vesicles were added to a solution containing EGTA ($\bigcirc$, $\bullet$) which gave 14 µM ionized Ca^{2+} by subsequent combination with 0.1 mM $CaCl_2$, or calcium/EGTA buffer with 14 µM Ca^{2+} ($\triangle$, $\blacktriangle$). The ATPase reaction was subsequently started by the addition of 10 M [γ-^{32}P]ATP and 0.1 mM $CaCl_2$ ($\bigcirc$, $\bullet$) or calcium/EGTA buffer ($\triangle$, $\blacktriangle$), respectively, through the rapid chemical quench flow apparatus, and the amount of EP formed was determined. (ref.(1))

resulted in a marked increase in the initial rate of EP formation (Fig. 1) (1). Thus, the value of $t_{1/2}$, which represents the reciprocal of the initial rate and is virtually independent of Ca^{2+} concentrations, was much shortened after phosphorylation of phospholamban; phosphorylated SR exhibited $t_{1/2}$ of 22 msec, compared with control value of 43 msec for determinations made at 6 different Ca^{2+} concentrations (Table 1).

<u>Functional implication of phospholamban in Ca pump ATPase.</u>

The alteration in kinetic properties of the ATPase by phospholamban phosphorylation can be interpreted in the light of the following equation of Ca^{2+}-dependent ATPase reaction (1):

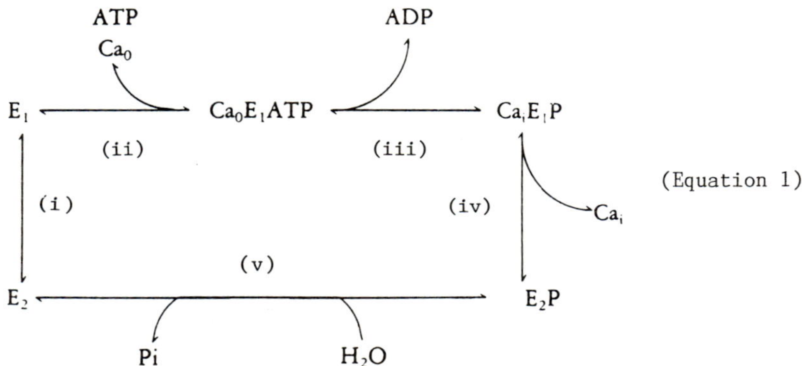

where E_1 and E_2 represent two different states of the ATPase, Ca^{2+}-bound and Ca^{2+}-free enzymes (see above); and i and o indicate the inside and outside of SR membranes, respectively. E_1P is the phosphorylated intermediate which has a high affinity for Ca^{2+}, while E_2P has a low affinity for Ca^{2+}. E_1P can react with ADP to form ATP, and is thus termed ADP-sensitive phosphoenzyme, while E_2P could not form ATP upon addition of ADP, and is thus termed ADP-insensitive phosphoenzyme. As usually measured, EP represents the sum of E_1P and E_2P. Like the step from E_2 to E_1 (Step i), the step at which E_1P is converted to E_2P (Step iv) is rate determining. Under the condition in which concentrations of Ca^{2+}, Mg^{2+} and K^+ are saturating, the phosphorylated enzyme is predominantly at E_1P form, since the decomposition of E_2P, but not that of E_1P, is accelerated under these conditions.

Kinetic data indicated that the rate of conversion from E_2 to E_1 (Step i), the rate-limiting step during EP formation, is enhanced by phospholamban phosphorylation (see above). The reversal rate of Step i ($E_1 \longrightarrow E_2$) is also augmented when phospholamban is phosphorylated. Also found was a marked enhancement in the rate of EP decomposition (see above), suggesting that either or both of Steps iv and v are accelerated. Circumstantial evidences are indicative of the possibility that Step iv ($E_1P \longrightarrow E_2P$) is probably accelerated, since transient state measurement of EP decomposition indicated that EP formed under these conditions largely represented ADP-sensitive E_1P whose decay was accelerated by phospholamban phosphorylation (6).

These findings are in support for the view that phospholamban could serve as a modulator of Ca pump ATPase. It is significant that both of the two key rate-determining steps (Steps i and iv) during the turnover of ATPase are enhanced when phospholamban is at the phosphorylated state. These are the major steps at which the affinity of the enzyme for divalent cations Ca^{2+} and Mg^{2+} is greatly altered, suggesting that phospholamban would probably exert its action by regulating the cation mediated conformational change of the ATPase enzyme. A direct protein-protein interaction has been proposed, with the assumption that the comformational state of a region of the ATPase molecule appeares to be under direct control of phospholamban.

STRUCTURAL CHARACTERISTICS OF PHOSPHOLAMBAN

<u>Purification</u> <u>of</u> <u>phospholamban</u>

Several attempts have been made to purify phospholamban. These procedures employed organic detergents, SDS, and non-ionic detergents like $C_{12}E_8$ and Zwittergent for fractionating hydrophobic membrane proteins. We overcame several difficulties by using $C_{12}E_8$ (octa-ethyleneglycol *n*-dodecylether) and obtained purified phospholamban with its inherent properties reasonably preserved (7). Judging from SDS-polyacrylamide gel electrophoresis and the extent of phosphorylation, our procedures yielded phospholamban with more than 99% purity. Table 2 compares the protein yield and extent of phosphorylation of phospholamban in the original SR preparation and in purified preparation of phospholamban. Approximately 0.06 mg of phospholamban was purified from 80 mg of canine cardiac SR. When amounts of cAMP-dependent phosphorylation were determined by incubating with the [γ-^{32}P]ATP and the catalytic subunit of cAMP-dependent

Table 2. Purification of phospholamban from cardiac SR

	Cardiac SR	Phospholamban
Protein (mg)	80	0.06
Protein-^{32}P (nmol/mg)	1.55	125
Total ^{32}P (nmol)	124	7.5
Recovery (%)	100	6.0

protein kinase, purified phospholamban incorporated about 125 nmol of
phosphate/mg protein, in contrast to the original SR vesicles which
incorporated about 1.55 nmol of phosphate/mg of SR protein. These findings
indicate an 80-fold purification with overall recovery of 6% from cardiac
SR.

Molecular assembly of phospholamban.

The molecular weight of phospholamban was originally reported to be
22,000 (8), based on electrophoretic mobility of ^{32}P-labeled phospholamban
on Weber & Osborn gel system. A number of reports indicated that the
molecular weight, determined by similar procedures, was in accord with our
original report (1).

Employing purified phospholamban in unphosphorylated form, we
demonstrated that the apparent molecular weight of phospholamban varied by
varying the gel system for electrophoresis. In the Weber & Osborn neutral
gel system, the molecular weight of phospholamban was 22,000 as originally
reported, against 27,000 in the Laemmli alkaline gel system, when either
gel system consisted of 15% polyacrylamide and 0.1% SDS (Fig. 2). A
similar shift of electrophoretic mobility on SDS-gel is reported in another
SR protein, calsequestrin, in which the molecular weight is 44,000 in
neutral system, against 55,000 in the alkaline system. In the subsequent
process to identify the phospholamban molecule, Laemmli gel system was
largely employed.

The purified phospholamban preparation exhibited unusual
electrophoretic behavior (Fig. 3)(9). While phospholamban migrated as
27,000-dalton component in the presence of SDS above the critical micelle
concentration, the heat treatment (90 °C or above) of phospholamban

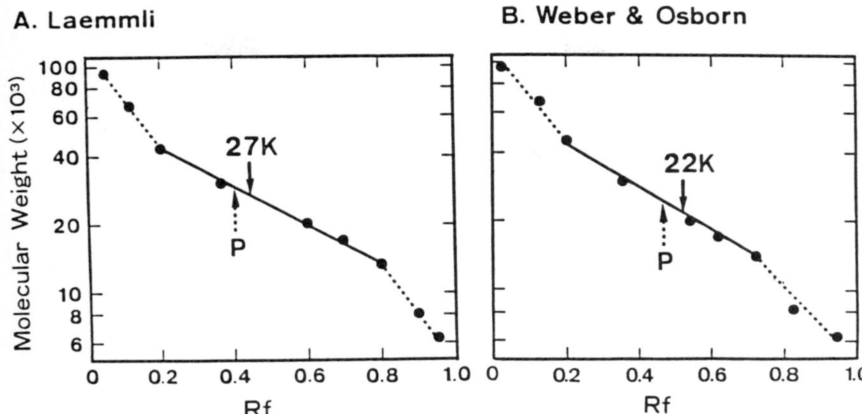

Fig. 2: Estimation of molecular weight of phospholamban by 0.1% SDS-15% polyacrylamide gel electrophoresis according to the method of Laemmli (A) and Weber and Osborn (B). **27K** and **22K** represent apparent molecular weight on the Laemmli (A) or Weber and Osborn (B) gel system, respectively. **P** shows the mobility of phospholamban phosphorylated by cAMP-dependent protein kinase in each gel system. (ref.(7))

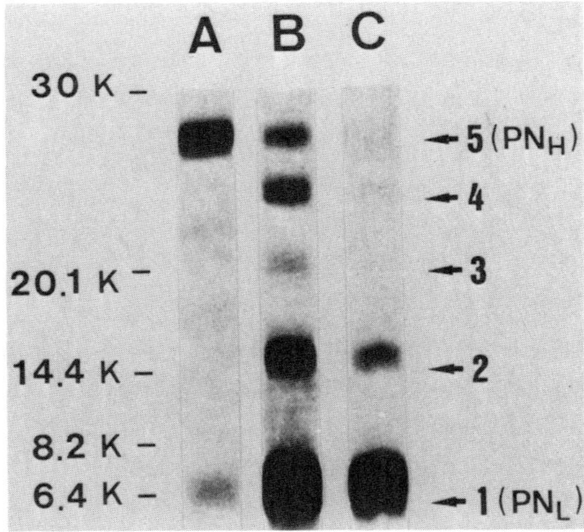

Fig. 3: Effect of heat treatment on purified phospholamban in SDS-polyacrylamide gel electrophoresis. Purified phospholamban was solubilized in 2% SDS and subjected to various heat treatment for 1 min prior to electrophoresis. Heat treatments were performed at low (lane **A**: 30 °C), moderate (lane **B**: 60°C), and high (lane **C**: 100°C) temperatures. Lane **B** represents the typical electrophoretic pattern exhibiting five bands, which were usually observed at the temperature ranging between 50 and 70°C. **PN_H** and **PN_L** designate the high and low Mr forms of phospholamban, respectively. (ref.(9))

preparation lowered the apparent molecular weight quite significantly. Thus, SDS-polyacrylamide gel electrophoresis of non-heated preparation gave a 27,000-dalton band and a trace band at 6,000-dalton component. Upon heat-treatment, the 6,000-dalton component was predominant. This temperature-dependent conversion was reversible, because the 27,000-dalton component was predominant when the heat-treated preparation was incubated at $-20\,°C$ over night. We tentatively designated the 27,000-dalton form of phospholamban as PN_H and the 6,000-dalton form as PN_L.

More precise examination of heat modifiability, performed by changing the temperature between 30 - 100 °C, demonstrated the existence of three intermediate electrophoretic bands between PN_H and PN_L, resulting in a total of five bands (Fig. 3)(9). Five bands were seen when the SDS concentration in the heat-treatment was lower or the temperature was mild (50-70 °C). Autoradiogram of phosphorylated phospholamban under these conditions indicated that all of five bands contained phosphorylation sites. Estimation by electrophoretic mobility suggested the possibility that PN_H and PN_L represents a pentamer and a protomer, respectively. It remains to be seen how the submolecular structure in phospholamban is controlled and how this structural regulation is related to its function.

The electrophoretic mobility of phospholamban also changed by changing the extent of the phosphorylation. While non-phosphorylated phospholamban exhibited 27,000 molecular weight, phospholamban fully phosphorylated by cAMP-dependent protein kinase exhibited 29,000 molecular weight (7). More peculiarly, such a shift of apparent molecular weight occurred in stepwise fashion, in that four intermediary bands were identifiable when the extent of phosphorylation was graded by altering incubation time (10, 11). In PN_L, the phosphorylation-induced shift in electrophoretic mobility of phospholamban showed only one step. This phenomenon also supported the view that holoprotein of phospholamban consists of five identical monomers.

<u>Primary structure of phospholamban monomer</u>

Phospholamban, purified by our standard procedures (7) utilizing non-ionic detergent $C_{12}E_8$, was subjected to amino acid sequencing (9). By direct Edman degradation, we could not detect significant PTH-amino acid derivative released from intact and S-aminoethylated phospholamban, indicating that the amino terminus of the protein is blocked. The intact protein was then cleaved by cyanogen bromide and two peptide fragments, CN1 and CN2, were fractionated by HPLC on a Phenyl 5PW-RP column. Edman

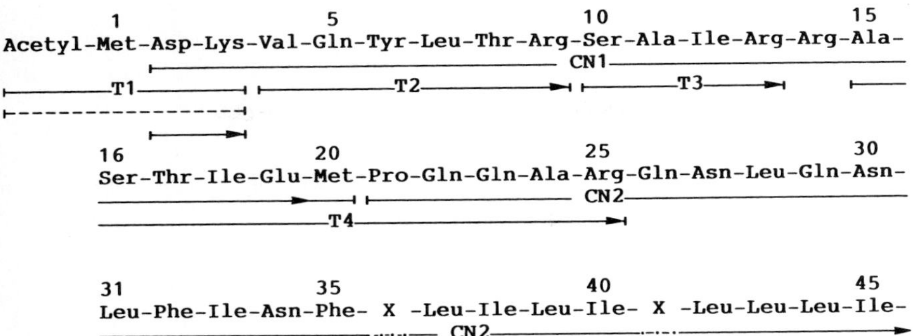

Fig. 4: Partial amino acid sequence of phospholamban from canine cardiac SR. Designations are; **CN**, cyanogen bromide cleaved peptide; **T**, tryptic peptide; **X**, unidentified residue; ├──┤, amino acid analysis; ──▶, automatic Edman degradation; ├──┤, fast atom bombardment mass spectrometry. (ref.(9))

degradation determined the first 18 amino acids of CN1, which are finally placed from Asp 2 to Glu 19 (Fig. 4). Although the C-terminal homoserine remained undetermined, Met 20 was placed at the C-terminus of CN1 from the sequence of T4 as mentioned later. Analysis of CN2 gave the unambiguous determination of the N-terminal 25 amino acids of which two of the residues were not identified.

The S-aminoethylated protein was digested with TPCK-trypsin and fractionated by Cosmosil columns, resulting in the separation of four tryptic fragments, T1 to T4 (Fig. 4). T1 was a tripeptide composed of Met, Asp, and Lys and could not generate the N-terminal PTH-amino acid, suggesting that T1 was originated from the blocked amino terminus of the protein. Fast atom bombardment mass spectrometry gave a major peak at M/Z 435.0 (Acetyl-Met-Asp-Lys-OH, MW = 434.5), indicating that T1 was N$^\alpha$-acetylated. Cyanogen bromide-cleaved T1 showed sequence Asp-Lys and acetylhomoserine was determined by reverse phase HPLC. The N-terminus of T1 was concluded to be Acetyl-Met. T4 provided sequential overlap for CN1 and CN2. It is likely that phospholamban with the free amino terminus as reported by Simmerman _et al._ (12) may represent a partially proteolyzed polypeptide. We could not obtain any peptide different from the sequence, indicating that the preparation contains homologous polypeptides. The observed amino acid sequence would represent the amino termini of homo-oligomer of phospholamban.

Recently we cloned and sequenced a cDNA of phospholamban from canine cardiac muscle (13). The protein derived from cDNA composed of 52 amino acid residues, with calculated molecular weight of 6,080. The deduced amino acid sequence completely included the sequence shown in Fig. 4. The cDNA derived sequence also showed that the two undetermined residues at positions 36 and 41 are cystein and that seven residues following Ile 45. These findings support the hypothesis that phospholamban consisits of homologous oligomers.

PHYSIOLOGICAL RELEVANCE OF PHOSPHOLAMBAN-ATPase SYSTEM

The two mechanical effects of catecholamines on the myocardium are the increased contractility, i.e., positive inotropic effect, and the abbreviation of systole, i.e., accelerated rates of contraction and relaxation. Such effects of catecholamines are considered to be produced during the E-C coupling by altering Ca fluxes across the two principal membrane systems, SR and sarcolemma, of the myocardial cells (Fig. 5). The cAMP and phospholamban-ATPase system in SR could alter the rate of Ca uptake, subsequently changing the rate of Ca release (see below). Ca influx across the sarcolemmal membrane was also found to increase during β-adrenergic stimulation of the myocardial cells (14), possibly due to the phosphorylation of a channel protein by cAMP-dependent protein kinase. In the presence of cAMP, the acceleration of Ca uptake by the ATPase-phospholamban system may explain the acceleration of relaxation, because the increased rate of Ca uptake by SR would increase the rate at which Ca^{2+} is removed from troponin. This effect could eventually increase the amount of Ca^{2+} stored within the SR, for some of the Ca^{2+} remaining within the SR might otherwise be lost during diastole. Catecholamine-induced enhancement of Ca influx across sarcolemma would produce the following two effects on the SR: (1) enhancement of Ca-induced Ca release from the SR and (2) increased amounts of Ca loading on SR. Increased amounts of Ca accumulation into the SR, brought out by the increases in Ca uptake in SR and Ca influx in sarcolemma, could add to the amounts of Ca^{2+} available for delivery to the myofibrillar proteins in subsequent contractions, thus promoting myocardial contractility. Increased Ca influx across sarcolemma could increase the Ca release, due to the Ca-induced Ca release mechanism, thus partly contributing to the latter effect. Increased Ca release from the SR could increase both the rate and extent of myofibrillar

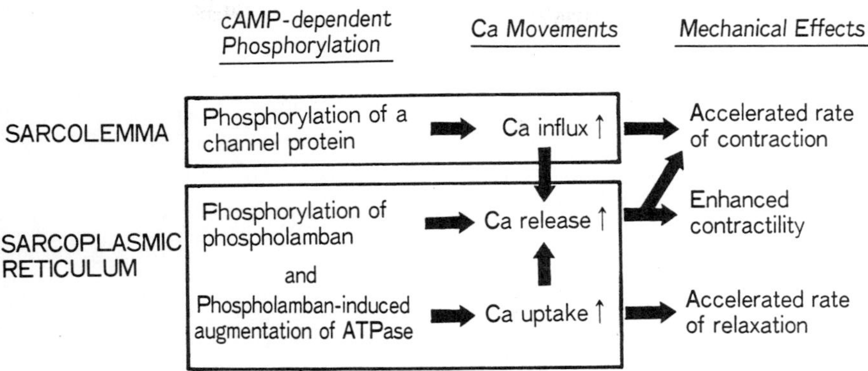

Fig. 5: Role of membrane phosphorylation in augmentation of Ca fluxes during catecholamine-induced mechanical responses of the myocardium. The β-adrenergic actions of catecholamines, inducing several mechanical responses on the heart, were interpreted to be mediated by cAMP-dependent phosphorylation and subsequent augmentation of Ca fluxes in two principal membranes, sarcolemma and SR. The chain of events taking place in SR was compared with those in sarcolemma. In the latter, an increased Ca influx associated with phosphorylation of a channel protein would cause an accelerated rate of contraction by either or both of the following mechanisms: (a) Increased Ca influx could directly augment the contraction by increasing the intracellular Ca^{2+}; (b) Increased Ca influx enhances Ca-induced Ca release in SR, thus augmenting the rate of contraction. (ref.(2))

contractions.

The _in vivo_ evidence supporting these intracellular mechanisms was obtained by several investigators (15, 16, 17), who documented that the addition of isoproterenol to the isolated heart or the sliced heart tissue perfused with $[^{32}P]P\underline{i}$ resulted in increased ^{32}P incorporation into phospholamban _in situ_, with the simultaneous increase in the rates of contraction and relaxation. Interestingly, cholinergic agonists are found to antagonize the isoproterenol-induced augmentation of phospholamban phosphorylation. Calmodulin inhibitor (fluphenazine) significantly reduced _in vivo_ phosphorylation of phospholamban (16), although the physiological relevance of such an effect is not entirely clarified.

There are other evidences that are consistent with the mechanism by which Ca^{2+} fluxes of SR are controlled by the cAMP-phospholamban system. Employing a skinned cardiac cell, which exhibits cycles of phasic contractions upon addition of Ca^{2+}, Fabiato and Fabiato (18) demonstrated that a brief preincubation with cAMP results in an increased amplitude of contraction and faster rates of tension development and relaxation. The more direct evidence is obtained by Allen and Blinks (19) who measured intracellular Ca^{2+} by aequorin, a Ca^{2+}-sensitive bioluminescent protein. They found that isoproterenol augments the initial rate of Ca^{2+} release from SR during the early phase of contraction, with the simultaneous enhancement in the rate of Ca^{2+} reduction at the onset of relaxation.

REFERENCES

1. Tada, M. and Katz, A.M. Annu. Rev. Physiol. 44: 401-423, 1982.
2. Tada, M. and Inui, M. J. Mol. Cell. Cardiol. 15: 565-575, 1983.
3. Tada, M., Ohmori, F., Yamada, M. and Abe, H. J. Biol. Chem. 254: 319-326, 1979.
4. Tada, M., Yamamoto, T. and Tonomura, Y. Physiol. Rev. 58: 1-79, 1978.
5. Tada, M., Yamada, M., Ohmori, F., Kuzuya, T., Inui, M. and Abe, H. J. Biol. Chem. 255: 1985-1992, 1980.
6. Tada, M., Yamada, M., Kadoma, M., Inui, M. and Ohmori F. Mol. Cell. Biochem. 46: 73-95, 1982.
7. Inui, M., Kadoma, M. and Tada, M. J. Biol. Chem. 260: 3708-3715, 1985.
8. Tada, M., Kirchberger, M.A. and Katz, A.M. J. Biol. Chem. 250: 2640-2647, 1975.
9. Fujii, M., Kadoma, M., Tada, M., Toda, H. and Sakiyama, F. Biochem. Biophys. Res. Commun. 138: 1044-1050, 1986.
10. Wegener, A.D. and Jones, L.R. J. Biol. Chem. 259:1834-1841, 1984.
11. Imagawa, T., Watanabe, T. and Nakamura, T. J. Biochem. (Tokyo) 99: 41-53, 1986
12. Simmerman, H.K.B., Collins, J.H., Theibert, J.L., Wegener, A.D. and Jones, L.R. J. Biol. Chem. 1986, in press.
13. Fujii, J., Ueno, A., Kitano, K., Tanaka, S., Kadoma, M. and Tada, M. J. Clin. Invest. 1986, in press.
14. Osterrieder, W., Brum, G., Hescheler, J., Trautwein. W., Flockerzi, V. and Hofmann, F. Nature 284: 576-578, 1982.
15. Iwasa, Y. and Hosey, M.M. J. Biol. Chem. 258: 4571-4575, 1983.
16. Le Peuch, C.J., Guilleux, J.-C. and Demaille, J.G. FEBS Lett. 114: 165-168, 1980.
17. Lindemann, J.P., Jones, L.R., Hathaway, D.R., Henry, B.G. and Watanabe, A.M. J. Biol. Chem. 258: 464-471, 1983.
18. Fabiato, A. and Fabiato, F. Nature 253: 556-558, 1975.
19. Allen, D.G. and Blinks, J.R. Nature 273: 509-513, 1978.

17

THE Ca^{2+} ATPase OF CARDIAC MUSCLE SARCOPLASMIC RETICULUM

CHRISTOPHER J. BRANDL[x], N. MICHAEL, GREEN[#] and DAVID H. MACLENNAN[x]
[x]Banting and Best Department of Medical Research, University of Toronto,
[#]C.H. Best Institute, 112 College Street, Toronto, Ontario, M5G 1L6 Canada
[#]National Institute for Medical Research, Mill Hill, London NW7 1AA, UK

INTRODUCTION

The sarcoplasmic reticulum of cardiac muscle is an internal membrane system which accumulates, sequesters and releases Ca^{2+}. The ability of this system to regulate cytoplasmic Ca^{2+} concentrations is central to the control of muscle contraction (1). The predominant protein of the sarcoplasmic reticulum is an integral membrane protein with a molecular weight of 110,000. This protein, a high affinity Ca^{2+} pump, utilizes the energy of ATP hydrolysis to transport Ca^{2+} against a concentration gradient into the lumen of the sarcoplasmic reticulum (2-4). Cytoplasmic Ca^{2+} concentration are thereby lowered to a level where Ca^{2+} dissociates from troponin C, permitting muscle relaxation (5-7).

The fast-twitch skeletal muscle form of the Ca^{2+} ATPase has been studied in more detail than the cardiac muscle enzyme but it is evident that their roles in muscle relaxation and their mechanisms of action are very similar (8,9). Functional differences have been observed between the two enzymes. The most important difference lies in the fact that the cardiac Ca^{2+} ATPase is sensitive to control by a pentameric, 5,000 dalton, phosphorylatable protein called phospholamban (10). When phosphorylated by cAMP or calmodulin-dependent kinases, phospholamban stimulates Ca^{2+} transport by the Ca^{2+} ATPase through an increase in the rate of turnover of the enzyme. Some models for the mechanism of action of phospholamban (10) suggest that phospholamban and the Ca^{2+} ATPase are closely associated within the membrane and that protein-protein contacts occur. Regulation by phospholamban has been proposed to explain the abbreviation of systole and increased contractility of the heart in response to catecholamines (10). Other functional differences exist between fast-twitch skeletal and cardiac Ca^{2+} ATPases. These include an increased K_{Ca}, altered rate constants for partial reactions and an increased nucleotide specificity (11-14).

The Ca^{2+} ATPase of cardiac muscle sarcoplasmic reticulum shares several

characteristics with the slow-twitch skeletal muscle enzyme. Their
concentrations in sarcoplasmic reticulum membranes are similar (1,2) their
specific activities are low (15) and characteristics of their partial reactions
are similar (16). Like cardiac sarcoplasmic reticulum, slow-twitch
sarcoplasmic reticulum contains the regulatory molecule, phospholamban (17-20).
The fast-twitch Ca^{2+} ATPase differs antigenically from both cardiac and slow
twitch enzymes (21-23). Jorgensen and Campbell (24) demonstrated that cardiac
and slow twitch ATPase enzymes share epitopes not present in the fast-twitch
enzyme.

We have used recombinant DNA techniques to begin to investigate the
primary structure of the cardiac and the two skeletal muscle forms of the Ca^{2+}
ATPase and to understand the relationship between slow-twitch and cardiac
muscle forms of the enzyme. In addition, we have studied the expression of
these molecules in developing skeletal muscle. This review will focus on our
findings as they apply to the cardiac form of the Ca^{2+} ATPase.

RESULTS AND DISCUSSION
Cloning of the Cardiac form of the Ca^{2+} ATPase

Neonatal rabbit skeletal muscle is a rich source of mRNA coding for the
Ca^{2+} ATPase (25). We initially used this source of mRNA to construct cDNA
libraries and, with synthetic oligonucleotide probes, isolated a cDNA clone
coding for the fast-twitch Ca^{2+} ATPase (26). When this was used to screen the
same cDNA libraries at lower stringency, a second group of clones was isolated
which encoded a protein of 997 amino acids with 84% sequence homology to the
fast-twitch enzyme (27) (see Fig. 1). The mRNA encoding this group of clones
was approximately 4200 bp in length and was present in neonatal rabbit mRNA in
about the same concentration as a transcript of about 3800 bp encoding the
fast-twitch enzyme (26). The amino acid sequence of this protein was identical
to that of the canine cardiac Ca^{2+} ATPase for 17 amino acids surrounding the
FITC binding site (28), providing the first indication that this second form of
the Ca^{2+} ATPase, expressed in neonatal muscle, might represent the cardiac form
of the enzyme. Northern blot analysis using a unique probe from the 3'
nontranslated region of this clone identified an mRNA of similar size and
sequence in adult slow-twitch and cardiac muscles but not in adult fast-twitch
skeletal muscle (26). We concluded that the cardiac and slow-twitch skeletal
muscle forms of the Ca^{2+} ATPase were identical and, moreover, that this form of
the enzyme was expressed in neonatal skeletal muscle.

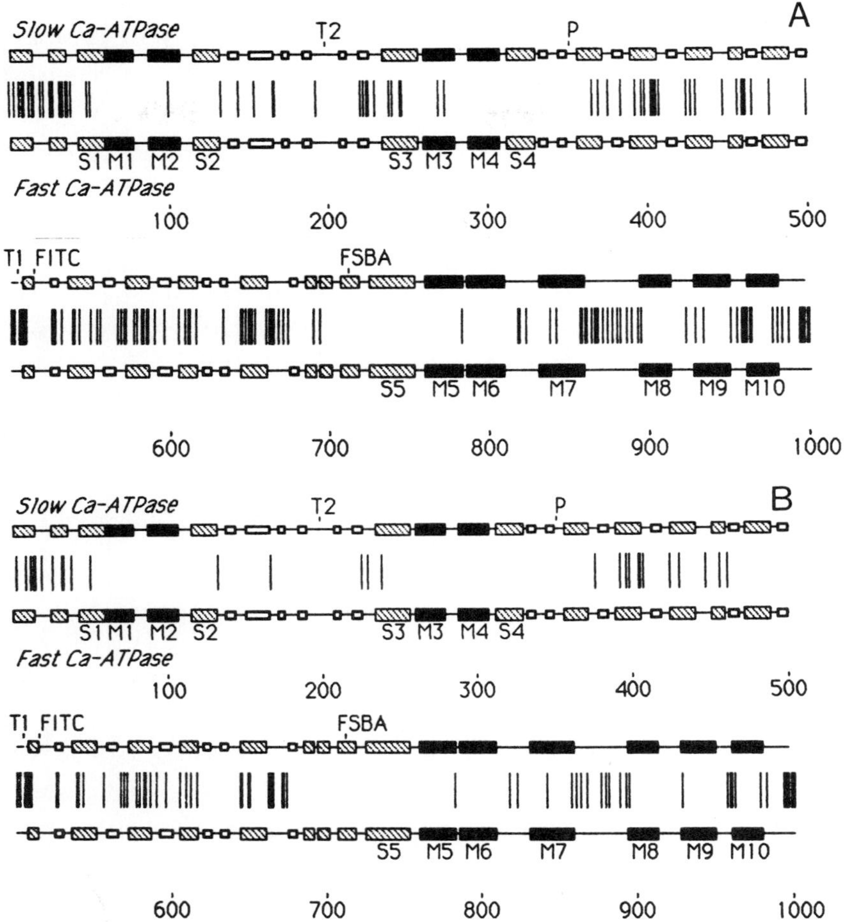

Fig. 1. Comparison of amino-acid sequences and structural predictions for fast-twitch and slow-twitch/cardiac Ca^{2+} ATPases. (■), transmembrane alpha helices; (▨), alpha helices; (▭), beta strands; (—), beta turns or undefined structures; (|||), amino acid differences. In A, all amino acid differences are shown: in B, conservative differences (Ser/Thr, Glu/Asp, Lys/Arg, Phe/Tyr/Trp, Ile/Leu/Val/Met) are not shown. Major tryptic cleavage sites of the fast-twitch Ca^{2+} ATPase (29) are indicated as T1 and T2; the phosphorylation site (30) as P; the site of fluorescein isothiocyanate binding (31) as FITC; and the site of 5' (fluorosulfonyl) benzoyladenosine binding (32) as FSBA. The transmembrane domain consists of hydrophobic helices M_1-M_{10}; the stalk sector consists of amphipathic helices S_1-S_5; the transduction domain encompasses residues 133-238; the phosphorylation domain, residues 330-505; the nucleotide-binding domain, residues 506-680 and the alpha-subdomain, residues 681-740, based on the numbering system for the slow-twitch/cardiac Ca^{2+} ATPase (27).

These observations suggested that there were at least two unique forms of the Ca^{2+} ATPase, one of which was expressed in fast-twitch muscle and the other in slow-twitch and cardiac muscles. Investigation of the number of closely cross-hybridizing genes in rabbit genomic DNA revealed that only two genes were present (26). These observations have been confirmed in the human genome where it has been found that these two genes reside on different chromosomes (H.F. Willard, C.J. Brandl, P.C. Holland and D.H. MacLennan, unpublished observations).

To verify the identity of cardiac and slow-twitch Ca^{2+} ATPases we constructed cDNA libraries from mRNAs from adult muscles in both these tissues and isolated the Ca^{2+} ATPase clones by colony hybridization (33). Restriction map and DNA sequence analyses show that adult cardiac and slow-twitch Ca^{2+} ATPase transcripts are identical and that they code for the same protein that is expressed in neonatal skeletal muscle (33). The cDNAs isolated from adult tissues differed from the neonatal cDNA in that they were extended by approximately 130 bases at their 3'ends.

A ribonuclease protection assay (34) using a complementary RNA probe from the 3' end of the adult cardiac message was performed in order to determine if alternative polyadenylation sites might be used and, if so, whether their use might be developmentally regulated (33). This assay revealed that several mRNA species with lengths ranging from approximately 4050 to 4222 bases exist in cardiac and slow-twitch muscles. Predominant forms of 4120 and 4222 bp exist and these follow perfect polyadenylation signals (AATAAA) while the others follow imperfect polyadenylation signals with one altered base in the signal sequence. No developmental pattern was observed for the appearance of the different mRNAs since the ratios were virtually constant at all stages of development.

We observed small amounts of fast-twitch Ca^{2+} ATPase transcripts in predominantly slow-twitch muscle (soleus), probably because this muscle contains a low percentage of fast-twitch fibers. We did not observe any fast-twitch Ca^{2+} ATPase transcripts in adult cardiac muscle, however (33).

The mRNA's of cardiac and fast-twitch skeletal muscle share approximately 76% nucleotide sequence homology in coding regions, but they display a pronounced difference in their pattern of codon usage (Table 1). The fast-twitch Ca^{2+} ATPase has a highly skewed codon usage, preferring those codons most commonly used in mammalian cells (35). By contrast, codon usage in the cardiac Ca^{2+} ATPase was found to be less highly selective and a wider range

Table 1. Codon usage in fast (F) and slow (S) twitch/cardiac Ca^{2+} ATPases

		F	S			F	S			F	S			F	S
UUU	Phe	11	20	UCU	Ser	12	18	UAU	Tyr	5	7	UGU	Cys	6	10
UUC	Phe	26	19	UCC	Ser	31	19	UAC	Tyr	17	11	UGC	Cys	18	16
UUA	Leu	0	5	UCA	Ser	3	8	UAA	Stp	1	1	UGA	Stp	0	0
UUG	Leu	5	8	UCG	Ser	4	1	UAG	Stp	0	0	UGG	Trp	13	13
CUU	Leu	6	14	CCU	Pro	5	20	CAU	His	1	4	CGU	Arg	2	2
CUC	Leu	23	14	CCC	Pro	22	7	CAC	His	11	9	CGC	Arg	20	7
CUA	Leu	2	5	CCA	Pro	9	10	CAA	Gln	2	2	CGA	Arg	4	3
CUG	Leu	57	48	CCG	Pro	10	8	CAG	Gln	21	24	CGG	Arg	18	14
AUU	Ile	4	34	ACU	Thr	4	19	AAU	Asn	7	13	AGU	Ser	2	4
AUC	Ile	64	32	ACC	Thr	38	15	AAC	Asn	29	30	AGC	Ser	5	8
AUA	Ile	4	8	ACA	Thr	6	19	AAA	Lys	7	21	AGA	Arg	1	10
AUG	Met	33	30	ACG	Thr	14	9	AAG	Lys	47	37	AGG	Arg	5	6
GUU	Val	4	15	GCU	Ala	14	27	GAU	Asp	11	22	GGU	Gly	7	20
GUC	Val	25	23	GCC	Ala	58	32	GAC	Asp	41	24	GGC	Gly	34	25
GUA	Val	0	10	GCA	Ala	3	17	GAA	Glu	16	36	GGA	Gly	4	11
GUG	Val	53	38	GCG	Ala	11	9	GAG	Glu	64	39	GGG	Gly	22	8

of codon usage was observed. This may be related to the lower level of
expression of the slow-twitch/cardiac Ca^{2+} ATPase gene as compared to the level
of expression of the fast-twitch form.

The identity of the Ca^{+} ATPase in cardiac and slow-twitch skeletal muscle
implies that a common regulatory signal for the expression of the enzyme exists
in both tissues. Since the regulatory molecule phospholamban is present in
both cardiac and slow-twitch muscle sarcoplasmic reticulum (17), the expression
of the cardiac/slow-twitch Ca^{2+} ATPase and phospholamban may prove to be
co-ordinately regulated.

Structure of the Cardiac Ca^{2+} ATPase

The cardiac Ca^{2+} ATPase is an integral membrane protein of 997 amino acids
with a molecular mass of 109,763 daltons (27). Our secondary structural
predictions, based on algorithms developed by Taylor and Thornton (36) suggest
that the molecule has a tripartite structure composed of three globular
cytoplasmic domains, connected to a transmembranous basepiece by a pentahelical
stalk (27). The molecule thus has a mushroom or inverted pear shape with a
height of approximately 12 nm and conforms with the shape identified for the
fast-twitch form by X-ray and neutron diffraction (37), three-dimensional

reconstruction from negatively-stained or frozen-hydrated, two-dimensional crystals induced by vanadate (38-40) and by electron microscopic studies (eg. 41). The model also positions tryptic cleavage sites and the ATP-binding site on the cytoplasmic surface where they were previously located by biochemical analyses (42).

The protein can be divided into several domains. Regions that interact directly with ATP and are responsible for the transduction of the energy of ATP hydrolysis into the formation of a Ca^{2+} gradient are found in the headpiece. A Ca^{2+} binding domain is located in the stalk and channel forming domains are located in the transmembrane section. We have named the headpiece domains the transduction domain, the phosphorylation domain, the nucleotide-binding domain and the alpha-subdomain. The transduction domain is a beta-sheet structure located in the cytoplasm between stalk sectors 2 and 3 (See Fig. 1 for the linear placement of these sites). Cleavage with trypsin in this region leads to loss of Ca^{2+} transport activity (43). The phosphorylation and nucleotide-binding domains are found in a long central cytoplasmic segment between stalk sectors 4 and 5. They are comprised of alternating alpha and beta structures. We have previously suggested that this region is actually composed of two domains (27) because of its structural similarity to phosphoglycerate kinase and hexokinase, both of which are made up of two hinged domains. This would suggest a similar mechanism of energy transfer and perhaps a common ancestry with these soluble kinases. The alpha-subdomain is a series of alpha-helices running from the end of the nucleotide-binding domain through stalk sector 5. This domain, together with stalk sectors 2, 3 and 4, may act to transfer conformational changes from the kinase-like headpiece domains into the transmembrane segments. The series of controlled conformational changes originating in the headpiece and extending through the stalk and transmembrane segments would, in our model, be responsible for the active transport of Ca^{2+}.

Since we did not observe any typical EF hand Ca^{2+} binding sites (44), we have predicted that the amphipathic stalk regions, which contain a total of 21 acidic amino acid residues, comprise the high affinity Ca^{2+} binding sites (27). This is in agreement with the localization of the Ca^{2+} binding sites at the amino-terminus of the molecule, (45-48) and the distance between Ca^{2+} binding and nucleotide binding sites (49-50). We visualize the energy transduction process as involving rotations of the stalk segments induced by conformation changes in the globular domains (26). Rotation would carry Ca^{2+} bound on cytoplasmic sites to an interior channel formed by the stalk and transmembrane segments. At the same time it would disrupt the Ca^{2+} binding sites, freeing

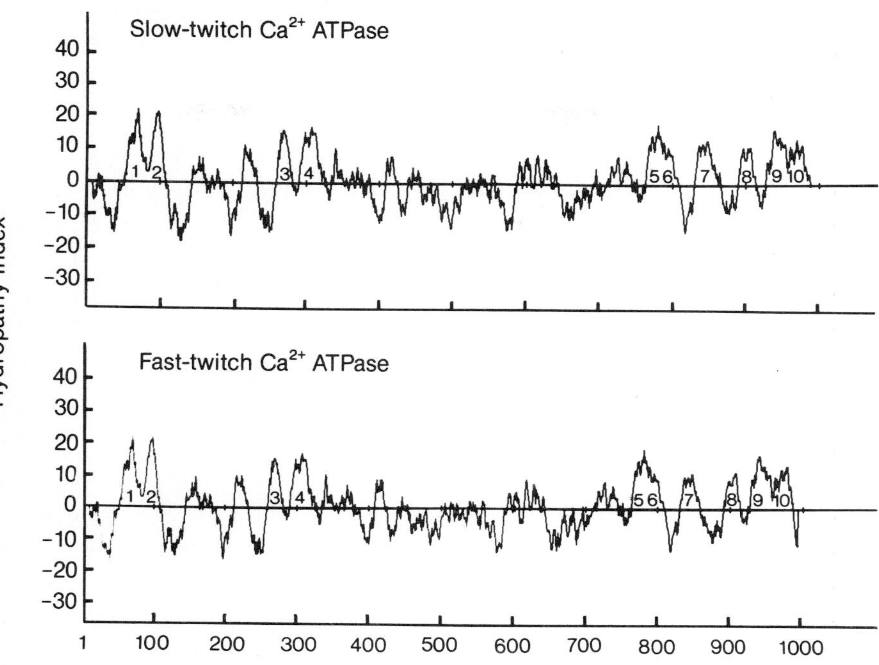

Fig. 2. Hydrophathy plots of the amino acid sequences of fast and slow-twitch/cardiac Ca^{2+} ATPases. The parameters for the analysis were those of Kyte and Doolittle (52). The hydropathy value was averaged over a window of 19 amino acid residues. Possible membrane traversing regions are numbered 1 through 10.

Ca^{2+} to move across the transmembrane channel. The localization of the Ca^{2+} binding sites among the helices of the stalk would permit slight helical rotations to bring about their re-orientation towards the lumen and their disruption (51).

From polarity and hydropathy plots (52) we have predicted that the Ca^{2+} ATPase has ten transmembrane passages (27) (Fig. 2). It is these sectors that must form the transmembranous Ca^{2+} channel. These transmembrane peptides contain approximately 25% polar amino acids which could allow translocation of Ca^{2+} through a relatively hydrophilic channel if the polar residues were aligned towards the interior of the channel. The three-dimensional folding pattern for the transmembrane segments is not yet clear. A single layer of helices surrounding a central channel, similar to bacteriorhodopsin (53), is one possibility, as is a two layer arrangement with a central core of helices lined on their outside by a second set. Blasie <u>et al.</u> (37) have observed changes in X-ray diffraction patterns of the Ca^{2+} APase induced by release of caged ATP which indicate penetration of up to 8% of the activated protein into the bilayer. The two layer structure could facilitate the penetration of the protein into the bilayer during the reaction cycle since it would provide an outer protein shell to buffer the interactions of the core helices with the hydrophobic lipid bilayer. The importance of the stalk sectors and transmembranous regions in the formation of the Ca^{2+} binding sites and the Ca^{2+} channel is evident from the fact that there is greater than 90% conservation of these regions between the two forms of Ca^{2+} ATPase (26).

The functional differences between the cardiac and fast-twitch skeletal muscle Ca^{2+} ATPase should be the result of primary sequence differences between the two forms. The amino acid differences are clustered with most of the variability at the amino-terminus, in the nucleotide and phosphorylation domains, between membranous passages 7 and 8, and at the carboxyl-terminus (Fig. 1). Variation is also more localized in regions predicted to be alpha-helices and bends as compared to beta-strands (26). The approximately 30 percent variability in the nucleotide-binding domain compares strikingly with the 5 percent variability seen in the alpha-subdomain which we believe is involved in transmitting conformational changes from the globular domains to the stalk. Variability in the nucleotide-binding domain is almost certainly reflected in changes in nucleotide specificity (54). Similarly, the other nonconserved regions will likely be linked to functional differences. Through the construction of chimaeric Ca^{2+} ATPase molecules and through site specific mutagenesis, it should be possible to locate those regions most important for creating these functional differences.

ACKNOWLEDGEMENTS
    This work was supported by grants to D.H.M. from the Heart and Stroke Foundation of Ontario, the Medical Research Council of Canada (MRCC) and the Muscular Dystrophy Association of Canada. C.J.B. was supported by a MRCC studentship. C.J.B. was supported by a MRCC studentship. The work of N.M.G was supported by the Medical Research Council (U.K.).

REFERENCES

1. Inesi, G., (1985) Ann. Rev. Physiol. 47, 573-601.
2. Suko, J., and Hasselbach, W. (1976). Eur. J. Biochem. 64, 123-130.
3. Affolter, H., Chiesi, M., Dabrowski, R., and Carafoli, E. (1976) Eur. J. Biochem. 67, 389-396.
4. Jones, L.R., and Cala, S.E. (1981) J. Biol. Chem. 256, 11809-11818.
5. Ebashi, S., Endo, M., and Ohtsuki, J., (1969) Quart. Rev. Biophys. 2, 351-384.
6. Solaro, R.J., and Briggs, F.N. (1974) Circ. Res. 34, 531-540.
7. Fabiato, A. and Fabiato, F. (1977) Circ. Res. 40, 119-129.
8. Tada, M., Yamamoto, T., and Tonomura, Y. (1978) Physiol. Rev. 58, 1-79.
9. Michalak, M. (1985) In: The Enzymes of Biological Membranes, Vol. 3 (A.N. Martonosi, ed.) Plenum Publishing Co. New York, pp. 115-155.
10. Tada, M., and Katz, A.M. (1982) Ann. Rev. Physiol. 44, 401-423.
11. Shigekawa, M., Finegan, J-A.M., and Katz, A.M. (1976) J. Biol. Chem. 251, 6894-6900.
12. Entman, M.L., Snow, T.R., Freed, D., and Schwartz, A. (1973) J. Biol. Chem. 248, 7762-7772.
13. Bick, R.J., Van Winkle, W.B., Tate, C.A., and Entman, M.L. (1983) J. Biol. Chem. 258, 4447-4452.
14. Harigaya, S. and Schwartz, A. (1969) Circulation Res. 25, 781-794.
15. Van Winkle, W.B., Pitts, B.J.R., and Entman, M.L. (1978) J. Biol. Chem. 253, 8671-8673.
16. Sumida, M., Wang, T., Mandel, F., Froehlich, J.P., and Schwartz, A. (1978) J. Biol. Chem. 253, 8772-8777.
17. Kirchberger, M.A., and Tada, M. (1976), J. Biol. Chem. 251, 725-729.
18. Heilman, C., Brdiczka, D., Nickel, E., and Pette, D. (1977) Eur. J. Biochem. 81, 211-222.
19. Schwartz, A., Entman, M.L., Kaniike, K., Lane, L.K., Van Winkle, W.B., and Bornet, E.P. (1976) Biochem. Biophys. Acta 426, 57-72.
20. Jorgensen, A.O., and Jones, L.R. (1986) J. Biol. Chem. 261, 3775-3781.
21. De Foor, P.H., Levitsky, D., Biryukova, T., and Fleischer, S. (1980) Arch. Biochem. Biophys. 200, 196-205.
22. Zubrzycka-Gaarn, E., MacDonald, G., Phillips, L., Jorgensen, A.O., and MacLennan, D.H. (1984) J. Bioenerg. Biomembr. 16, 441-464.
23. Damiani, E., Betto, R., Salvatori, S., Volpe, P., Salviati, G., and Margreth, A. (1981) Biochem. J. 197, 245-248.
24. Jorgensen, A.O., and Campbell, K.P. (1986) Biophys. J. 49, 589a.
25. Reithmeier, R.A.F., de Leon, S., and MacLennan, D.H. (1980) J. Biol. Chem. 255, 11839-11846.
26. Brandl, C.J., Green, N.M., Korczak, G., and MacLennan, D.H. (1986) Cell 44, 597-607.
27. MacLennan, D.H., Brandl, C.J., Korczak, B., and Green, N.M. (1985) Nature 316, 696-700.
28. Briggs, F.N., Cable, M.B., Geisow, M.G., and Green, N.M. (1986) Biochem. Biophys. Res. Commun. 135, 864-869.
29. Thorley-Lawson, D.A., and Green, N.M. (1973). Eur. J. Biochem. 40, 403-413.
30. Allen, G., and Green, N.M. (1976) FEBS Lett. 63, 188-192.
31. Mitchinson, C., Wilderspin, A.F., Trinnaman, B.J., and Green, N.M. (1982) FEBS Lett. 146, 87-92.
32. Ohta, T., Nagano, K., and Yoshida, M. (1986). Proc. Natl. Acad. Sci. USA. 83, 2071-2075.
33. Brandl, C.J., de Leon, S., Martin, D.R., and MacLennan, D.H. (1986) J. Biol. Chem. (submitted).

34. Melton, D.A., Krieg, P.A., Rebagliati, M.R., Maniatis, T., Zinn, K., and Green, M.R. (1984) Nucl. Acids Res. 12, 7035-7056.

35. Grantham, R., Gauthier, C., Gouy, M., Jacolzone, M., and Mercier, R. (1981). Nucl. Acids Res. 9, r43-r74.

36. Taylor, W.R., and Thornton, J.M. (1984) J. Mol. Biol. 173, 487-514.

37. Blasie, J.K., Herbette, J.G., Pascolini, D., Skita, V., Pierce, D.H., and Scarpa, A. (1985) Biophys. J. 48, 9-18.

38. Taylor, K. Dux, L., and Martonosi, A. (1984) J. Mol. Biol. 174, 193-204.

39. Dux, L., Taylor, K.A., Ting-Beall, H.P., and Martonosi, A.N. (1985) J. Biol. Chem. 260, 11730-11743.

40. Ho, M.-H., Taylor, K.A., and Martonosi, A.N. (1986) Biophys. J. 49, 570a.

41. Greaser, M.L., Cassens, R.G., Hoekstra, W.G., and Briskey, E.J. (1969) J. Cell Physiol. 74, 37-50.

42. MacLennan, D.H., and Reithmeier, R.A.F. (1985) In: Structure and Function of Sarcoplasmic Reticulum, (S. Fleischer and Y. Tonomura, ed). Academic Press, London, pp 91-100.

43. Scott, T.L., and Shamoo, A.E. (1982) J. Memb. Biol. 64, 137-144.

44. Kretsinger, R.H. (1976) Ann. Rev. Biochem. 45, 239-266.

45. Shamoo, A.E., Ryan, T.E., Stewart, P.S., and MacLennan, D.H. (1976) J. Biol. Chem. 251, 4147-4154.

46. MacLennan, D.H., Reithmeier, R.A.F., Shoshan, V., Campbell, K.P., and LeBel, D. (1980) Ann. N.Y. Acad. Sci. 358, 138-148.

47. Pick, U., and Racker, E. (1979) Biochemistry 18, 108-113.

48. Ludi, H., and Hasselbach, W. (1984) FEBS Lett. 167, 33-36.

49. Highsmith, S.R., and Scales, D. (1984) Z. Naturforsch. 39C, 177-179.

50. Scott, T.L., (1985) J. Biol. Chem. 260, 14421-14423.

51. Tanford, C. (1982) Proc. Natl. Acad. Sci. USA 79, 2882-2884.

52. Kyte, J., and Doolittle, R.F. (1982) J. Mol. Biol. 157, 105-132.

53. Henderson, R., and Unwin, P.N.T. (1975) Nature 257, 28-32.

54. Tate, C.H., Bick, R.J., Chu, A., Van Winkle, W.B., and Entman, M.L. (1985) J. Biol. Chem. 260, 9618-9623.

E. CONTRACTILE PROTEIN FUNCTIONS

18

CONTRACTILE AND REGULATORY PROTEINS IN CARDIOVASCULAR SYSTEM

S. EBASHI

National Institute for Physiological Sciences
Myodaiji, Okazaki, Japan

INTRODUCTION

The contractile proteins of cardiac muscle are distinct
from those of fast white skeletal muscle, but akin to those
of slow red one. This indicates that marked functional
differences between cardiac and skeletal muscles mainly reside
in the neural control and the excitable membrane. Even so,
comparative studies on contractile proteins will provide us
with some important informations necessary for a thorough
understanding of cardiac muscle functions.

In 1976 Kitazawa (1) presented an important paper from
physiological points of view on cardiac muscle. The main aim
of his paper was to make it clear that the contraction-
relaxation cycle of cardiac muscle is chiefly controlled by
the sarcoplasmic reticulum, not by mitochondria. Incidentally,
two other remarkable facts were noted in this paper. One is
that cardiac and slow skeletal glycerinated fibers exhibit
higher sensitivities to Sr^{2+}.

Already in 1927, Ono (2) had shown that cardiac muscle
retained its rhythmical contractility for a long time in the
bathing solution in which Ca^{2+} is replaced by Sr^{2+}. Since
smooth muscle soon loses its contractility in a similar medium,
keeping its electrical activity (3), it is quite probable that
Sr^{2+} can support the contractility of cardiac system as does
Ca^{2+}. The result of Kitazawa has given a concrete basis for
the classical observation. From the molecular viewpoints,
however, the matter is not so simple and has required further
investigation, which will be described later.

Another notable fact is that while the tension developed

by fast skeletal muscle reaches plateau at around 10^{-5}M Ca^{2+}, that by cardiac muscle is still increasing with increase in the Ca^{2+} concentration beyond 10^{-5}M. This is rather reasonable because every twitch in skeletal muscle has to attain maximally activated state, whereas the physiological contraction in the heart is carried out at Ca^{2+} concentrations far lower than those to produce maximum contraction. Consequently, there must be some device corresponding to this difference in function. In this connection, the interaction of two troponin subunits, troponin T and troponin C, was proposed as the candidate to explain this difference (4). This explanation will find a further justification in this article.

In addition to the above a brief reference will be made to the regulatory mechanism of vascular smooth muscle. Attention will be paid on its distinct point from that of visceral smooth muscle.

RESULTS AND DISCUSSION

Sr^{2+} sensitivity of cardiac contractile system

Prior to the observations with glycerinated fibers (1) (Fig. 1), the sensitivities of natural actomyosin or myosin B

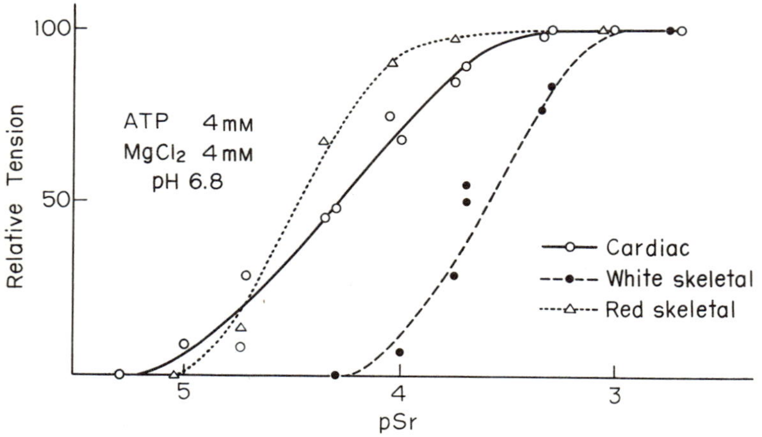

Fig. 1 Relationships between Sr^{2+} concentrations and tensions developed by glycerinated cardiac, fast white skeletal and slow red skeletal muscle fibers [quoted from Kitazawa (1)]

to alkaline earth metal ions were studied using superprecipitation as the index of in vitro contraction (5) (Table 1).

Table 1. Sensitivities of various myosin B (natural actomyosin)
preparations to alkaline-earth metal ions

	Sensitivities (relative to Ca^{2+})	
	Sr^{2+}	Ba^{2+}
Fast white skeletal (rabbit)	1/34	<1/600
Slow red skeletal (rabbit)	1/7	1/250
Cardiac (bovine)	1/5	1/32
Gizzard (chicken)	1/20	1/210
Aortic (bovine)	1/22	<1/200

The reciprocal ratio of the concentration of Sr^{2+} or Ba^{2+} to
that of Ca^{2+}, the concentration which induces the same degree
of superprecipitation, was considered as the sensitivity of
the actomyosin system to Sr^{2+} or Ba^{2+}, respectively. In the
above case, $9 \times 10^{-7}MCa^{2+}$ was adopted as the reference.

Thus the high sensitivity of cardiac muscle to Sr^{2+} seemed to
be well demonstrated on the molecular level. Interestingly,
smooth muscle system is rather close to white skeletal muscle,
and as expected, the cardiac system, which is very sensitive
to Sr^{2+} compared with other two kinds of muscle, is also
sensitive to Ba^{2+}.

As a whole, it appeared as if the matter were finally
settled. Berson (6) showed, however, that such a remarkable
difference could not be observed if the actomyosin ATPase
activity was used as the index of in vitro contraction.

In the meantime, Kohama was working on the divalent
cation binding to troponins, especially cardiac troponin.
Unexpectedly, he found no difference in the Sr^{2+} concentration
to produce half saturation of Sr^{2+} binding (7)(Fig. 2). He

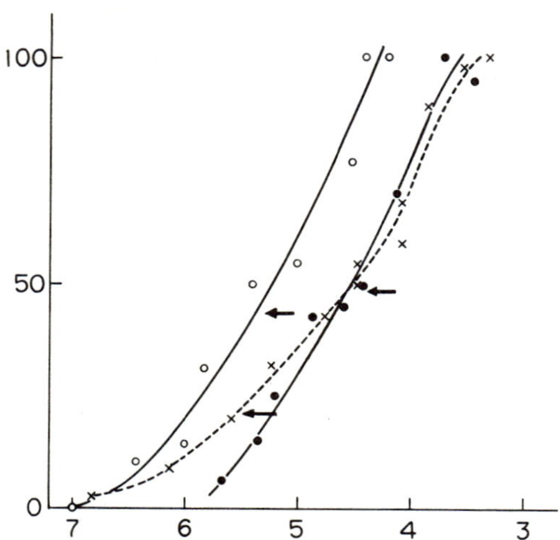

Fig. 2   Relationships between pSr^{2+} and Sr^{2+} binding to
troponins derived from cardiac (x), fast white skeletal (●)
and slow red skeletal (O) muscles.
Arrows indicate the threshold concentrations derived from Fig.
1 [for other details, see Kohama (7); quoted from Kohama (7)].

wondered if troponin in the isolated state might not be
different from that situated in the myofilament. The result
under the latter condition was, however, the same as that in
the former one. This compelled him to work on Sr^{2+} sensitivity
of actomyosin ATPase activities and the result was essentially
the same as that of Berson (6). The overall results obtained
by him and his collaborators are listed in Table 2, of which
the data include also those derived from other laboratories.

Now a definite tendency has emerged. Although no
difference can be detected in half maximum Sr^{2+} binding, a
little difference is noticed in the case of the ATPase
activities. This difference becomes more notable in the case
of superprecipitation and most remarkable in glycerinated
fibers. If we compare the profiles of the curves for the
tension and the ATPase activity, it is clear that at relatively
low Sr^{2+} concentrations, tension does not develop in spite of
considerable sizes of ATPase activities.

Table 2. Sr^{2+} sensitivities of various actomyosin systems

	Ratios of Sr^{2+} sensitivities of cardiac system to those of skeletal system[a]
Glycerinated fibers	4.1 (1) 5.9[b] (1)

Superprecipitation
  natural actomyosin
 	
  desensitized actomyosin
   with native tropomyosin
	7[b] (5)
	3.0 (8, 10)
	5.7[b] (5)

ATPase
  desensitized actomyosin
   with native tropomyosin
 	
  natural actomyosin
 	
  desensitized actomyosin
   with tropomyosin and
   reconstituted troponin
	1.6 (6)
	
	2.0 (8, 10)
	
	2.9 (9)

Sr^{2+} binding to troponin
  troponin alone
  troponin bound to
   desensitized actomyosin
	1.0 (7)
	1.0 (10)

Figures in parentheses indicate the number of references.
a) Sr^{2+} concentrations to give half maximum activities were compared, unless otherwise stated.
b) Sr^{2+} concentrations to give 30% of maximum activities were compared.

Since the result with Sr^{2+} should be the matter with Ca^{2+}, it is now clear that in the range of low Ca^{2+} concentrations, where some actin-myosin-ATP interaction certainly exists, the energy derived from ATP breakdown cannot be converted to contraction. Superprecipitation behaves essentially in the same way as the tension development of glycerinated fibers.

There is no doubt that actomyosin ATPase activity is the fundamental process underlying muscle contraction, but if the matter is concerned with the event in living muscle, superprecipitation is more akin to the physiological contraction,

being a better in vitro model for contraction. This is
particularly so in dealing with such a complicated phenomenon
as regulatory mechanism.

A question then arises why such a discrepancy could take
place. The difference between Sr^{2+} binding and the ATPase
activity can be partially explained, if we assume that the high
affinity sites of troponin be mainly utilized for the ATPase
activity; at lower Sr^{2+} (and Ca^{2+}) concentration, cardiac
troponin shows significantly higher affinity than skeletal
troponin. This may partly explain the difference between the
Sr binding and the ATPase activity, but not the remarkable
discrepancy between the ATPase activity and the contraction.

The fact that some ATPase is not expressed as contraction
but dissipated as the heat, is not a new thing but has already
been noticed by many researchers. Famous Solandt's effect(11)
may be considered as the first indication of this phenomenon.

A schematic illustration to represent the relationship
among contraction, superprecipitation, ATPase and Ca binding
is presented in Fig. 3.

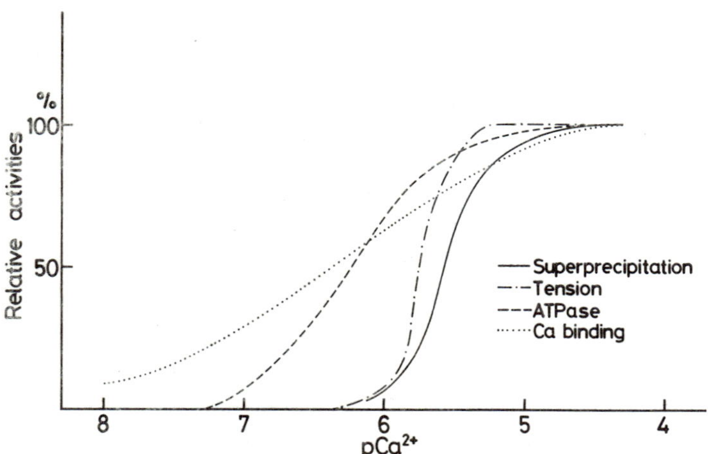

Fig. 3 Schematic illustration of relationships in skeletal
muscle systems between Ca^{2+} concentrations and tensions
developed by glycerinated fibers, superprecipitation of natural
actomyosin, its ATPase activities or Ca binding to troponin.

In this connection it is worthy of note that in the presence of some agent like quercetin, the tension development at lower Ca^{2+} concentrations is enhanced and as a result the profile of its relation to Ca^{2+} concentrations becomes very much like that of the ATPase activity (12); no change in the Ca^{2+} binding is observed and the ATPase activity is rather repressed (Y. Ogawa, personal communication). To be more interesting, the velocity of tension development is elevated in all the range of Ca concentrations (12).

We are apt to think that higher the activity is, the more akin to living state. As indicated above, however, there is a remarkable gap between Ca^{2+} binding or ATPase activity and the real contraction. This means that in the native state a kind of negative control is exerted on the contractile system and some amount of energy is dissipated apparently in vain. It is of profound interest whether such a waste indicates an incompleteness of the natural device, or it has a substantial importance to the physiological regulation of the contractile system.

Lack of inhibitory mechanism at high Ca^{2+} concentrations in cardiac muscle

The relationship between the Ca^{2+} concentration and the tension development shown in Fig. 4 is a modification of a

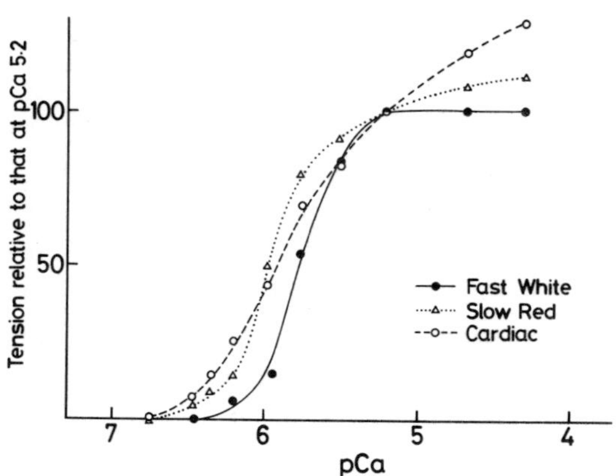

Fig. 4 Relationships between Ca^{2+} concentrations and tensions developed by glycerinated cardiac, fast white skeletal, slow red skeletal muscles, relative to those at 5×10^{-5} M Ca $^{2+}$, respectively.
This figure was derived from Fig. 11 in the paper of Kitazawa (1)

figure presented in Kitazawa's paper (Fig. 11 in ref. (1)).
It is notable that the contraction of fast white skeletal
muscle reaches maximum around $5 \times 10^{-6}M$ Ca^{2+} and then forms a
plateau in spite of the increase in Ca^{2+} concentrations. Since
it is probable that low affinity sites for Ca^{2+} play a major
role in muscle contraction (but high affinity sites undoubtedly
participate in the activation of the actomyosin ATPase at low
Ca^{2+} concentrations where tension does not develop; in cardiac
muscle, the role of the high affinity site may be more important
(13)), there must be some mechanism to repress further tension
development. It has been asserted that the interaction of
troponin T and troponin C is responsible for this mechanism
based on the observations with the eight hybrid troponins
composed of either cardiac or skeletal troponin subunits (14);
the troponin T-troponin C interaction opposes the activating
interaction of troponin C and troponin I.

The excellent paper of Yamamoto (9) has made it possible
to compare the maximum ATPase activities of hybrid troponins
with the interactions of subunits. The result is summarized
in Table 3. It is concluded that maximum ATPase activities
are related to the Ca^{2+} dependent interactions of troponin I
and troponin C and inversely related to that of troponin T and
troponin C (the data listed are still semiquantitative; this
should become more quantitative if the information about the
interaction of troponin I and troponin T is furnished).

Now we can more definitely state that cardiac muscle
virtually lacks the mechanism to protect myofilaments from
their decomposition due to vigorous contraction. There is a
plenty of circumstantial evidence that the thin filament is
liable to be decomposed by its interaction with myosin (F.
Oosawa, personal communication). The contractile system of
skeletal muscle is always activated to a full extent, so that
without a self-defense system such as the interaction of troponin
T and troponin C, the thin filament should have been destroyed.
Since cardiac muscle operates at low Ca^{2+} concentrations under
physiological conditions, there may be no necessity for such a
self-defense system, but in pathological conditions where Ca^{2+}

concentration can reach much higher values, the matter should be serious because of the lack of such protecting mechanism. The stiffness of skeletal muscle is our daily events, but that of cardiac muscle perhaps means the death of the tissue.

Table 3. Actomyosin ATPase activity in relation to the troponin T - troponin C interaction and the troponin C - troponin I interaction.

Origins of muscle from which troponin subunits were derived			Degrees of T-C inter-actions (a) (inhibiting)	Degrees of C-I inter-actions (b) (activating)	Maximum ATPase activities expected from a and b	Actual maximum ATPase activities
T	C	I				
c	c	c	C	B	B	114
c	s	s	C	A	A	153
s	s	c	A	C	D	73
s	s	s	A	A	C	(100)

s: skeletal origin   c: cardiac origin   T,C and I: troponin T, C and I
A,B,C and D: the grades of respective activities in the order from A to D (the quantitative aspects of the ATPase activities were derived from ref. 9).
Expected maximum ATPase activities were estimated under the assumption that the ATPase activity was mainly dependent on the C-I interaction, but that the T-C interaction counteracts the C-I interaction repressing the maximum ATPase activity (i.e., the maximum ATPase should be something like b divided by a). As a result a good correlation between expected and actual ATPase activities was demonstrated.

Ca^{2+} regulation in vascular smooth muscle

It has been claimed by many researchers that the Ca^{2+} regulation in smooth muscle is carried out by a Ca^{2+} dependent myosin light chain kinase (MLCK) and a phosphatase specific for the dephosphorylation (15, 16, 17). In addition to this, many subsidiary factors have been reported.

Our research group has quite a distinct opinion from this. An actin-linked factor, called leiotonin, is responsible for the activation of actomyosin system of smooth muscle. We once believed that we had obtained pure leiotonin (18), but it was

later found to be a proteolytic product. Search for the
original leiotonin has reached a preliminary result that
leiotonin is a protein physicochemically akin to MLCK (19).

Since it is certain that the protein isolated as MLCK has
an activating effect on the actin-myosin ATP interaction as
MLCK group asserts, the investigation whether or not this
protein fraction exerts its effect through MLCK activities was
carried out. The protein fraction prepared from bovine stomach
by the routine method of our laboratory (20) was the main
material of this research. It should be emphasized that in
all the experiments natural actomyosin or its desensitized
actomyosin was used; reconstituted actomyosin composed of
separately purified myosin and actin does not necessarily give
rise to the following results: a) Two kinds of fractions,
155K and 130K daltons in their molecular weights, respectively,
exhibiting MLCK activities (MLCK) as well as actomyosin-
activating effect (AMA), are obtained (cf. Fig. 6); b) The
ratio of AMA to MLCK is very high in 155K protein; it is more
than 10 times that of 130K (cf. Fig. 6); c) If 155K protein is
treated with a low concentration of trypsin, almost all AMA is
lost, retaining more than 80% of MLCK (21); d) Some of
polyclonal antibodies and one monoclonal antibody against 130K
gizzard protein, represses AMA, without affecting MLCK
activity (21); e) At pH 8, MLCK falls to less than 20% of that
at pH 6.8, retaining AMA almost intact (21); f) Suppression by
NEM is more marked on MLCK than on AMA (this has confirmed the
result with gizzard crude leiotonin (22)); g) Michaelis
constants for AMA and MLCK of bovine stomach actomyosin systems,
viz., desensitized actomyosin plus 155K protein or natural
actomyosin, are about 10μM and more than 0.5mM, respectively;
at 50μM, almost full AMA with a trace of MLCK (Fig. 5).

Thus it appears more definite that the actomyosin-activating
effect of 155K fraction is not exerted through MLCK activity
but some other mechanism, which has remained to be solved.

Although the studies on vascular smooth muscle are still on
a preliminary stage, the results so far obtained with bovine
aorta (Fig. 6) are essentially the same as those with bovine

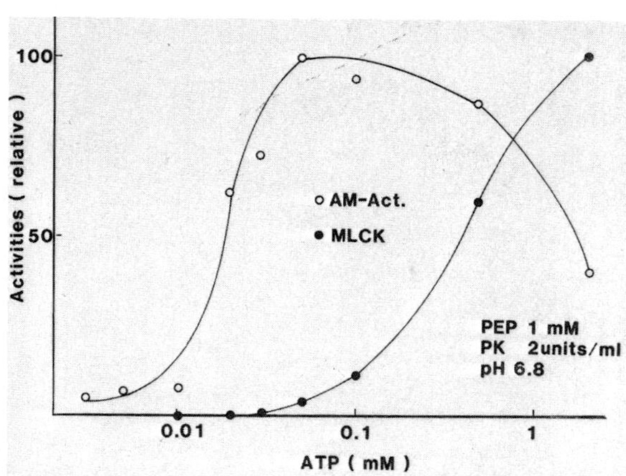

Fig. 5   Relationships between ATP concentrations and activities of AMA (superprecipitation) and MLCK of bovine stomach natural actomyosin.   Crude leiotonin fraction (the fraction between 20 and 28 g ammonium sulfate per 100 ml of bovine stomach extract) was assayed by desensitized gizzard actomyosin (quoted from ref. 20).

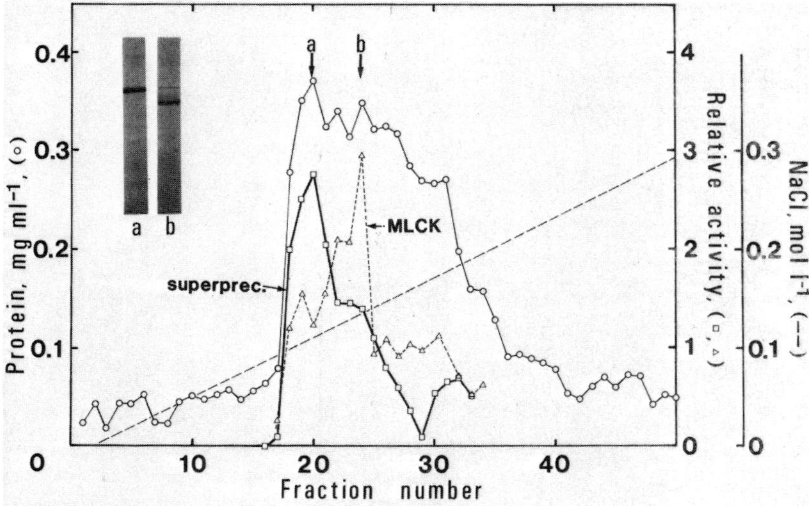

Fig. 6   Elution pattern of DEAE cellulose (DE 32) chromatography of bovine aorta extract.
This followed the procedures used for bovine stomach extract.   Ratios of AMA/MLCK of fraction number 20 is more than 10 times as that of the number 29.   The difference between stomach and aorta is that the MLCK elution pattern assumes a wide plateau in stomach, but a rather sharp peak in aorta (quoted from ref. 20).

stomach (cf. Ebashi, in press). Notable points of aorta
smooth muscle is that its 130K component has a slightly larger
molecular weight and a considerably lower AMA/MLA ratio than
does the corresponding bovine stomach component.

Thus the research of smooth muscle regulation is still
on a preliminary stage. The concept that it is mainly
operated by MLCK has not yet attained full credit. Further
penetrating studies are urgently needed.

SUMMARY

Some properties of cardiac contractile system distinct
from those of fast white skeletal muscle were noted and
discussed.

One of such properties is its high sensitivities to Sr^{2+}.
Investigation into this property has incidentally revealed the
discrepancy between the actomyosin ATPase activity and the
contraction of glycerinated fibers; the latter is far more
sensitive to Sr^{2+} than is the latter. The result with
superprecipitation is close to that with glycerinated fibers,
indicating that superprecipitation is an <u>in vitro</u> index for
contraction more akin to living muscle than is the ATPase
activity. The presence of an inhibitory control in converting
the energy of ATP to contraction under physiological
conditions is pointed out.

Another property is virtual lack in the cardiac system of
the mechanism to prevent the muscle from excess contraction at
higher Ca^{2+} concentration; this mechanism is based on the Ca-
dependent interaction of troponin T and troponin C and is
pronounced in fast white skeletal muscle.

The mechanism of Ca^{2+} regulation in vascular smooth muscle
is not essentially different from that in visceral smooth
muscle.   In any case, its contraction is controlled by a
factor(s), of which the function is not mediated by myosin
light chain kinase action.

291

REFERENCES

1. Kitazawa, T. J. Biochem. 80: 1129-1147, 1976.
2. Ono, R. Fol. Pharmacol. Jap. 4: 389-411, 1927.
3. Hotta, Y. and Tsukui, R. Nature 217: 867-869, 1968.
4. Ebashi, S. J. Mol. Cell. Cardiol. 16: 129-136, 1984.
5. Ebashi, S., Kodama, A. and Ebashi, F. J. Biochem. 64: 465-477, 1968.
6. Berson, G. In: Calcium Binding Proteins (Eds. W. Drabikowski, H. Strzelecka-Golaszewska and E. Carafoli), PWN-Polish Scientific, Warszawa, 1974, pp. 197-201.
7. Kohama, K. J. Biochem. 86: 811-820, 1979.
8. Ebashi, S., Nonomura, Y., Kohama, K., Kitazawa, T. and Mikawa, T. In: Molecular Biology Biochemistry and Biophysics, 32 Chemical Recognition in Biology (Eds. F. Chapeville and H.-L. Haenni), Springer-Verlag, Berlin, Heidelberg, 1980, pp. 183-194.
9. Yamamoto, K. (1983) J. Biochem. 93: 1061-1069, 1983.
10. Kohama, K., Saida, K., Hirata, M., Kitaura, T. and Ebashi, S. Jap. J. Pharmacol. in press
11. Solandt, D.Y. J. Physiol. 86: 162-170, 1936.
12. Kurebayashi, N. and Ogawa, Y. J. Mus. Res. Cell. Motil. 6: 189-196, 1985.
13. Kohama, K. J. Biochem. 88: 591-599, 1980.
14. Ebashi, S. In: Lipmann Symposium, Energy, Biosynthesis and Regulation in Molecular Biology (Ed. D. Richter), Walter de Gryter, Berlin, New York, 1974, pp. 165-178.
15. Bruemel, R.D., Sobieszek, A., and Small, J.V. In: The Biochemistry of smooth muscle (Ed. N.L. Stephens), University Park Press, Baltimore, 1977, pp. 413-443. (in this article Sobieszek and Small first presented the MLCK concept).
16. Hartshorne, D.J., and Siemankowski, R.F. An. Rev. Physiol. 43: 519-530, 1981.
17. Stephens, N.L. (Ed.), Smooth Muscle Contraction. Marcell Dekker, Inc., New York, 1984.
18. Mikawa, T., Toyo-oka, T., Nonomura, Y. and Ebashi, S. J. Biochem. 81: 273-275, 1977.
19. Ebashi, S. and Nonomura, Y. In: Calcium Regulation in Biological Systems (Eds. S. Ebashi et al.), Academic Press, New York, 1984, pp. 59-69.
20. Kuwayama, H., Suzuki, M., Koga, R. and Ebashi, S. Submitted to J. Biochem.
21. Ebashi, S., Koga, R., Suzuki, M and Ishizaki, Y. Submitted to J. Biochem.
22. Ebashi, S. and Nakasone, H. Proc. Japan Acad. 57: 217-221, 1981.

19

DISTRIBUTION OF CARDIAC MYOSIN ISOZYMES IN HUMAN AND RAT
HEART-IMMUNOHISTOCHEMICAL STUDY USING MONOCLONAL ANTIBODIES

Y. YAZAKI[*], Y. KIRA[**] and Y. ITO[***]

[*]The Third and [**]Fourth Department of Internal Medicine,
The University of TOKYO, [***]Sanraku Hospital, TOKYO, Japan, 101.

INTRODUCTION

Recent studies using enzymatic(1-7), electrophoretic(8-14) and immunohistochemical(15-21) analysis have demonstrated the existence of 2 distinct cardiac myosin heavy chains, $HC\alpha$ and $HC\beta$. It has also been shown that cardiac ventricular myosins are composed of 3 different isozymes designated as V_1, V_2 and V_3. V_1 and V_3 correspond to homo-dimers of $HC\alpha$ and $HC\beta$, respectively, while V_2 is a heterodimers of $HC\alpha$ and $HC\beta$. V_1 has higher Ca^{2+}- and actin-activated ATPase activity than V_3, while V_3 generates force more efficiently than V_1. However these studies have been restricted to ventricular myosin and also mainly to experimental animals until recently because of technical difficulties.

This paper consists of 2 parts. Part 1 is the results on human hearts concerning the distribution and its changes of $HC\alpha$ and $HC\beta$ not only in ventricle but also in atrium and in conduction system by means of immunohistochemical technic using monoclonal antibodies. Part 2 consists of the redistribution of myosin isozymes in right and left ventricles of monocrotaline-induced right ventricular hypertrophy in rats.

MATERIALS AND METHODS

Human cardiac specimens were obtained at autopsy from 5 subjects without heart diseases within 3hr after death and by biopsy during cardiac surgery from 30 subjects suffering from various cardiac diseases consisting of valvular heart diseases and ischemic heart disease. Cardiac catheterization had been performed in all these patients within 4 wk prior to cardiac surgery.

Monoclonal antibodies specific for $HC\alpha$ or $HC\beta$ were obtained from cloned hybridomas as previously reported (19). In brief, myosins used as $HC\beta$ or $HC\alpha$ antigen were obtained from human ventricles and bovine atria by a dilution technic. Hybridomas producing anti-myosin antibo-dies were obtained essentially according to the protocol of Köhler and Milstein (22). Anti-myosin activity in the medium from hybridoma colonies was screened by enzyme-linked immunosorbent assay (ELISA) (23). Two colonies (CMA 19 and HMC 14) of hybrid cells secreting anti-myosin antibodies were selcted for discriminating the antigenic difference between $HC\alpha$ and $HC\beta$. For indirect immunofluorescence, cryostat sections were first incubated with anti-myosin antibodies and then stained according to the usual method. Purification of myosins by affinity chromatography using CMA 19 for $HC\alpha$ or HMC 50 for $HC\beta$, transfer of myosins to nitrocellulose sheets, immunological staining, preparative electrophoretic elution and proteolytic digestion of myosin heavy chains in the experiment to determine the characteristics of myosin heavy chain, $HC\alpha$ and $HC\beta$, of canine hearts were reported previously (24).

For the monocrotaline experiment, male Sprague-Dawley young adult rats (body weight ca. 200g) were used. Rats were killed at 1, 2,3, 4 and 6 week after one subcutaneous injection of monocrotaline 40 mg/kg, respectively and compared with corresponding control rats. Each group consisted of 5 to 9 rats. The pressures of both ventricles were measured before kill. The hearts were removed atria and separated into free walls of left and right ventricle and inter-ventricular septum and these 3 specimens were weighed. The polyacryl-amide gel electrophoresis with pyrophosphate buffer was carried out on each specimen as usual. The serum thyroxine levels in some rats were also measured by radioimmunoassay. The non-paired Student's t-test was used for statistical analysis.

RESULTS

Part 1. Human Study

In the ELISA test, monoclonal antibody CMA 19 reacted with human atrial myosin specifically and HMC 14 selectively reacted with human ventricular myosin as reported previously (19). They showed no reaction with light chains. The negligible reaction between CMA 19 and ventricular myosin and the reduced amount of cross-reactivity between HMC 14 and atrial myosin were explained by the presence of a very small amount of atrial type myosin in the ventricle and significant amount of ventricular type myosin in the atrium, respectively. Then we used CMA 19 as a monoclonal antibody specific for $HC\alpha$ and HMC 14 as a monoclonal antibody specific for $HC\beta$, respectively.

The staining pattern of normal human ventricular myofibers was quite different from that of atrium in the immunofluorescence study using CMA 19 and HMC 14 (Fig. 1). All myofibers of ventricle were stained strongly and homogeneously with HMC 14 (Fig. 1A), whereas only a small numbers of them were labeled with CMA 19 (Fig. 1B). On the other hand, only moderate numbers of atrial myofibers were stained with HMC 14. It was noteworthy that the staining intensity of labeled myofibers was highly variable and divided into at least 4 grades, namely strongly positive (a), positive (b) and "pseudonegative" (c) or "completely negative" (d) (Fig. 1C), while almost all atrial myofibers were strongly stained with CMA 19 (Fig. 1D)

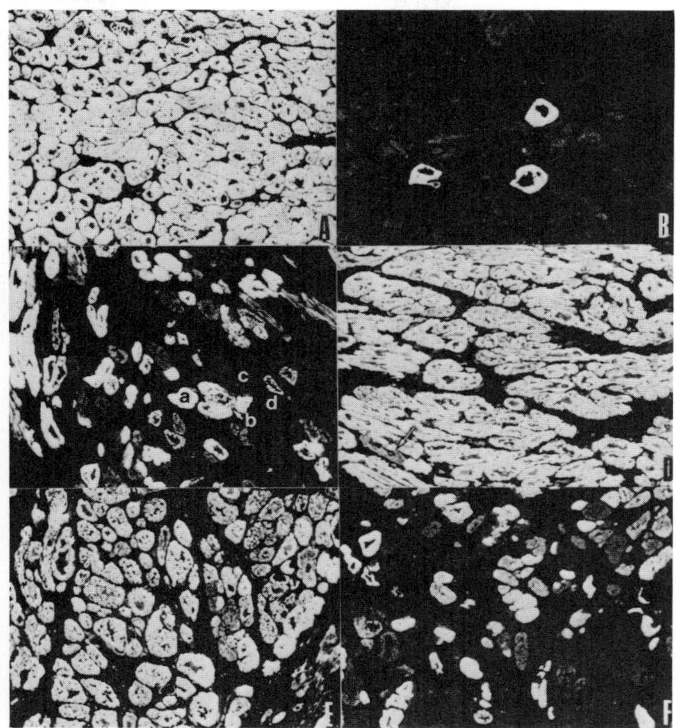

Fig. 1. Cryostat section of normal human ventricle stained by HMC 14
(A) and by CMA 19 (B). Cryostat section of normal human atrium
stained by HMC 14 (C) and by CMA 19 (D). Cryostat section of a
pressure-overloaded atrium stained by HMC 14 (E) and by CMA 19 (F).
Specimen was obtained from a patient with mitral stenosis and regurgitation. See text. Arrow in D indicates a myofiber, which shows a
weak reaction with CMA 19 (Reprinted with permission from ref. 19)

In the next step, we investigated left atrial appendages of
mitral valvular heart diseases obtained by biopsy during cardiac
surgery. In these pressure overloaded left atria, there was the
marked increase of HCβ-containing myofibers (Fig. 1E) concomitant with
the marked decrease in HCα-containing myofibers (Fig. 1F). This
figure showed a sharp contrast with that of normal atrium (Fig. 1C and D).

To quantify the changes in the amount of HCα- or HCβ-containing
myofibers of atria more clearly, we counted the number of myofibers,
which reacted with CMA 19 or HMC 14 in various valvular heart diseases
and ischemic heart disease. We graded the staining patterns into 4
classes above mentioned and scored as 1, 0.5 and 0 for (a), (b) and

(c) or (d), respectively. Then the total scores of HCα- or HCβ-
containing myofibers were calculated per 1,000 myofibers in 10 left
atria and 20 right atria. Each total score per 1,000 myofibers was
plotted against respective mean atrial pressure or mean pulmonary
wedge pressure. The total score of HCα per 1,000 myofibers had significant negative correlation with mean presures (r=-0.75, p<0.01),
while that of HCβ correlated positively with mean pressures (r=0.78,
p<0.01). Thus it was indicated that the decrease of HCα concomitant
with the increase of HCβ occured according to the elevation of
pressure in atria (Fig. 2).

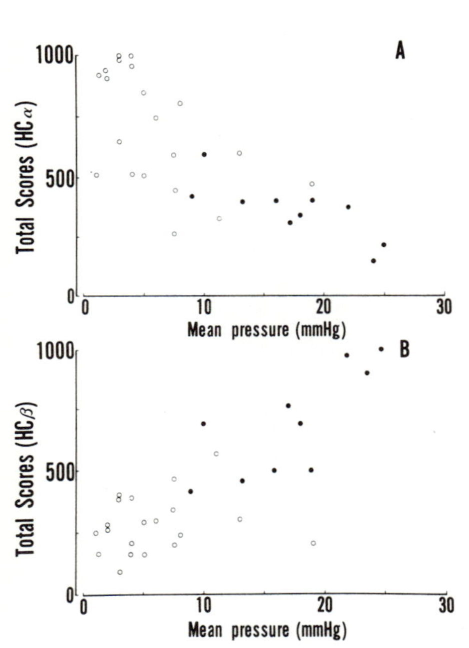

Fig. 2.
The total scores per
1,000 myofibers of HCα
(A) or HCβ(B) plotted
against the mean atrial
or pulmonary wedge
pressures
○ right atrium
● left atrium
(Reprinted with per-
mission from ref. 19)

Then we studied the regional distribution of CMA 19-labeled
myosin, namely HCα-containing myofibers in normal human ventricle.
The amount of myofibers containing HCα was greater in the subepicardial region and the central portion of the interventricular septum (10
– 15% of myofibers) than in the subendocardial region, where few HCα
-containing myofibers (0 – 2% of myofibers) were found. This distri-

bution pattern was similar in both ventricles. The papillary muscles
also showed similar regional variation of lesser degree to that of
interventricular septum.

We calculated the total scores of HCα per 1,000 myofibers in 27
left ventricular papillary muscles obtained during mitral valve
replacement as mentioned above and plotted against left ventricular
systolic pressures. There was a significant negative correlation between them (r=-0.67, p<0.01), namely HCα-containing fibers in left
ventricular papillary muscles diminished with the increase of pressure
load. It was noticed that HCα-containing fibers were hardly found in
the papillary muscles of left vevntricles when systolic pressure
exceeded 170 mmHg. On the other hand, there were no significant
correlations betweeen the total scores of HCα per 1,000 myofibers in
papillary muscles and endodiastolic volumes or ejection fractions of
left ventricles, which were measured by left ventriculography or echocardiography.

It is interesting to make clear whether HCα and HCβ found in
atria by this study have the same characteristics as HCα and HCβ present in ventricles, respectively. We isolated 2 purified myosin heavy
chain isozymes from canine atria by affinity chromatography using the
monoclonal antibodies, CMA 19 and HMC 50, specific for HCα and HCβ,
respectively and compared the characteristics with those of ventricular HCα and HCβ. One-dimentional gel analysis of partial α-chymotryptic
digests of myosin isozymes showed that the peptide maps
of HCαs from atrium and ventricle were indistinguishable as previous
reports (12, 14, 17). The peptide maps of HCβs from atrium and
ventricle were also very similar. There were definite differences
between the peptide maps of HCα and HCβ. It was demonstrated that HCα
and HCβ possessed several common specific peptides, respectively (Fig.3).
Also in 2 dimentional gel analysis of peptides produced by complete
cyanogen bromide digestion, the peptide map of HCβ from atrium was
very similar to that of HCβ from ventricle, if not indential, while
the map of HCα from atrium was clearly different from those of HCβs
from atrium and ventricle (24). Furthermore the Ca^{2+}-activated ATPase
activities of both HCαs from atrium and ventricle were above 2 times
higher than those of both HCβs from them, although the K$^+$-EDTA-activated
ATPase activities of HCα and HCβ showed no difference (24).

The human conduction system was investigated in the autopsy
materials, since it has not been elucidated precisely, while a few
data were reported in animals (16, 25).

All myofibers of sinus node cells were strongly stained by anti
HCα, CMA 19, whereas a very small proportion of them were reacted with
anti HCβ, HMC 14. In the A-V node, all myofibers were labeled with
anti HCβ homogenously. The staining patterns with anti HCα were

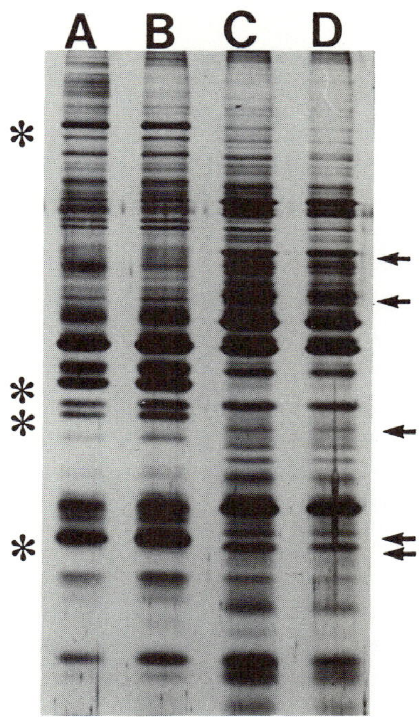

Fig. 3.
One-dimentional gel ana-
lysis of partial chy-
motryptic digests of
myosin isozymes.
Affinity-purified myosin
isozymes, ventricular HCα
(A), atrial HCα (B),
atrial HCβ (C) and
ventricular HCβ (D), were
cleaved with
α-chymotrypsin at a myosin
to protease ratio of 4 :
1 for 30 min and
electrophoresed at a 10
mA constant current for
12 hr.
The asterisks and arrows
indicate HCα-specific and
HCβ-specific peptides,
respectively. (Reprinted
with permission from ref.
24)

variable, namely all myofibers in the central portion and in the transitional zone to atrial myocardium were stained homogeneously with
anti HCα, but that of the transitional zone to the bundle of His
showed a decreased number of cells stained by anti HCα. As to the
bundle of His and bundle branches, all fibers were stained by anti HCβ
homogeneously and a considerable proportion of myofibers also were
stained by anti HCα in variable intensities. The Purkinje fibers contained moderate amount of HCα (Fig. 4A) besides HCβ (Fig. 4B). This
staining pattern showed a great contrast to the ordinary working
myocardial cells in the subendocardial region, which were stained
exclusively with anti HCβ (Fig. 4A,B).

Table 1 indicates the summary of the distribution of HCα and HCβ
in normal human heart. In the atrium, all myofibers contained HCα and
20 - 60% of the myofibers in the auricle had HCβ, while almost all
myofibers in the crista terminalis and the lower portion of the
interatrial septum were labeled by HCβ antibody. In the ventricle, HCβ
was distributed throughout the myocardium. As to HCα, up to 15% of

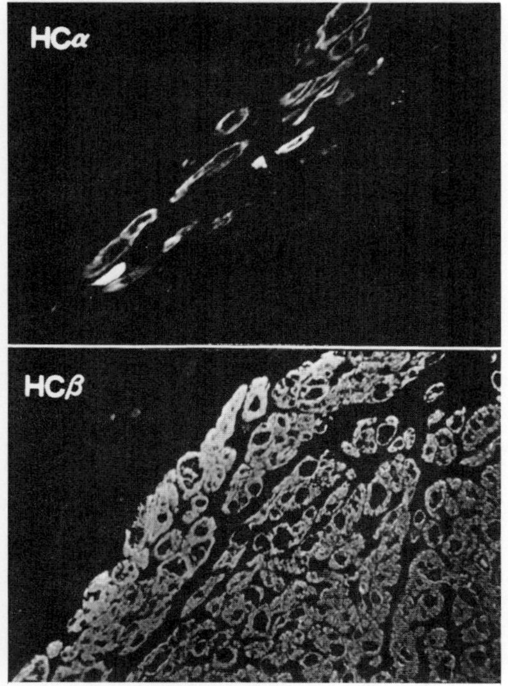

Fig. 4.
Cryostat sections of Purkinje fibers and ventricular myocardium.
Upper: stained with CMA 19
Lower: stained with HMC 14
Note the different staining patterns of Purkinje fibers and ordinary working myocardial cells by CMA 19 and HMC 14 (Reprinted with permission from ref. 26)

myofibers in the subepicardial region had HCα, while the subendocardial myocardial fibers contained few HCα. Concerning conduction system, almost all cells of sinus node contained HCα and decrease in HCα content with corresponding increase of HCβ occured in the lower conduction system, in roughly parallel with the decreasing rate of electrical automaticity.

Table 1. Distribution of isoforms of myosin heavy chain in human cardiac muscle   *Mean±SD n=5

Fiber type	CMA 19-reactive myofibers (%)	HMC 14-reactive myofibers (%)
Sinus node	100	4.7 ± 1.8*
Atrium	100	20 - 100
AV node	100	100
Bundle of His		
Bundle branches	55.2 ± 10.2*	100
Purkinje fibers		
Ventricle	0 - 15	100

(Reprinted with permission from ref. 26)

Part 2. Monocrotaline Experiment

The monocrotaline-induced pulmonary hypertensive rats showed the marked elevation of right ventricular systolic pressure along with the definite increase of weight ratio of right ventricular free wall to whole ventricle. The increases of the 2 parameters became significant at 2 wk reaching to almost maximal value 4 wk after monocrotaline injection (Fig. 5). On the other hand, those of left ventricle did not show any significant difference from the control rats.

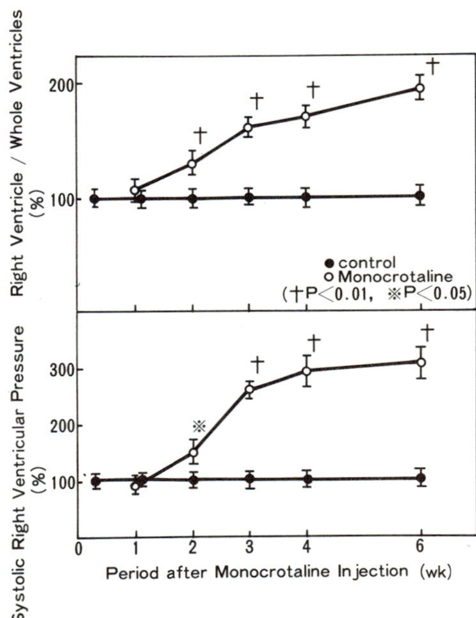

Fig. 5.
Changes of weight ratio of right ventricular free wall to whole ventricle (top) and right ventricular systolic pressure (bottom) in rats after monocrotaline injection. The figures are expressed in percentage to the corresponding control values, which are regarded as 100%.
● Control
○ monocrotaline
● mean ± S.E.

In the study of polyacrylamide gel electorophoresis with pyrophosphate buffer, it was demonstrated that myosin isozyme V_1 decreased not only in the right but also in the left ventricle just 4 wk after injection of monocrotaline (Fig. 6), although the weight and systolic pressure of right ventricle increased significantly by 2 wk after injection. Almost all myosins (around 92% of whole myosins) of

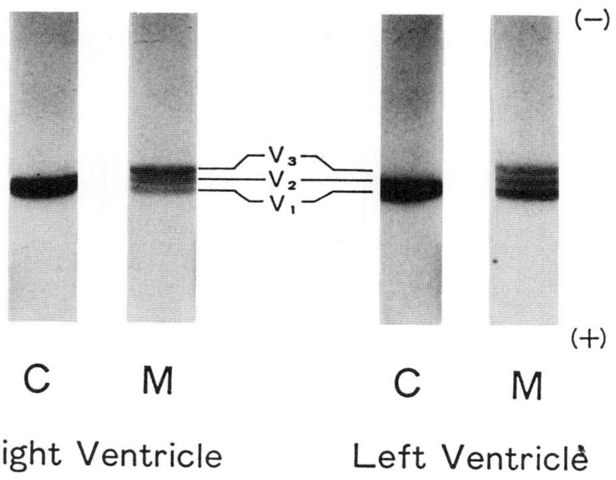

Fig. 6. Electrophoretic analysis of cardiac myosin isozymes in a rat 6 wk after monocrotaline injection. Note the decrease of V1 isotype along with the increase of V2 and V3 isotypes in both ventricles of monocrotaline rat, while the decrease of V1 isotype in left ventricle was of lesser degree. C: control M: monocrotaline

both ventricular free walls and interventricular septum in control rats were V1 isotypes throughout the experimental period and did not show any significant change, although V_1 isotype content in 6 wk rats showed a slight decline up to 84% of whole myosins. The contents of V1 isotype in right ventricle, interventricular septum and also left ventricle significantly ($p < 0.01$) decreased to 58, 62 and 72% of the corresponding control values at 4 wk, respectively, when hypertrophy of right ventricle was induced by monocrotaline. These values further declined to 39, 55 and 64% of the control values after 6 wk, respectively ($p < 0.01$). In addition, the difference in content of V_1 isotype between right and left ventricle became significant after 4 wk ($p < 0.01$) (Fig. 7). The serum thyroxine (T_4) levels diminished significantly ($p < 0.01$) at 6 wk after monocrotaline injection (3.4 µg/dl) compared with control (4.4 µg/dl).

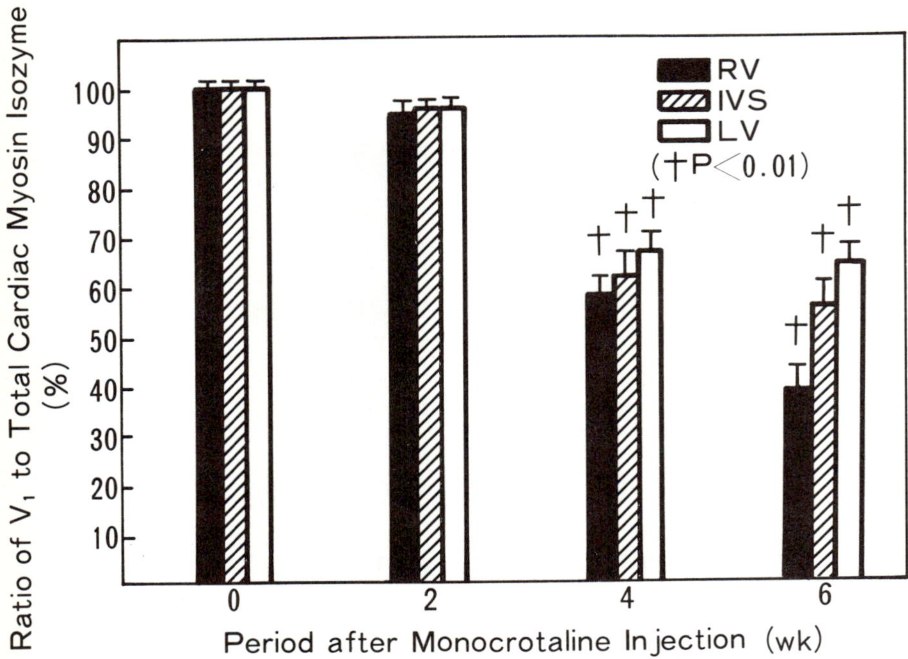

Fig. 7. Changes in ratio of V_1 isotype to total myosin isozymes in right ventricle, interventricular septum and left ventricle of rats injected monocrotaline. Figures are expressed in percentage to the corresponding control values, which are regarded as 100%.
RV right ventricular free wall   IVS interventricular septum
LV left ventricular free wall   mean ± S.E.

DISCUSSION

We have presented in this paper using monoclonal antibodies that there were 2 myosin isozymes, namely HCα and HCβ also in human hearts and redistribution of these isozymes occured in the cases of pressure overload. A considerable amount of HCβ existed in normal human atrium, although all myofibers of it also contained HCα. We found that human left auricle contained rather more HCβ than right auricle (data not shown). This finding was contrary to that of Gorza et al (17) in bovine heart using polyclonal antibodies. The reason of difference was not clear. It may be a species difference or due to different method of using monoclonal or polyclonal antibodies. However our results in normal human atria seem to be reasonable, since the pressure of left atrium is higher than that of right atrium and pressure load induces the increase in the amount of HCβ. The amount of HCα-containing myofiber in atria decreased concomitant with the increase of HCβ-containing fibers, according to pressure elevation

(Fig. 1 and 2). This fact indicates that cardiac adaptation for
pressure overload is expressed also in human as the redistribution of
myosin isozymes from $HC\alpha$ to $HC\beta$, which develops force more efficiently. In this context, the distribution of myosin isozymes in the
ventricular myocardium is easy to understand. The stress across the
ventricular wall decreases from subendocardial to subepicardial region
so that the amount of $HC\alpha$-containing fibers in subspicardial region is
greater than that in the subendocardial region. The distribution of
$HC\alpha$ in right ventricle is similar to that of left ventricle, since the
stress on each contractile unit seems to be almost equal if corrected
by total muscle mass, despite the great difference of pressure between
both ventricles exists.

All myofibers of the upper conduction system (sinus node and AV
node) and about half of myofibers in the lower conduction system
(bundle of His, bundle branches and Purkinje fibers) contained $HC\alpha$
(Table 1). Moderate content of $HC\alpha$ in the Purkinje fibers, in sharp
contrast with the ordinary working myocardium in subendocardial
region, may be due to their non-contracting characteristic despite of
their locating in the subendocardial region. The suggestive evidence
that the $HC\alpha$ content is likely to correlate inversely with the rate of
spontaneous electrical automaticity of conduction system is needed to
investigate further physiologically and biochemically.

Peptide map of $HC\beta$ found in atrium was very similar to that of
ventricular $HC\beta$, but both peptide maps were quite different from
ventricular and atrial $HC\alpha$, which also again were indistinguishable
each other in accordance with the previous reports (12, 14, 17).
There was a significant great difference in the Ca^{2+}-activated ATPase
activity between $HC\alpha$ and $HC\beta$ as reported earlier (1-7).

In the rats with right ventricular hypertrophy induced by
monocrotaline injection (27), it was demonstrated that the significant
decrease of V_1 content occured after 4 wk not only in right ventricle
but also in left ventricle, although that in the latter was of lesser
degree. The predominant content of V_1 in both ventricles of control
rats sustained during the experimental period. The decrease of V_1
content was 2 wk behind the significant elevation of right ventricular
pressure indicating the delay of adaptation to pressure overload,
while the left ventricular pressure did not show any definite changes.
One of the most important factors for changing from V_1 to V_2 or V_3
myosin isozymes in the hearts was pressure overload as reported
earlier. However some other factors besides it had to be functioning in
this experiment, since V_1 contents in the left ventricles of normal
pressure in monocrotaline rats also declined. The decrease of V_1 contents in both ventricles after 6 wk might be brought about in part by
low serum level of thyroxine, which was significantly lower at this

period compared with that of control rats. However serum thyroxine
level alone could not explain the results at 4 wk after monocrotaline
injection, since it was not different from the control rats. It may
be influenced by serum catecholamines, although we did not measure
them in this study. The aging was unlikely a cause, since V1 contents
in control rats did not change significantly during the experimental
period. Further investigations were needed to clarify the factors
other than above-mentioned.

SUMMARY

In studies of human hearts using monoclonal anti-myosin antibodies with indirect immunofluorescence method, we showed the existence of 2
distinct myosin isozymes HCα and HCβ not only in atria but also in
ventricles. Myofibers of normal human atria had a considerable amount
of HCβ, while HCα was distributed in all fibers. The marked increase
of HCβ along with the remarkable decrease of HCα occured in response to
pressure overload like mitral valvular heart dieases. All of the
ordinary working ventricular myofibers contained HCβ. There were
scarce myofibers containing HCα in the subendocardial region, while
those in the subepicardial region contained some amount of HCα. The
amount of HCα in the papillary muscles of left ventricle also
decreased in pressure overload. In the conduction system, the amount
of HCα-containing myofibers decreased from sinus node to the Purkinje
network, namely from 100% to 55% of all myofibers.

Atrial and ventricular HCαs (HCβs) each other were very similar
in their peptide maps as well as Ca^{2+}-activated ATPase activities,
while those of HCα and HCβ were quite different.

The content of V_1 type myosin isozymes decreased significantly
not only in right but also in left ventricle of rats, which developed
right ventricular hypertrophy by monocrotaline injection, although
these changes were 2 wk behind the elevation of right ventricular
pressures and the decreases in left ventricles were of lesser degree,
where the pressures were normal. The other factors than pressure
overload were suggested.

REFERENCES

1. Yazaki, Y. and Raben, M. S. Circ. Res. 35: 15-23, 1974.
2. Yazaki, Y. and Raben, M. S. Circ. Res. 36: 208-215, 1975.
3. Yazaki, Y., Ueda, S., Nagai, R. and Shimada, K.
                    Circ. Res. 45: 522-527. 1979.
4. Syrovy, I., Delcayre, C. and Swynghedauw, B.
          J. Mol. Cell. Cardiol. 11: 1129-1135, 1979
5. Pope, B., Hoh, J. F. Y. and Weeds, A.
                    FEBS Lett. 118: 205-208, 1980.
6. Martin, A. F., Pagani, E. D. and Solaro, R. J.
                    Circ. Res. 50: 117-124, 1982.
7. Mercadier, J. J., Bouveret, P., Gorza, L., Schiaffino, S., Clark,
     W. A., Zak, R., Swynghedauw, B. and Schwartz, K.
                    Circ. Res. 53: 52-62, 1983.

8. Hoh, J. F. Y., McGrath, P. A. and Hale, P. T.
J. Mol. Cell. Cardiol. 10: 1053-1076, 1977
9. Hoh, J. F. Y., Yeoh, G. P. S., Thomas, M. A. W. and
Higginbottom, L.   FEBS Lett. 97: 330-334, 1979.
10. Flink, I. L., Rader, J. H. and Morkin, E.
J. Biol. Chem. 254: 3105-3110, 1979.
11. Chizzonite, R. A., Everett, A. W., Clark, W. A., Jakovic, S.,
Rabinowitz, M. and Zak, R.
J. Biol. Chem. 257: 2056-2065, 1982.
12. Clark, W. A., Chizzonite, R. A., Everett, A. W., Rabinowitz, M.
and Zak, R.   J. Biol. Chem. 257: 5449-5454, 1982.
13. Schwartz, K., Lompre, A. M., Bouveret, P., Wisnewsky, C. and
Whalen, R. G.   J. Biol. Chem. 257: 14412-14418, 1982.
14. Chizzonite, R. A., Everett, A. W., Prior, G. and Zak, R.
J. Biol. Chem. 259: 15564-15571, 1984.
15. Gorza, L., Pauletto, P., Pessina, A. C., Sartore, S. and
Schiaffino, S.   Circ. Res. 49: 1003-1009, 1981.
16. Sartore, S., Gorza, L., Pierobon-Bormioli, S., Dalla Libera, L.
and Schiaffino, S.   J. Cell. Biol. 88: 226-233, 1981.
17. Gorza, L., Sartore, S. and Schiaffino, S.
J. Cell. Biol. 95: 838-845, 1982.
18. Gorza, L., Mercadier, J. J., Schwartz, K., Thornell, L, E.,
Sartore, S. and Schiaffino, S.
Circ. Res. 54: 694-702, 1984.
19. Tsuchimochi, H., Sugi, M., Kuro-o, M., Ueda, S., Takaku, F.,
Furuta, S., Shirai, T. and Yazaki, Y.
J. Clin. Invest. 74: 662-665, 1984.
20. Yazaki, Y., Tsuchimochi,H., Kuro-o, M., Kurabayashi, M., Isobe,
M., Ueda, S., Nagai, R. and Takaku, F.
Eur. Heart J. 5 Suppl. F, 103-110, 1984.
21. Bouvagnet, P., Leger, J., Pons, F., Dechesne, C. and Leger, J, J.
Circ. Res. 55: 794-804, 1984.
22. Köhler, G. and Milstein, C.
Nature (London) 256: 495-497, 1973.
23. Guesdon, J., Ternynck, T. and Avrameas, S.
J. Histochem. Cytochem. 27: 1131-1139, 1979.
24. Komuro, I., Tsuchimochi, H., Ueda, S., Kurabayashi, M., Seko, Y.,
Takaku, F. and Yazaki, Y.
J. Biol. Chem. 261: 4504-4509, 1986.
25. Sartore, S., Pierobon-Bormioli, S. and Schiaffino, S.
Nature (London) 274: 82-83, 1978.
26. Kuro-o, M., Tsuchimochi, H., Ueda, S., Takaku, F. and Yazaki, Y.
J. Clin. Invest. 77: 340-347, 1986.
27. Rupp, H., Popova, N. and Jacob, R.   In: Cardiac Adaptation to
Hemodynamic Overload, Training and Stress (Eds. R. Jacob,
R. W. Gülch and G. Kissling) Steinkopf Verlag, Darmstadt.
1983, p. 46.

20

REMODELLING OF THE MYOCYTE AT A MOLECULAR LEVEL — RELATIONSHIP
BETWEEN MYOSIN ISOENZYME POPULATION AND SARCOPLASMIC RETICULUM

H. RUPP, R. WAHL[+] and R. JACOB

Physiologisches Institut (II) and [+]Medizinische Klinik,
Universität Tübingen, 7400 Tübingen, F.R.G.

INTRODUCTION

There is increasing evidence that the molecular structure
of the myocyte is variable, critically depending on the functional
load to which the heart is subjected on a long-term basis.
The potential of the myocyte to adapt its functionally important
structural elements to a given load represents an important
means by which the heart can cope with a variety of loads ranging
from those arising during physical exercise or increased blood
pressure (1). Although such remodelling of the myocyte is of
great functional relevance, only little is known at present
in terms of the trigger reactions involved at the cellular or
molecular level. In view of the great number of variable
elements of the myocyte, it is unlikely that for each one there
is a selective trigger signal. Rather, it can be assumed that
a given stimulus affects a number of functionally coherent
structures of the myocyte in a concerted manner. An understanding
of mechanisms involved in the remodelling is the prerequisite
not only for a rational description of myocardial performance
but also for tracing the causes of pathological processes such
as decompensation of the pressure loaded heart issuing in pump
failure. The present approach describes the effect of different
functional loads on myosin isoenzyme populations and the rate
of Ca^{2+}-uptake of sarcoplasmic reticulum. The myosin isoenzyme
population is the main determinant of myofibrillar ATPase (2,3),
maximum speed of shortening (4,5) and of the economy of tension
generation (6-8). Changes in sarcoplasmic reticulum are expected
to be reflected in altered excitation-contraction coupling (9)
or energetics (10) and to influence particularly the rate of
relaxation.

MATERIALS AND METHODS

Male Wistar/WU rats and spontaneously hypertensive rats
(SHR) were obtained from Ivanovas, Kissleg, F.R.G. Rats were
fed ad libitum, fed intermittently (feeding every other day),
fed a sucrose-rich diet (8 g/l sucrose in drinking water) or
were swim-exercised (max. 2 x 90 min/d, 35°C water (11)). After
4 – 5 weeks of a given routine, rats were injected with isoproterenol (i.p.) 20 min prior to sacrifice (decapitation).
Quantitative analysis of the myosin isoenzyme population was
carried out using pyrophosphate gel electrophoresis as described
previously (12). Ca^{2+}-uptake of fragmented sarcoplasmic reticulum
was determined in crude homogenate using arsenazo III and an
Aminco DW-2a dual wavelength spectrometer (675 – 685 nm). The
assay medium contained 100 mM KCl, 5 mM $MgCl_2$, 5 mM NaN_3,
20 mM Hepes, 10 mM sodium oxalate, 300 mM sucrose, 10mM Tris-Cl,
0.03 mM arsenazo III, 0.02 mM $CaCl_2$, 1 mM MgATP; pH 7.4;
temperature 37°C. Triiodothyronine in serum was determined
using a commercial radio immunoassay (Immophase, Corning).
Statistical comparisons were performed using Student's t-test.

RESULTS

To depict changes in the myosin isoenzyme population, a
triangular diagram was used (Fig. 1). The curve describing the
theoretical distribution of the myosin isoenzymes was derived
from a statistical model. In this approach, a lower probability
for formation of the heterodimer VM-2 (VM, ventricular myosin)
had to be assumed in order to account for the proportion of
VM-2 which was lower than that expected from a random distribution.
Given that the interval between imposing a load resulting in an
altered gene expression of myosin heavy chains and examination
of the myosin isoenzyme population is longer than approximately
5 days, then all possible isoenzyme profiles have to conform to
the curve which spans from a point of 100% VM-1 to a point of
100% VM-3 (Dietz and Rupp, unpublished). Using this plot a
change in isoenzyme population can be ascertained by only one
data point without having to use 3 values for the respective
isoenzymes. In contrast to the three-dimensional presentation

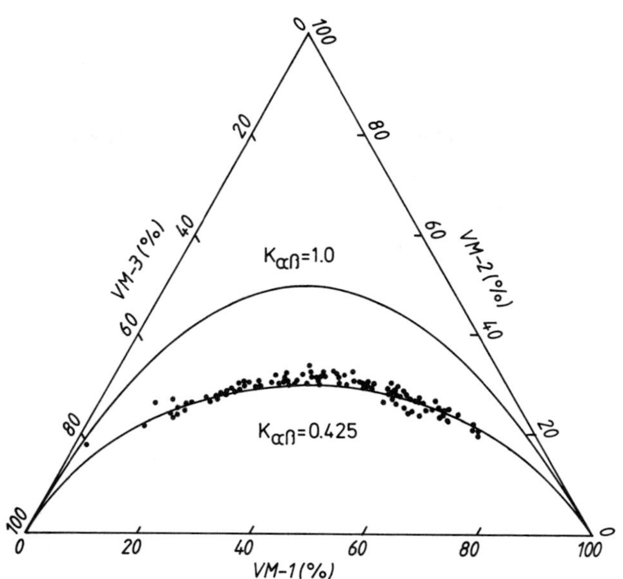

Fig. 1. The theoretical distribution of the 3 myosin isoenzymes VM-1, VM-2 and VM-3 is based on a statistical model (13) which assumes a lower probability (0.425) for formation of the hetero-dimer VM-2 with alpha, beta heavy chains (lower curve). Equal probability for the formation of homodimers and heterodimers would result in the upper curve which does not fit the experimental data points.

we used previously, the triangular plot has the advantage of unequivocally describing the isoenzyme population in one plane.

In order to trace changes in sarcoplasmic reticulum, the rate of Ca^{2+}-uptake of crude homogenate rather than of a purified preparation was determined. In the present correlative approach, it was thought necessary to avoid the possibility of different recoveries from various groups during purification of sarco-plasmic reticulum. Furthermore, to detect functionally comparable changes in myosin isoenzyme population and sarcoplasmic reticulum, an extreme state of phospholamban phosphorylation must be reached. Different degrees of adrenergic drive before or during sacrifice of the rat would result in a variable extent of phospholamban phosphorylation and thus to differences in rate of Ca^{2+}-uptake. The rats were, therefore, injected with isoproterenol before sacrifice to assure maximum adrenergic drive of the heart.

In the pressure-loaded heart of SHR with compensated
hypertrophy, the proportion of VM-3 was increased compared to
Wistar rats which exhibit an identical isoenzyme population
at an age when both strains have the same ventricular mass.
Furthermore, rate of Ca^{2+}-uptake was reduced in SHR (Fig. 2).
In the compensated stage of SHR and in Wistar rats, ventricular
mass correlated with the proportion of VM-3 and inversely with
rate of Ca^{2+}-uptake (not shown). Thus, increase in ventricular
mass is correlated with rate of cross bridge cycling and rate
of Ca^{2+}-uptake in a concerted manner, indicating a transformation
of the myocardium in the direction of a slow-type muscle.

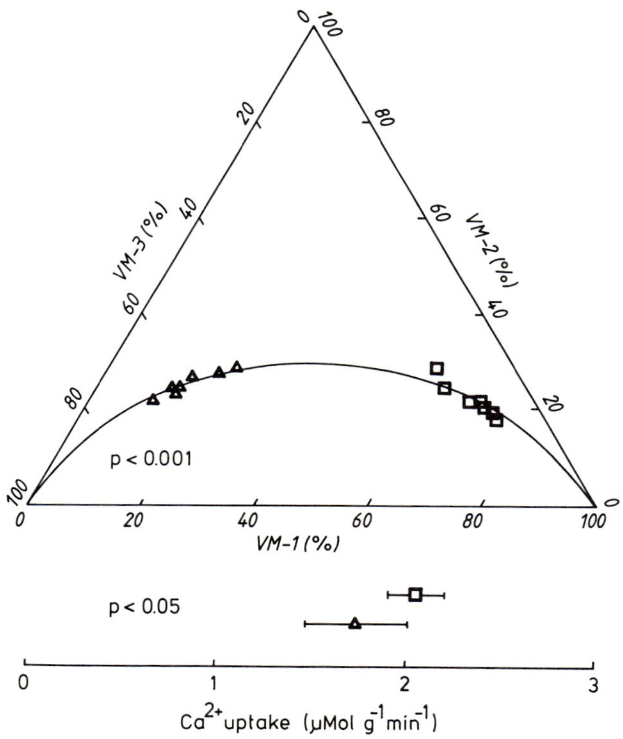

Fig. 2. Myosin isoenzyme population and rate of Ca^{2+}-uptake
of sarcoplasmic reticulum (mean ± S.D. of individual rats)
in pressure-loaded left ventricles of SHR ($\triangle$) as compared
to Wistar rats ($\square$). Note, the VM-1 (%) axis is not linked
to the lower axis which depicts rate of Ca^{2+}-uptake.

The effect of increasing ventricular mass can be experimentally mimicked by altering the schedule from ad libitum to intermittent feeding, whereby the rats are fed ad libitum only every other day. Such a routine induced an increase in the proportion of VM-3 and a reduced rate of Ca^{2+}-uptake (Fig. 3). Although ventricular mass is less than that of rats fed ad libitum, two important parameters of myocardial performance change in a manner that is typical for ventricles of higher mass.

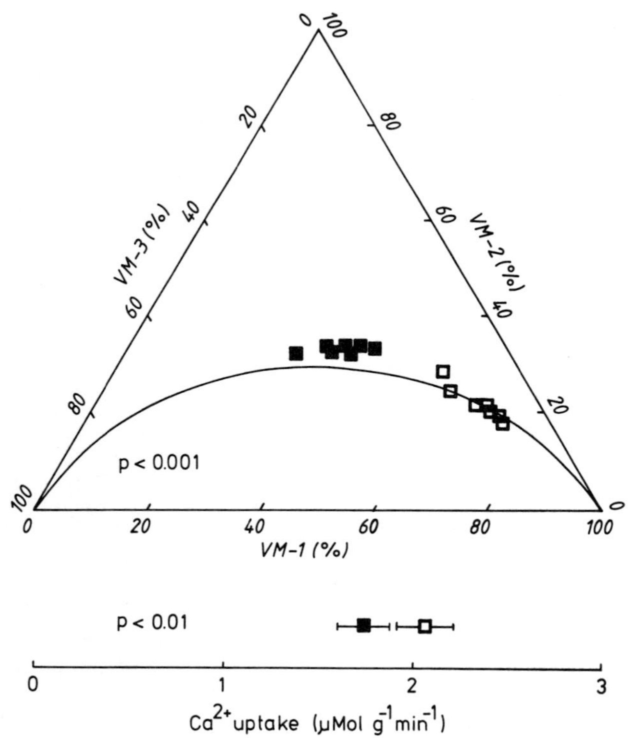

Fig. 3. Myosin isoenzyme population and rate of Ca^{2+}-uptake of sarcoplasmic reticulum (mean ± S.D. of individual rats) in intermittently (■) and ad libitum (□) fed Wistar rats.

A redistribution in the direction of VM-1 can be induced by feeding rats ad libitum a diet rich in sucrose. As in the previous cases, rate of Ca^{2+}-uptake was again affected in a functionally comparable manner, when determined after maximal adrenergic stimulation (Fig. 4).

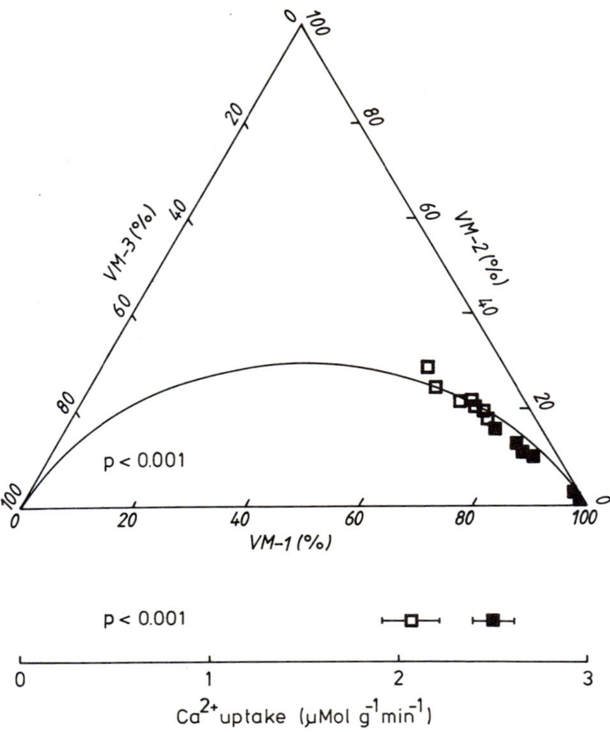

Fig. 4. Myosin isoenzyme population and rate of Ca^{2+}-uptake of sarcoplasmic reticulum (mean $\pm$ S.D. of individual rats) of Wistar rats fed a sucrose-rich diet (■) or a standard diet (□).

By contrast, a dissociation was observed following intense exercise in the form of swimming. Although the proportion of VM-1 was increased, rate of Ca^{2+}-uptake was not significantly altered. Thus, in the exercised heart, the potential for fast contraction is increased, whereas sarcoplasmic reticulum remains unaffected. It should, however, be noted that in contrast to myosin, the activity of sarcoplasmic reticulum can acutely be modulated via phospholamban phosphorylation. Although sarco-plasmic reticulum in the exercised heart apparently does not seem to be adapted to the period of physical activity, this cannot be interpreted as a mismatch between molecular structure and functional demands. It is our working hypothesis that the

increased proportion of VM-1 arises from the high adrenergic
drive during the exercise routine. The unchanged activity of
sarcoplasmic reticulum is most probably a result of the time
average of the high adrenergic drive during exercise and the
markedly reduced tone at rest.

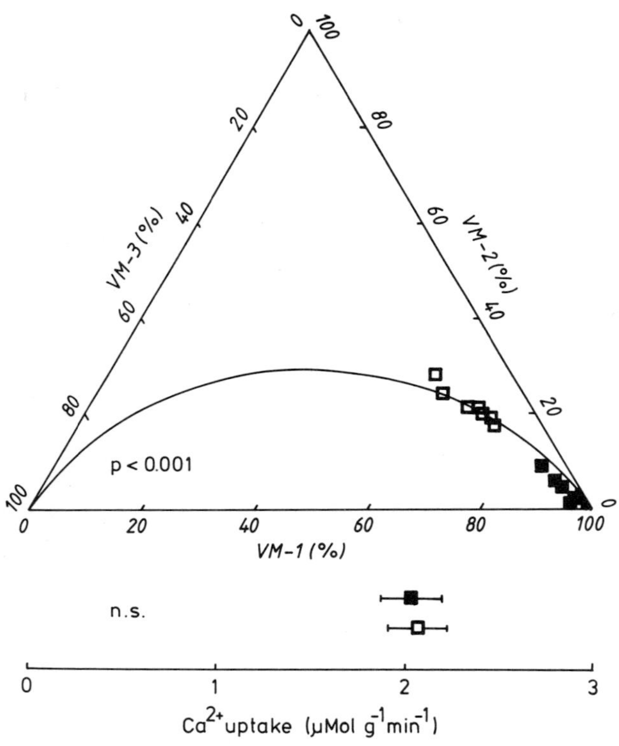

Fig. 5. Myosin isoenzyme population and rate of Ca^{2+}-uptake
of sarcoplasmic reticulum (mean ± S.D. of individual rats)
in swim-exercised (■) and sedentary (□) Wistar rats.

As regards possible trigger mechanisms involved in the
changes seen in myosin and sarcoplasmic reticulum, thyroid
hormone status is most important. For example, an increase in
the concentration of circulating thyroid hormones results in
a higher proportion of VM-1 and faster Ca^{2+}-uptake (not shown).

Concentrations of triiodothyronine (T_3) in the serum are given in the following table for different functional states:

Functional state	n	T_3 (ng/dl)
Wistar, control	7	96 ± 5
SHR, control	7	109 ± 5^x
Wistar, intermittently fed	7	68 ± 4^x
Wistar, fed a sucrose diet	7	110 ± 10^x
Wistar, swim-exercised	7	74 ± 12^x

^{x} $P < 0.05$, SHR and experimental Wistar groups versus Wistar control group; for determination of T_3, the sera of individual rats within a given group were pooled; n, number of rats

From these data, it follows that the increased proportion of VM-3 in the hypertrophied myocardium of SHR cannot be accounted for by a reduced serum concentration of T_3. SHR exhibited even an increase in T_3 which has to be counteracted by the still unknown mechanism responsible for the redistribution in the direction of VM-3. In intermittently fed rats, T_3 concentration was markedly reduced which is considered to be the main cause for the increased proportion of VM-3 and the reduced rate of Ca^{2+}-uptake. Also in the case of the rats fed a sucrose-rich diet, there was a change in both parameters which could be at least partially accounted for by the higher T_3 concentration. In the swim-exercised rats, T_3 concentration was reduced, which, however, was neither reflected in myosin nor in sarcoplasmic reticulum. Thus, the mechanisms operating in the exercised heart can overcome the reduced T_3 concentration and induce a higher proportion of VM-1 and maintain the activity of sarcoplasmic reticulum.

DISCUSSION

The present data demonstrate that the myocyte can be
remodelled by a number of functional loads involving concerted
and non-concerted reactions. Concerted reactions affect both
the myosin isoenzyme population and sarcoplasmic reticulum in
a functionally comparable manner. For example, the potential
for fast contraction and for fast relaxation are enhanced.
Concerted reactions arise from factors involved in altered
ventricular mass, from intermittent feeding, from pharmacological
interference with thyroid status and from a sucrose-rich diet.
The latter case fulfills the criteria for a concerted reaction
only when the heart has been subjected to a high adrenergic
drive, but not after in vitro dephosphorylation of phospholamban
with a phosphoprotein phosphatase preparation. Under these
conditions rate of Ca^{2+}-uptake was not significantly increased,
indicating that thyroid hormones cannot solely explain the
changes in myosin and sarcoplasmic reticulum. Following intense
exercise, a non-concerted reaction has been observed which is
present also after dephosphorylation of phospholamban. The
effect of swimming exercise on sarcoplasmic reticulum has been
a controversial issue (14,15) probably due to the uncontrolled
extent of phosphorylated phospholamban. The dissociation between
myosin and sarcoplasmic reticulum demonstrates that trigger
mechanisms exist which can selectively affect gene expression
of myosin.

Regarding the mechanisms involved in concerted and non-
concerted reactions, one has to distinguish between reactions
which are mediated by altered circulating thyroid hormones and
those which cannot be accounted for by altered thyroid status.
In the latter case, there still exists the possibility of
altered nuclear T_3 receptors in heart (Wahl and Rupp, unpublished).
Concerted reactions are mediated by thyroid hormones in the
case of pharmacologically induced hyper- or hypothyroidism and
most probably after intermittent feeding. There is no evidence
that they are mediated by circulating thyroid hormones in the
case of a change in ventricular mass and mechanisms in addition
to thyroid hormones have to be implicated in rats fed a sucrose-
rich diet. Non-concerted reactions are expected not to be

mediated by altered thyroid hormones, as is demonstrated by
the example of the swim-exercised heart. Thus we can state that,
if the concentration of circulating T_3 is altered, most probably
concerted reactions ensue. However, this argument cannot be
reversed. The fact that concerted reactions are observed does
not necessarily imply an altered T_3 concentration in the blood,
as is demonstrated by SHR with compensated hypertrophy.

In reactions not arising from altered circulating thyroid
hormones, adrenergic drive seems to be a decisive factor. Thus,
administration of the beta-blocker atenolol and the drugs
guanethidine and reserpine which deplete norepinephrine from
the adrenergic nerve terminal induce a higher proportion of
VM-3 and a reduced rate of Ca^{2+}-uptake when determined after
dephosphorylation of phospholamban (Rupp, unpublished). Whether
the adrenergic system is solely responsible for the changes
seen in the above reactions which cannot be accounted for by
altered thyroid hormone concentrations, remains to be established.
As regards the intracellular trigger responsible for mediating
the effect of the adrenergic system, one has to consider by
which mechanism changes in myosin isoenzyme population and rate
of Ca^{2+}-uptake arise. A change in myosin isoenzyme population
can be traced to a selective expression of genes coding for
alpha- or beta-heavy chains (16). The putative trigger has,
therefore, to influence gene expression at the nuclear level.
As regards the changes in sarcoplasmic reticulum, there are a
number of ways of affecting the rate of Ca^{2+}-uptake (17). Since
in the present approach the activity was determined in crude
homogenate, a reduction in rate of Ca^{2+}-uptake might be due
to dilution of sarcoplasmic reticulum membranes by other
organelles when ventricular mass increases. This possibility
can, however, be ruled out, since it was previously shown that
in SHR, Ca^{2+}-uptake was reduced even when using a purified
preparation (18,19). It is more plausible that the number of
pump sites per unit surface area of the membrane varies (19)
and thereby affects total activity, or that the lipid matrix
of the membrane is modified affecting the activity of the Ca^{2+}-
pump. In view of the existence of myosin isoenzymes, one should

not dismiss the idea that also the Ca^{2+}-pump exists in isoforms
which differ in their enzymatic activity. Despite the fact that
the intracellular mechanisms that regulate the activities of
myosin and sarcoplasmic reticulum are not necessarily the same,
it is noteworthy that a number of different loads induce
functionally comparable changes. The elucidation of the respective
trigger reactions at a cellular and molecular level presents a
great challenge which necessitates the application of molecular
biology as well as knowledge of regulatory aspects operating
in the whole organism.

SUMMARY

In a comparative approach, the potential of the myocyte
to react to different loads by remodelling of the functionally
important structures of myosin and sarcoplasmic reticulum was
studied. The myosin isoenzyme population was determined using
pyrophosphate gels and rate of Ca^{2+}-uptake was measured by the
arsenazo III method. In order to achieve a high degree of
phospholamban phosphorylation, rats were injected with 40 mg/kg
isoproterenol before sacrifice. The following loads affected
the myosin isoenzyme population and sarcoplasmic reticulum in
a functionally comparable manner. Both compensated hypertrophy
in SHR and intermittent feeding (ad libitum feeding every other
day over 4 weeks) increased the proportion of VM-3 and reduced
rate of Ca^{2+}-uptake. Feeding rats a sucrose-rich diet for 4
weeks increased the proportion of VM-1 and led to a higher
rate of Ca^{2+}-uptake. A dissociation between changes in myosin
and sarcoplasmic reticulum were observed following intense
exercise in the form of swimming (max. 2 x 90 min/d, 4 weeks).
Although the proportion of VM-1 increased, rate of Ca^{2+}-uptake
was unaltered, demonstrating a non-concerted reaction. The
concentration of triiodothyronine (T_3) in serum was altered
in a manner which could account for the observed changes in
myosin and sarcoplasmic reticulum only in the case of intermittent feeding and the sucrose-rich diet. For the effect of
increasing mass and exercise, other mechanisms have to be
involved. Since pharmacological interference with the adrenergic

318

drive of heart can influence both myosin and sarcoplasmic
reticulum, it is an attractive possibility that adrenergic
activity plays an important role in reactions not mediated
by circulating thyroid hormones, particularly in those
operating in the exercised heart.

ACKNOWLEDGEMENTS

     This study was supported by the Deutsche Forschungsgemein-
schaft. The expert work of Mr.L.Schwarz and the valuable
suggestions of Prof.K.Dietz on myosin distribution are grate-
fully acknowledged.

REFERENCES

1. Rupp, H. (Ed.) Regulation of Heart Function — Basic Concepts
    and Clinical Applications, Thieme Inc., Stuttgart-New York,
    1986.
2. Rupp, H. Basic Res. Cardiol. 77: 34-46, 1982.
3. Rupp, H. Mol. Physiol. 3: 249-263, 1983.
4. Ebrecht, G., Rupp, H. and Jacob, R. Basic Res. Cardiol.
    77: 220-234, 1982.
5. Schwartz, K., Lecarpentier, Y., Martin, J.L., Lompré, A.M.,
    Mercadier, J.J. and Swynghedauw, B. J. Mol. Cell. Cardiol.
    13: 1071-1075, 1981.
6. Alpert, N.R. and Mulieri, L.A. In: Regulation of Heart
    Function — Basic Concepts and Clinical Applications (Ed. H.
    Rupp), Thieme Inc., Stuttgart-New York, 1986, pp. 292-304.
7. Kissling, G., Rupp, H., Malloy, L. and Jacob, R. Basic
    Res. Cardiol. 77: 255-269, 1982.
8. Jacob, R., Ebrecht, G., Kissling, G., Rupp, H. and Takeda,
    N. In: Regulation of Heart Function — Basic Concepts and
    Clinical Applications (Ed. H. Rupp), Thieme Inc., Stuttgart-
    New York, 1986, pp. 305-326.
9. Fabiato, A. Am. J. Physiol. 245: C1-C14, 1983.
10. Hasselbach, W. and Oetliker, H. Ann. Rev. Physiol. 45:
    325-339, 1983.
11. Rupp, H. and Jacob, R. Can. J. Physiol. Pharmacol. 60:
    1098-1103, 1982.
12. Rupp, H., Felbier, H.-R., Bukhari, A.R. and Jacob, R.
    Can. J. Physiol. Pharmacol. 62: 1209-1218, 1984.
13. Rupp, H. Basic Res. Cardiol. 80: 608-616, 1985.
14. Malhotra, A., Penpargkul, S., Schaible, T. and Scheuer, J.
    Am. J. Physiol. 241: H263-H267, 1981.
15. Pagani, E.D. and Solaro, R.J. Am. J. Physiol. 247: H909-
    H915, 1984.
16. Mahdavi, V., Chambers, A.P. and Nadal-Ginard, B. Proc.
    Natl. Acad. Sci. USA 81: 2626-2630, 1984.
17. Limas, C.J. In: Regulation of Heart Function — Basic
    Concepts and Clinical Applications (Ed. H. Rupp), Thieme
    Inc., Stuttgart-New York, 1986, pp. 145-158.
18. Limas, C.J. and Cohn, J.N. Circ. Res. 41: I-62 - I-69, 1977.
19. Heilmann, C., Lindl, T., Müller, W. and Pette, D. Basic
    Res. Cardiol. 75: 92-96, 1980.

21

ISOMYOSINS AND ISOACTINS IN MAMMALIAN MYOCARDIUM

J.J. MERCADIER, A.M. LOMPRE, D. de la BASTIE, J.L. SAMUEL, B. SWYNGHEDAUW, L. RAPPAPORT and K. SCHWARTZ.

Unité 127 I.N.S.E.R.M., Hopital Lariboisière, 75010 Paris, France.

INTRODUCTION

Myosin and actin are the major components of the thick and the thin filaments of the sarcomere, respectively. The existence of several isomyosins with different heavy chains and different enzymatic activities was demonstrated more than 20 years ago when adult fast-twitch and slow-twitch muscles were compared to cardiac ventricular tissue and it is clear now that the sarcomeric myosin heavy chains (MHC) are coded by a highly conserved multigene family (1). The classical experiments of Barany (2) who showed that maximal velocity of a given muscle fiber is correlated to the ATPase activity of its constituent myosin, and of Buller, Eccles and Eccles (3) in which the nerve was shown to modulate the properties of a muscle, opened an exciting new era in muscle research and neurobiology. Much less was known concerning cardiac isomyosins, but the applications of recent advances in molecular and cell biology have made the past few years a period of rapid development in this field. After the pioneer work of Hoh et al. (4) it is clear now that in a number of animal species, the ventricular tissue contains several isomyosins whose relative amounts change depending on the developmental, physiological and pathological state of the animal (see ref. 5 for review) and that these changes contribute markedly to the regulations of ventricular contractility (6, 7). The atrial myocardium which is characterized by higher contractile performance - or at least higher contractile reserve

(8) - and higher myosin ATPase activity (9) than those of the corresponding ventricle, has been less studied.

Actin, although a highly conserved protein, is also encoded by a multigene family, consisting of at least six different members in mammalian tissue (see ref. 10 for review). It now appears that the spectrum of actin isotype expression within various tissues is more complex than was previously thought, and that most tissues express more than a single actin isotype. Two sarcomeric actins exist, the skeletal and the cardiac isoforms, which are transiently coexpressed in the striated muscles during ontogenic development (11, 12). Thus far, relatively little is known about the variability of their expression in the heart in pathological conditions.

The purpose of this paper is to present recent work from our laboratory which was undertaken to improve our knowledge of i) the tissue specific expression of the different myosin heavy chain genes within the heart, i.e. a comparison between atria and ventricles and ii) the coexpression of the sarcomeric actin pair in the cardiac tissue.

COMPARATIVE MYOSIN-HEAVY CHAIN EXPRESSION IN ATRIA AND VENTRICLES.

Immunological peptide mapping, amino acid sequence analyses as well as recombinant DNA technology have demonstrated the existence of two closely related, but distinct isoforms of myosin heavy chain, in mammalian cardiac tissues. Those two types of myosin heavy chain, α and β, give rise to $\alpha\alpha$ and $\beta\beta$ homodimers, which correspond respectively to the V_1 and V_3 isomyosins with high and low ATPase activity, and to an $\alpha\beta$ heterodimer (V_2)

with intermediate activity (4). Increased pressure or volume loading of the ventricles results in the development of ventricular myocytes which demonstrate a transition from the α to the β myosin heavy chain (13, 14). As a consequence, overall myosin ATPase activity is reduced which in turn leads to slower (6) but more efficient myocardial contraction (7). The potential for this transition depends on the initial ventricular phenotype and is therefore species specific since rat and to a lesser degree rabbit ventricles contain predominantly α, whereas human ventricle contains predominantly β, and therefore, the transition can only be very small (15). In contrast, in human atria, which are composed essentially of α-MHC, a dramatic change was found by immunocytochemistry in the chronically overloaded human left atrium (16-18).

By an enzyme-linked immunosorbent assay (19). We have now quantitated the true proportion of α-MHC present in the normal and chronically overloaded left atrium and have tested a possible relationship between this proportion and atrial size. The study included 25 patients, who had a history of long-standing left atrial overload secondary to rheumatic lesions of the mitral valve i.e. mitral stenosis and mitral regurgitation. Almost all of them had been receiving digitalis and diuretic drugs. Four patients were also included who suffered from a Wolff - Parkinson - White syndrome, and underwent section of an accessory pathway. To avoid variations due to a possible regional heterogeneity, the same surgeon sampled intra-operative biopsies in the same left atrial area located in the postero-lateral wall, at the time of left atrial incision. Atrial size was estimated by planimetric analysis of the scans obtained by two-dimensional echography.

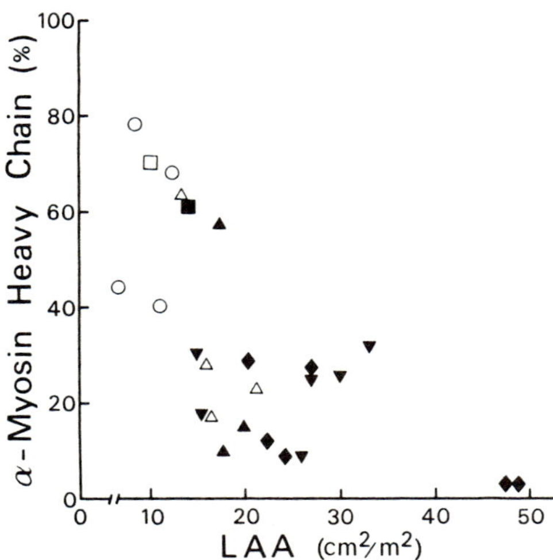

Fig. 1. Relationship between indexed left atrial area (LAA) and the proportion of α -MHC in the atrial tissue (r = 0.66, p < 0.001). Patients with Wolff - Parkinson - White syndrome (○), pure tight mitral stenosis (△ , ▲), mitral stenosis plus mild regurgitation (▽ , ▼), severe chronic mitral regurgitation (◆). Open symbols : sinus rhythm ; closed symbols, atrial fibrillation.

Figure 1 shows that the proportion of α-MHC in the atrial

tissue varied from one patient to the other. α-MHC was the

predominant isoform of the patients with Wolff - Parkinson - White

syndrome, whereas it was a minor component of all patients with

rheumatic valve dysfunction. A highly significant negative linear

correlation was found between α -MHC proportion and left atrial

area (r = 0.66, p <0.001), which was in very good agreement with

previous data showing an analogous correlation with left atrial

diameter (Mercadier et al., submitted). Our present results confirm

that α-MHC is the essential myosin isoform of human atrium

submitted to normal hemodynamic conditions and are consistent with

previous immunocytochemical observations (16-18); we show also that
the isomyosin shift that takes place (from α-MHC to β MHC) is
related to the degree of atrial dilation, which indicates that
human atrial and rat ventricular myocardium seem to behave
identically to a mechanical overload, whatever the trigger.

In addition to work overload, several other factors affect the
ventricular isomyosin pattern. Among them, the effect of thyroid
hormone is very well documented, both at the protein and the gene
level : hypothyroidism induces β , whereas thyroxine induces α
(4). These transitions are regulated at the level of the respective
messenger RNA (mRNA) availability, which in turn is probably
transcriptionally regulated (20). The isomyosin pattern of
hypothyroid atria is drastically different from that of ventricles
since the α-MHC is still present in rats (21) as well as in
rabbits (22).

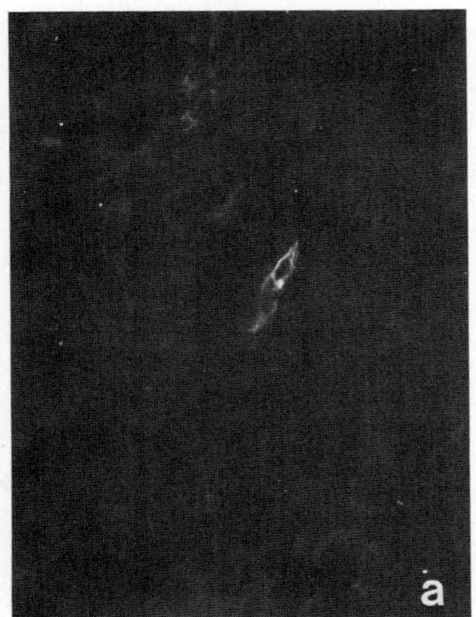
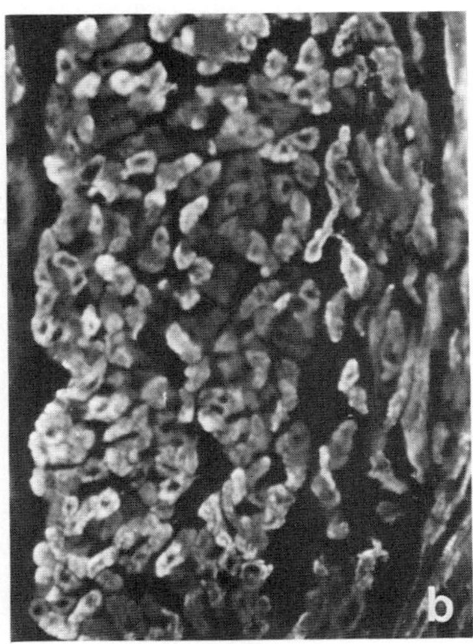

Fig. 2. Indirect immunofluorescence of a left atrial myocardium of
a control rat (a) and of one hypothyroid rat (b). Sections were
stained with anti - β myosin heavy chain immunoglobulin (x 300).

As shown in Figure 2, we recently observed (23) that in those hypothyroid atria, all cells were also labeled with a polyclonal antibody specific to β-MHC. The relative amount of β-MHC, determined by the same quantitative ELISA test as above, was however, less than 5%. These data thus show that thyroid hormones modulate the expression of β-MHC as in ventricles, but at a very low level. As in ventricles also, the atrial transitions at the protein level are regulated at a pre-translational level, since α-MHC gene transcripts are not markedly modified in the hypothyroid atrium, where a small amount of β-MHC mRNA is present (20). Taken together, these data clearly indicate that the extent of hormonal regulation of α- and β-MHC is very different in the two cardiac tissues.

CO-EXPRESSION OF SKELETAL AND CARDIAC ACTIN GENES IN THE HEART

The determination of actin isoform expression in sarcomeric tissues is difficult because these proteins are nearly identical (24). The nucleotide sequences are more divergent, especially in the 3' untranslated regions which allowed several teams to develop cloned DNA probes specific for skeletal and cardiac actin mRNA (11, 12, 25). In rats (11) and mice (12) the skeletal gene encodes the major actin species in adult skeletal muscle, whereas the cardiac gene encodes the major actin species in the adult heart. Both genes are developmentally regulated, since they are transiently coexpressed at birth in developing skeletal and cardiac muscles. We have thus addressed the question whether hypertrophy of the adult rat heart is also associated with such a coexpression (26).

The experimental model of cardiac hypertrophy that we chose was that of pressure overload of the left ventricle produced by coarctation of the upper abdominal aorta using a partially occluded Weck Hemoclip (13). Detection and quantification of the skeletal and cardiac gene transcripts was performed by Northern blot analysis of cardiac RNAs with two cDNA probes, one to determine the amount of total striated actin mRNA and the other that of skeletal actin mRNA (27). This procedure circumvented all errors inherent to the RNA transfer.

A summary of results obtained at different times after aortic stenosis is presented in Figure 3.

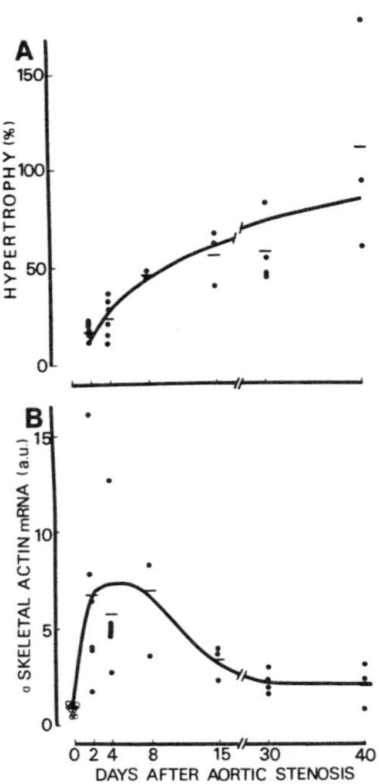

Fig. 3. Time course of expression of skeletal actin mRNA and cardiac hypertrophy after a pressure overload of rat left ventricle. a.u.: arbitrary units.

There was a significant accumulation of skeletal actin mRNA during the first post-operative week, at the beginning of the hypertrophic process, followed by a slow decline. A month after the aortic constriction, in hearts which were markedly hypertrophied, the relative amount of skeletal actin messages returned to control values. These results clearly demonstrate that the skeletal actin gene can be induced in the cardiac tissue of adult rats in response to an altered functional condition. Since the physiological significance of the different actin isoforms is not known, it is not known whether this induction occurs in response to a requirement for this actin isoform or whether during this period of fast growth, the cardiac gene is not sufficient for the synthesis of enough actin. In humans, the basal level of skeletal actin is much higher than in rats (20 - 30%), and it is not clear whether this level changes depending on the pathological conditions since thus far only two patients have been studied and the results do not agree (24, 25).

CONCLUSION

The specificity in expression of myosin and actin multigene families in the atria and in the ventricles is striking : the same myosin heavy chain gene is responsive to thyroid hormone in a very different mode in the two tissues and to hemodynamic load in an identical mode. On the other hand, the same trigger, hemodynamic overload, regulates myosin and actin multigene families in a completely incoordinate fashion in the same tissue, viz, the ventricle. Moreover, each member of both families is under different programs, depending on the cardiac tissue, and these

programs are species specific, since rat and human do not express
the same sets of myosin and actin genes. The physiological
significance of isomyosin shifts is clear, but that of isoactins is
not, and in a more general way, the role of differentially
expressed actin isotypes is one of the central problems of actin
biology. Nevertheless, our results show that the thin filament
participates as well as the thick filament in the response of
cardiac muscle to new functional requirements.

ACKNOWLEDGEMENTS

We thank P. Bouveret, C. Wisnewsky and P. Oliviero for their
skillfull technical assistance and M. de Villedon for the
secretarial work. We are indebted to Dr. P. Menashé for the human
biopsies, to Dr. S. Sartore and Prof. S. Schiaffino for the gift of
the anti- MHC immunoglobulins and to S. Alonso and M. Buckingham
for the gift of the actin cDNA probes.

This work was supported by I.N.S.E.R.M. and by a grant from the
Caisse Nationale d'Assurances Maladies des Travailleurs Salariés.
D. de la Bastie is a recipient of a Contrat Industriel de Formation
pour la Recherche (Roussel Laboratory).

REFERENCES

1. Nguyen, H.T., Gubits, R.M., Wydro, R.M. and Nadal-Ginard, B. Proc.
   Natl. Acad. Sci. USA 79: 5230-5234, 1982.
2. Barany, M. J. Gen. Physiol. 150: 197-216, 1967.
3. Buller, A.J., Eccles, J.C. and Eccles, R.M. J. Physiol. 150:
   417-439, 1960.
4. Hoh, J.F.Y., Mc Grath, P.A. and Hale, P.T. J. Mol. Cell. Cardiol.
   10: 1053-1076, 1978.
5. Schwartz, K. and Mercadier, J.J. In: The Developing Heart (Ed. M.
   Legato), Martinus Nijhoff Publishing, Boston, The Hague, Dordrecht,

Lancaster, 1984, pp. 149-171.
6. Schwartz, K., Lecarpentier, Y., Martin, J.L., Lompré, A.M., Mercadier, J.J. and Swynghedauw, B. J. Moll. Cell. Cardiol. 13: 1071-1075, 1981.
7. Alpert, N.R. and Mulieri, L.A.   Circ. Res. 50: 491-500, 1982.
8. Goldman, S., Olajos, M. and Morkin, E. Cardiovasc. Res. 18: 604-612, 1984.
9. Yazaki, Y., Ueda, S., Nagai, R. and Shimada, K. Circ. Res. 45: 522-527, 1979.
10. Buckingham, M.E. Essays in Biochemistry 20: 77-109, 1985.
11. Mayer, Y., Czosnek, H., Zeelon, P.E., Yaffe, D. and Nudel, U. Nucleic Acids Res. 12: 1087-2000, 1984.
12. Minty, A.J., Alonso, S., Caravatti, M. and Buckingham, M.E. Cell 30: 185-192, 182.
13. Lompre, A.M., Schwartz, K., d'Albis, A., Lacombe, G., Van Thiem, N.G. and Swynghedauw, B. Nature 282: 105-107, 1979.
14. Litten, R.Z., Martin, B.J., Low, R.B. and Alpert, N.R.   Circ. Res. 50: 856-864, 1982.
15. Mercadier, J.J., Bouveret, P., Gorza, L., Schiaffino, S., Clark, W.A., Zak, R., Swynghedauw, B. and Schwartz, K. Circ. Res. 53: 52-62, 1983.
16. Gorza, L., Mercadier, J.J., Schwartz, K., Thornell, L.E. Sartore, S. and Schiaffino, S. Circ. Res. 54: 694-702, 1984.
17. Tsuchimochi, H., Sugi, M., Kuro-o, M., Ueda, S., Takaku, F., Furuta, S.I., Shirai, T. and Yazaki, Y. J. Clin. Invest. 74: 662-665, 1984.
18. Bouvagnet, P., Léger, J., Dechesne, C.A., Dureau, G., Anoal, M. and Léger, J.J.   Circulation 72: 272-279, 1985.
19. Schwartz, K. and Mercadier, J.J. In: Methods of Enzymatic Analysis (Ed. U.V. Bergmeyers), VHC, Weinheim, vol.IV, 1986, pp. 225-238.
20. Izumo, S., Nadal-Ginard, B. and Mahdavi, V. Science 231: 597-600, 1986.
21. Chizzonite, R.A., Everett, A.W., Prior, G. and Zak, R. J. Biol. Chem. 259: 15564-15571, 1984.
22. Banerjee, S.K. Circ. Res. 52: 131-136, 1983.
23. Samuel, J.L., Rappaport, L., Syrovy, I., Wisnewsky, C., Marotte, F., Whalen, R.G. and Schwartz, K. Am. J. Physiol. 250: 331-341, 1986.
24. Vandekerckhove, J., Bugaisky, G. and Buckingham, M. J. Biol. Chem. 241: 1836-1843, 1986.
25. Gunning, P., Ponte, P., Blau, H. and Kedes, L. Molec. Cell. Biol. 3: 1985-1995, 1983.
26. Schwartz, K., de la Bastie, D., Bouveret, P., Oliviero, P., Alonso, S. and Buckingham, M. Circ. Res. in press.
27. Alonso, S., Minty, A., Bourlet, Y. and Buckingham, M.E. J. Mol. Evol. 23 in press, 1986.

22

CROSSBRIDGE MECHANISMS OF CONTRACTION IN VASCULAR SMOOTH MUSCLE

N.L. STEPHENS, S.K. KONG AND G. MORGAN
Department of Physiology, Faculty of Medicine, Univ. of Man.,
770 Bannatyne Ave., Winnipeg, Man., R3E OW3

Not more than ten years ago it would have been wellnigh impossible to envisage discussion of the topic of this chapter. Smooth muscle research was very much a second rate activity and lay under a cloud. Yet one could not fault the critics, for smooth muscle seemed deserving of its sobriquet "the headache muscle." The principal objection lay in the fact that no symmetrical organized structural substrate existed to which to relate the results of biophysical experiments on smooth muscle.

Since then the scene has changed and evidence is accruing that smooth muscle is perhaps not smooth at all but in fact striated and possessed of sarcomeres. There is of course, no doubt, that crossbridges must be shown to exist in smooth muscle before we can begin to talk about crossbridge mechanisms of contraction. Furthermore organization into homogeneous symmetric sarcomeres within homogeneneous fibres must be demonstrated before one can analyze smooth muscle bundle mechanics in terms of crossbridges.

Smooth Muscle Structure

The first part of this chapter deals with presentation of the evidence that supports the idea that sarcomeres exist in smooth muscle. It must be pointed out en passant, that indirect evidence of the similarities in smooth and striated muscle function exists. For example the qualitative similarities in the length tension, stimulus-response, and force-velocity relationships of these two muscles is evident on comparing the appropriate data (1,2,3,4).

Figure 1 is a light micrograph, published by Groeschel-Stewart (5), showing smooth muscle fibres treated with antimyosin antibodies and stained appropriately. The cross-striation pattern is striking and provides strong support for the belief that smooth muscle is really striated. Admittedly the picture only shows surface patterns and the entire muscle bundle needs to be explored.

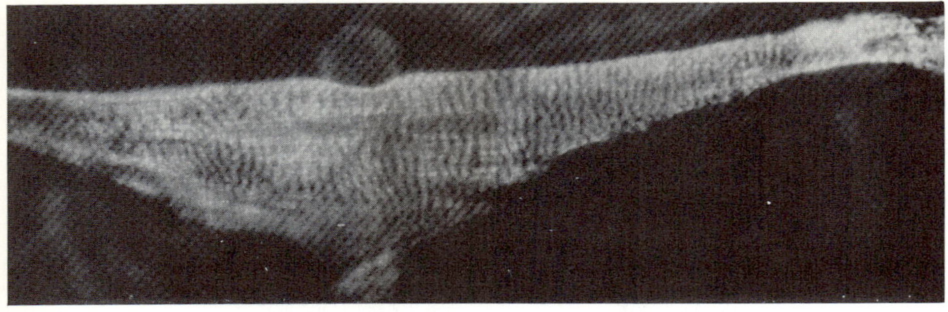

Fig. 1 Antismooth muscle myosin immunofluorescence of guinea pig vas deferens in culture. Note the appearance of cross-banded fibrils. There is considerable alignment of the cross-bands across the cell. (Magnification x 1670) (From Groeschel-Stewart et al. Histochem 50:271, 1977).

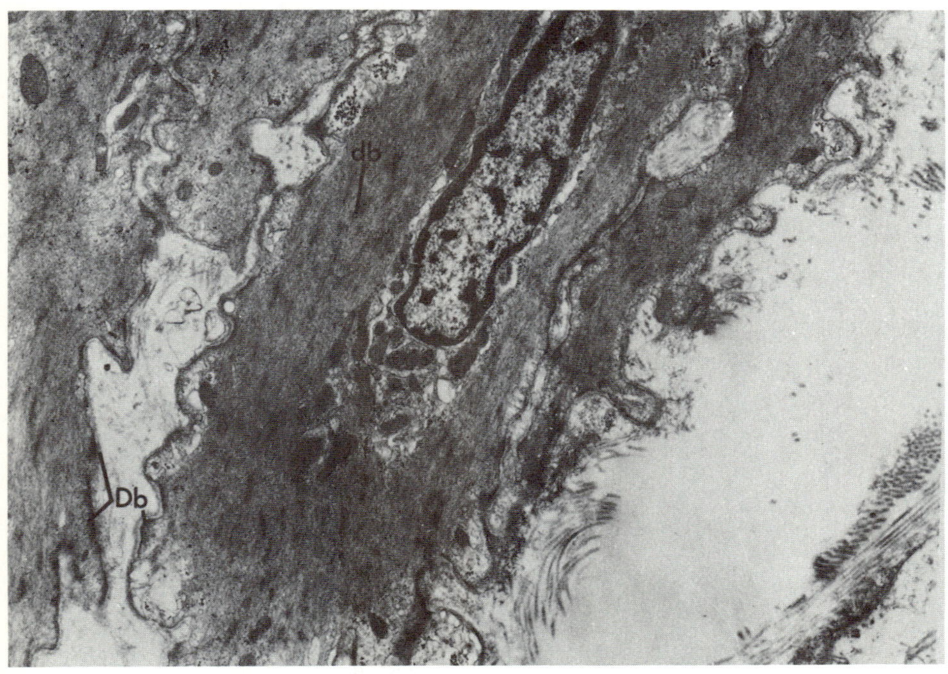

Fig. 2 Low power electron micrograph of canine tracheal smooth muscle in longitudinal secion. db=dense body, Db=dense band.

331

Additional support has been provided by Somlyo et al (6) by a different approach. Figure 2 shows a low power electon micrograph of longitudinal canine tracheal smooth muscle obtained by us, and for present purposes, is reproduced to only demonstrate the presence of dense bodies (DB's) scattered, seemingly randomly, throughout the cytoplasm. Electron dense areas akin to the DB's, are also seen in the sarcolemma. These are known as dense bands and resemble the dense bodies. It was long thought that these structures were analogues of the Z-discs of striated muscle but their random

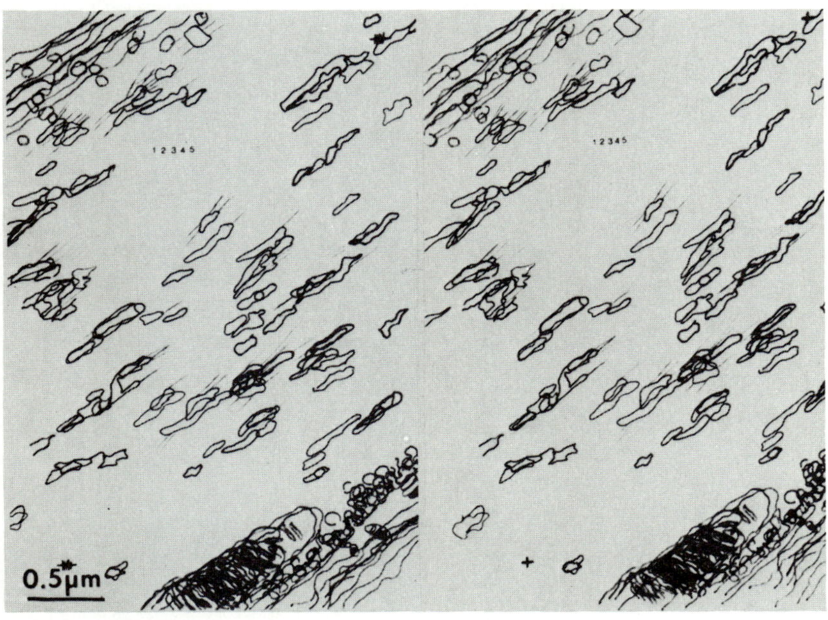

Fig. 3 Stereoview of reconstruction of dense body traces made from 5 consecutive longitudinal 50 nm sections. When viewed in stereo the sections appoear as if there is a spacer between them due to the placement of the traces for obtaining stereo pairs. Dense bodies which overlap are in fact continuous from one section to the next. Note that the dense bodies tend to be elongated and obliquely oriented with respect to the long axis of the cell. Actin filaments have been drawn in for only those dense bodies which were examined at high magnification (x115,000) and where parallax measurements showed them to enter into the dense body. (From Somlyo, A.V. et al. In: Smooth Muscle Contraction. Ed. N.L. Stephens, Publ. Marcel Dekker, New York, 1984).

organization seemed to preclude a similar role. However using anti-actinin antibodies, and analysing the micrographics so obtained (Fig 3), Somlyo et al demonstrated that dense bodies are arrayed in some order, and by careful

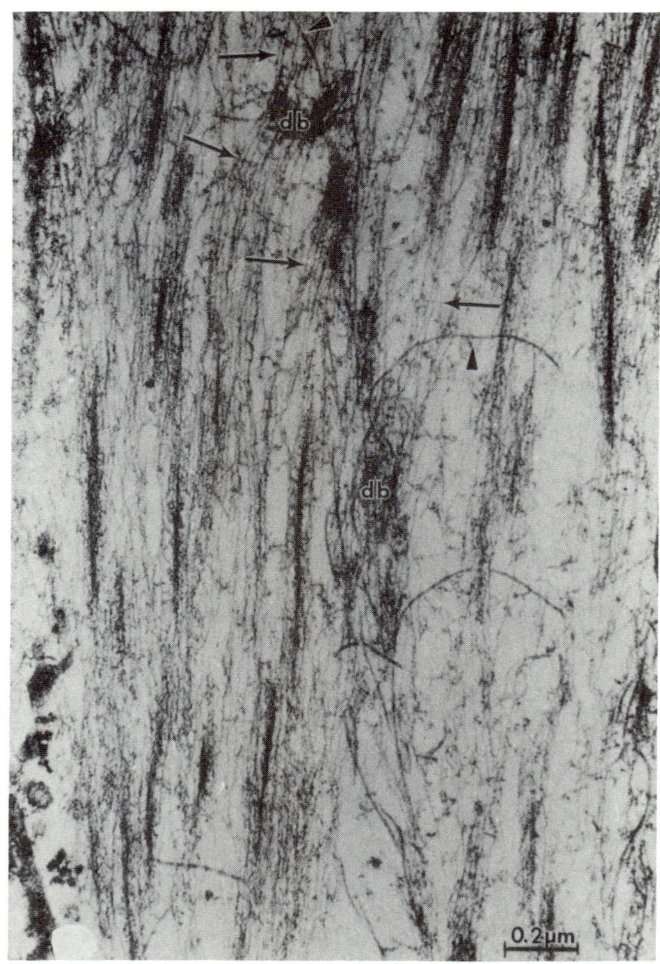

Fig. 4 Longitudinal section of a portal vein smooth muscle cell briefly skinned with saponon and fixed in the presence of tannic acid. Actin filaments (small arrows) insert on both sides of the dense bodies (db) and run to the myosin filaments. The 10 nm filaments (arrowheads) are closely associated and surround the dense bodies (see db on the right). The 10 nm filaments connect to the dense bodies rather than running paralell to the sarcomere unit. (From Somlyo A.V. et al. In: Smooth Muscle Contraction. Ed: N.L. Stephens, Publ: Marcel Dekker Inc. New York, 1984).

measurements they were able to deduce that sarcomeric units existed in smooth muscle. Figure 4 depicts a high power electron micrograph of vascular smooth muscle. This is also taken from the work of Somlyo's group(6). Dense bodies are seen. The actin filaments can be clearly seen running into the dense bodies and this strengthening the Z-disc analogy. Employing myosin sub-fragment 1 (SF1) the Somlyos have shown "decoration" of actin filaments and polar reversal of the orientation of the arrow heads produced by SF1 at either end of the dense body is clearly visible.

Arcuate filaments are also seen in Fig.4 and are described as stretching from one dense body to another. These 100 Å filaments are components of the cytoskeleton, and are, in all likelihood, vimentin filaments. By linking dense bodies they are said to confer structual support to the sarcomere.

In between the thin actin filaments, myosin filaments are seen. These are homogeneous in their length dimensions. However they are longer (2u) than striated myosin filaments which are 1.6u long. The ratio of actin to myosin filaments in smooth muscle is about 15 to 1 which differs mmarkedly from the 6 to 1 ratio of striated muscle. It must also be pointed out that smooth muscle contains only about one fifth the amount of myosin that striated does and yet exerts the same maximum isometric tetanic force (Po). This bespeaks the considerately greater economy of contraction of the former.

To sum up this discussion of the structure of vascular smooth muscle it may be stated that fairly good evidence of sarcomeric (or mini-sarcomeric, as the Somlyos state) organization exists. Parallel arrays of thick and thin filaments are present and myosin cross-bridges are clearly seen. Thus all the elements for the sliding filament, crossbridge theory of contraction are present.

Mechanical Properties of Crossbridges

For long the only measurements made of smooth muscle mechanical function were those of isometric force development. Notable and pioneering exceptions were those of Bozler (7) and of Csapo (1). Over the years length-tension and force-velocity data have been reported for a variety of smooth muscles (8,9,10,11). While their validity has never been established nor has it been refuted. It is noteworthy that because the so-called a constant of Hill's equation is load-dependent and not truly a constant, the equation is no longer a valid way of analysing subcellular mechanisms of contraction. It nevertheless still provides a good phenomenological description of the force-velocity relationship. Woledge (8) has shown that in slow muscle from tortoise, _a_ is constant and hence interpretation of the force-velocity equation in terms of subcellular mechanisms for this muscle is meaningful. Since mammalian smooth muscle is a slow muscle, the assumption has been made that similar validity obtains in this muscle. However, experimental evidence showing that _a_ is load-independent is badly needed..

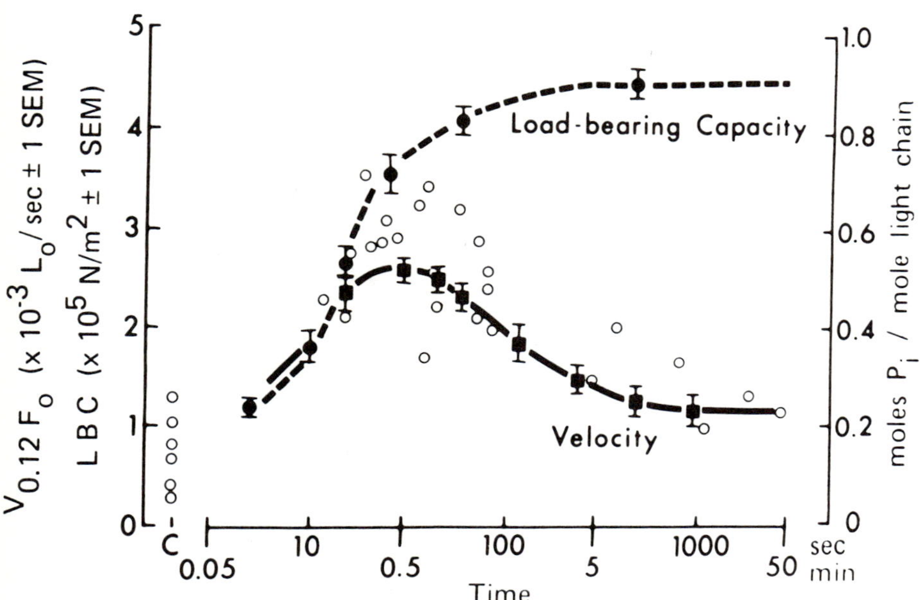

Fig. 5 Time course of changes in number of attached crossbridges (load bearing capacity, their average cycling rate (shortening velocity) and phosphorylation of the 20,000 dalton myosin light chain in swine carotid media. The tissues were stimulated by 109 mMK+ substituted for Sodium. Load bearing capacity is the total passive stress at which the contractile system yields when the tissue is subjected to a quick-stretch. Shortening velocities were measured at a constant afterload of 0.12 F_0. The active stress (F_0) developed at the optimum length (Lo) was 2.84×10^5 N/M^2. Phosphorylation (open circles) was determined in tissues quick-frozen at the indicated times (N=30; C designates unstimulated tissues; note log scale for abscissa). Reprinted from Dillon et al; 1981 by permission).

335

Newer techniques have demonstrated that analysis of mechanical smooth muscle function in terms of crossbridge mechanisms is now possible. Figure 5 is taken from a report of Dillon et al(9) dealing with vascular smooth muscle. The solid line curve is a plot of quasi-maximal velocity of shortening at different points in time. It shows clearly that peak velocity is attained early in contraction and then falls to low basal levels. To account for this behaviour they measured the stoichiometry of myosin light chain phosphorylation since it was known that this phosphorylation regulated smooth muscle contraction(9). A linear relationship between actomyosin ATPase activity and myosin light chain phosphorylation was also known to exist. The open circles in the figure represent the time course of phosphorylation and demonstrate a striking similarity with the phasic velocity curve. From this they postulated that the velocity of crossbridge cycling is controlled by the degree of phosphorylation. They also postulated that as a consequence of dephosphorylation via specific myosin light chain phosphatases (9,10) latch bridges, that barely cycled at all,

were produced. These retarded the motion of the normally cycling crossbridges resulting in overall slowing of the muscle's isotonic shortening. Siegman et al (11) on the other hand feel that latch bridges do not exist, and slowing of muscle shortening is the result of progressive slowing of all the activated bridges that started out cycling at a normal rate. Whatever the true mechanism may turn out to be, all are agreed, that quite unlike striated muscle, from a mechanical point of view in smooth muscle velocity falls as shortening progresses.

We now present some of our own data (12,13) dealing with crossbridge mechanics in airway smooth muscle to provide a foundation for discussing data we have obtained to date from vascular smooth muscle. Figure 6 is a record from a single experiment. The uppermost double line represents the time course of the supramaximal electrical stimulus employed. The lowermost sigmoidal solid line represents isotonic shortening of a lightly preloaded strip of canine tracheal smooth muscle. The load was exactly that required to stretch the muscle to its pre-determined optimal length (l_0). At selected intervals the load was abruptly (within 3 msec) reduced to zero with the help of an electro-magnetic lever system adapted from one designed by Brutsaert et al (14). A rapid transient emanating from the series elastic component (SEC) of the muscle develops followed by a slow transient.

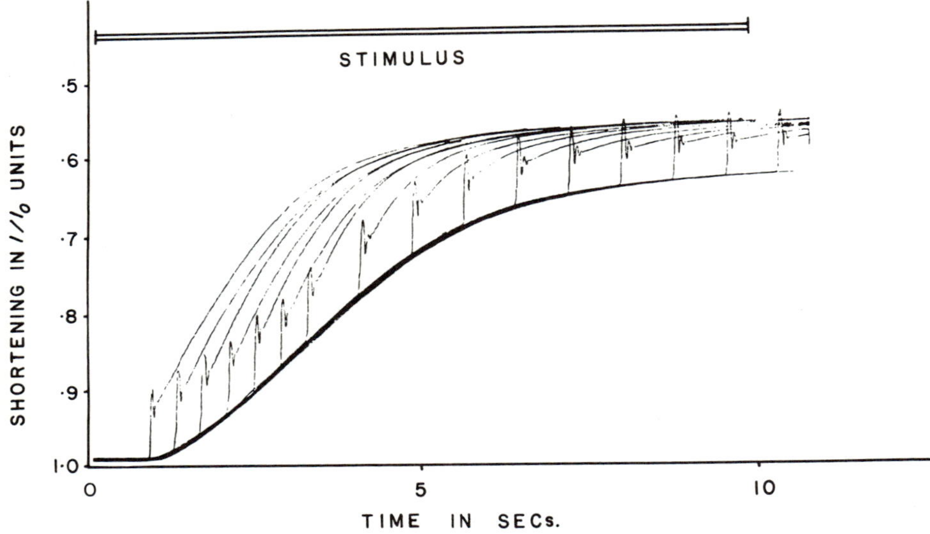

Fig. 6 Oscilloscopic records obtained from a single typical experiment (n=20). (From Stephens et al. Am. J. Physiol. in press).

The latter represents shortening of the contractile element (CE). The maximum slope of this transient is attained very early and represents the maximum velocity of shortening (Vo) for that contraction. Since the muscle is shortening with a zero load, this velocity is a good index of actin activated myosin ATPase activity. Inspection of the various slow transients reveals that V_0 progressively decreases with time.

Figure 7 shows a plot of the V_0's obtained in the previous figure as a function of time. Using high resolution oscilloscopic records at a fast time sweep we have shown that from a mechanical point of view the earliest onset of muscle activation is at 600 msec (15), this implies says that causal biochemical processes must be measured before this. We have published a preliminary report that shows myosin light chain phosphorylation is almost fully complete 400 msec after onset of electrical stimulation. The figure shows peak V_0 (Vmax) is attained 1.75 sec after stimulus onset. We surmise that this represents activation of early crossbridges cycling at a normal (for smooth muscle) rate. The low velocity prior to Vmax is due to

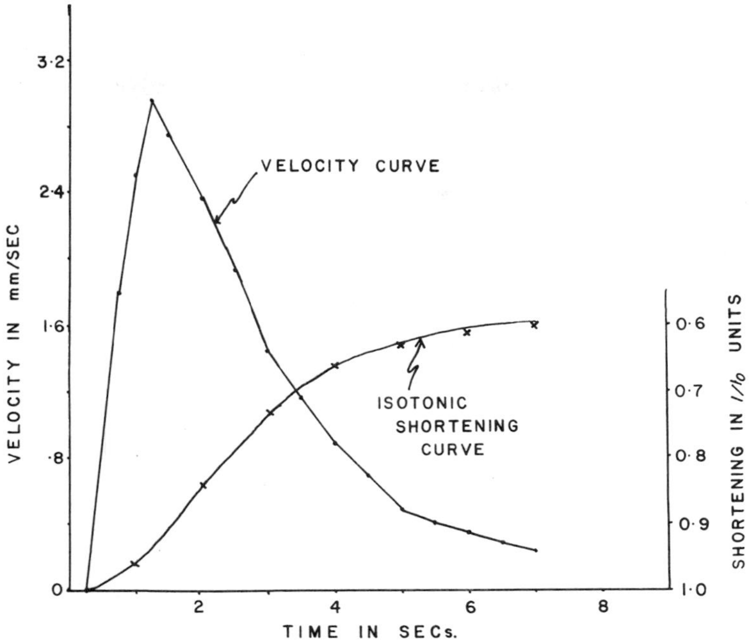

Fig. 7 Plot of Vo's (obtained from fig 6) vs time. From Stephens et al. Am. J. Physiol. in press).

incomplete activation of energy liberating reactions. After 1.75 sec the V_0 curve displays a curvilinear decline much like that in figure 5. This could represent recruitment of latch bridges and shortening at low velocity. Because of the current controversy between the latch bridge and slowly cycling crossbridge schools of thought, it is perhaps safest to term them as early and late crossbridges, recognizing the late bridges are much stronger than the early.

In Figure 8 a conventional compartmental analysis of the descending limb of the velocity curve of fig 7 is depicted. An equation incorporating two exponential terms has been fitted with a significant goodness of fit. Inspection of the equation reveals that the rate constant of the fast compartment (early crossbridges) is almost three times faster than that of the slow (late crossbridges). We have thus succeeded in quantitating the

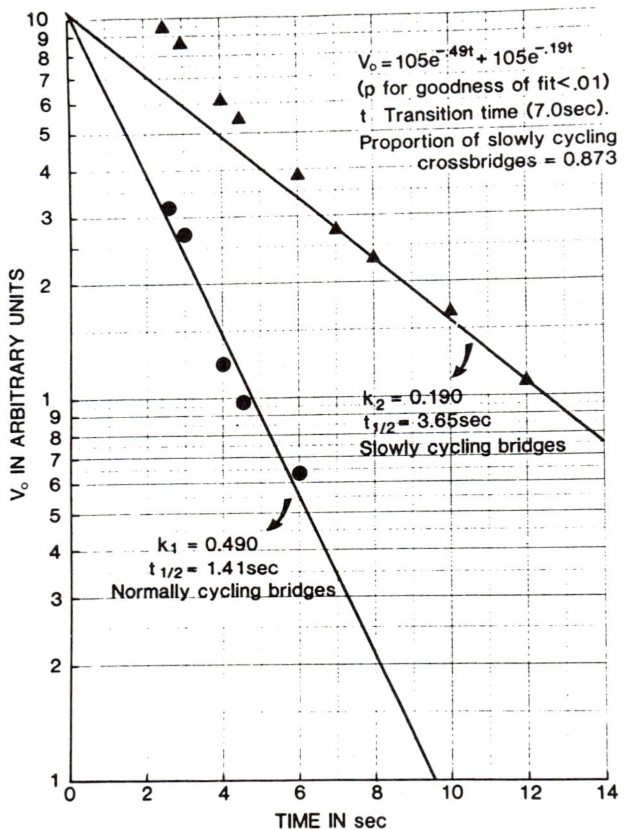

Fig. 8 Semi-logarithmic plot of zeroload velocity (V_O) versus time. A conventional "curve-peeling" analysis has been carried out.

velocities of these two types of crossbridges and are currently addressing ourselves to determining the relative properties of the two types of crossbridges active at any given instant in time. We are also employing pharmacological methods to study these two types of crossbridges seperately. Preliminary, unpublished reports indicate that if tracheal smooth muscles is equilibrated in zero calcium-containing Krebs-Henseleit solution and then stimulated with histamine a phasic contraction is seen; no tonic phase develops. Zero load clamps applied early and late in this phasic response show evidence of only early, i.e. relatively fast, crossbridge activity. Thus this provides a method for isolating a seemingly pure population of early crossbridges. If now 2.0mM calcium is added back to the bathing medium, in the presence of histamine, only a slow contraction develops and zero lead clamps elicit only late crossbridge activity. These experiments are, however, hampered by the fact that we obtain them only in 40% of the experiments we have conducted; as yet we have no explanation for this variability.

We now proceed to consideration of the possible causes for the production of slow bridges. The latch versus slowly cycling crossbridge controversy has already been alluded to. The controversy is further compounded by the fact that not all investigators agree that slow or latch bridges are caused by dephosphorylation of the myosin light chain.

Chatterjee and Murphy (16) have suggested that latch bridge development is highly calcium sensitive in addition to requiring myosin light chain dephosphorylation. However Siegman et al (11) and we (15) find no dephosphorylation please. This represents yet another controversial area in smooth muscle research.

With respect to other possible causes of crossbridge slowing, we conducted experiments in which zero load clamps were applied during the course, not of an isotonic, but, of an isometric contraction a V_0 versus time plot was obtained. The major difference in these two modes is that minimal shortening occurs in the former. Figure 9 shows plots of V_0 versus time for these two types of experiments. At the 10 sec point it is clear that the reduction in V_0 is much less for the isometric mode. This deficit, which amounts to almost 70%, can be ascribed to the obligatory shortening of the isotonic experimental mode. The mechanism for this has not been directly investigated but we have shown (17) by delineating length-tension curves for smooth muscle bathed in 1.9mM and 4.75mM Calcium containing solutions, that as the muscle shortens it deactivates itself. This deactivation could easily account for the decrease in isometric force production. Similar phenomena have been reported for single skeletal muscle fibres (18) and for cat heart papillary muscle (18). Siegman et al (19) have reported similar data for aciothe smooth muscle. Their structural

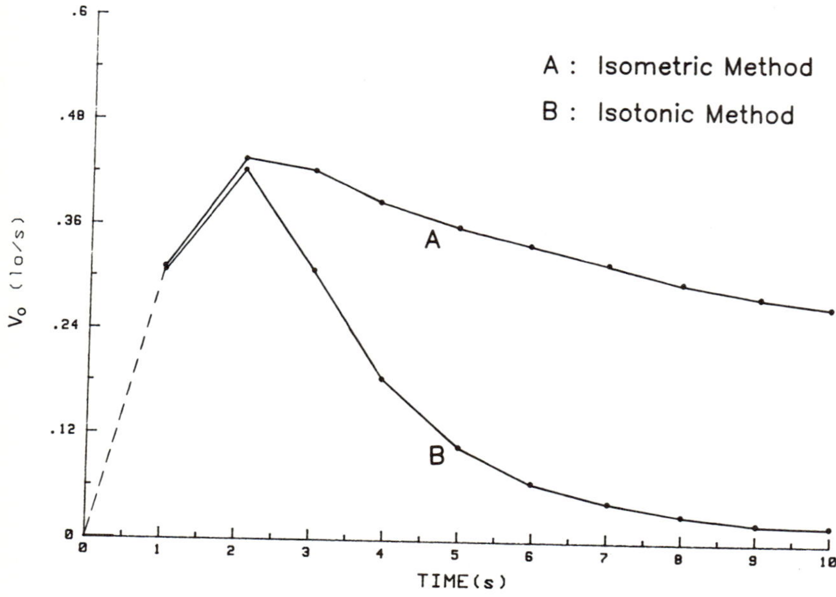

Fig. 9 Vo versus time plots obtained by zero load in the clamping course of isotonic (lower curve) and isometric experiments.

studies indicate that as the muscle shortens its central fibres are inactivated. However the germane issue is what happens to V_0 as the muscle shortens. We have reported (20) that V_0 is unaffected by 20% shortening of the muscle from l_0; thereafter it falls. At the 10 sec point in the contraction the isotonic muscle has shortened considerably more than this, and thus reduced activation could account for the 70% difference in V_0 at 10 sec, between isotonic and isometric contractions. This also enables us to conclude that the 30% reduction between Vmax at 1.75 sec and V_0 at 10 sec is due to non-shortening related causes among which could be included latch bridge mechanisms. In figure 5 a considerably greater drop in V_0 is evident. The experiment was conducted in isometric mode and the fall off is surprising. Possible explanations are that the tissues are different (hog carotid versus dog trachealis) as are the stimuli (pharmacologic for the carotid and electrical for the dog trachealis) employed.

Another possible explanation for the 30% drop in V_0 alluded to above for isometric mode experiments is the development of intra-cellular acidosis towards the end of a tetanus. Since smooth muscle (especially multi-unit type, to which category belongs the trachealis) relies more on the anaerobic glycolytic pathway for energy production (21,22) accumulation of lactic acid is greater. The development of fatigue, and compartmentalized changes in osmolarity or temperature, could be other possible causes. A final speculation stems from the notion that muscle contraction could be produced by phophorylation dependent on protein kinase-C activation. Using phorbol esters Rasmusse et al (23) have shown an action like diacylglycerol in activating protein kinase C. The contracture resulting from this is of a slow type. It is therefore possible that the faster crossbridge is recruited by calcium-calmodulin dependent mechanisms and the slower by protein-kinase C dependent processes.

In concluding this section the point we would like to make is that a variety of mechanisms exist that could slow down normally cycling crossbridges without involving any specific dephosphorylation mechanism. The dephosphorylation could therefore be merely an epiphenomenon. Reduced activation due to shortening, development of intracelluar acidosis, fatigue, and recruitment of slow bridges by protein kinase C dependent phosphorylation, will all have to be accounted for before one can identify to what extent latch bridges contibute to slowing of shortening.

Alterations in Vascular Smooth Muscle Crossbridge properties in Pathophysiologic states

We now pass to a consideration of how the physiological insights discussed above may be applied to the elucidation of disease processes affecting smooth muscle. Two of the commonest are asthma and essential hypertension. In conditions such as these and in a variety of mechanical dysfunctions affecting gastro-intestinal, uterine and uretero-vesical structures the major parameter affected is that of resistance. All the smooth muscles mentioned encircle hollow organs and carry out their regulatory functions by decreasing cross-sectional areas and luminal volumes. Thus circulation of blood, passage of air down airways, or of a food bolus down the gastro-intestinal tract and of the conceptus down the uterine passages, all involve alterations in resistance. Hence in studying these smooth muscles it is shortening parameters that must be studied. Yet the commonest variable measured _in vitro_ is that of isometric tetanic force. While this provides information regarding the stiffness properties of smooth muscle which affects flow in a relatively minor way, it tells us nothing about resistance and conductance. To re-iterate, the maximum capacity of isotonic shortening (Δlmax) tells us more about what we want to know about airway smooth muscle from asthmatic patients and animal models of asthma than isometric force development. We have reported that in both ovalbumen (24) and ragween pollen (25) sensitized airway smooth muscle Δlmax is increased; this is the _in vitro_ analogue to increased _in vivo_ bronchoconstriction. Measurement of V_O is also useful because it provides a clue as to what alteration has developed in the contractile machinery. We have also reported that V_O is increased in sensitized airway smooth muscle when compared to that of littermate controls (24,25). It must be remembered that with respect to asthma, Δlmax is the parameter of prime importance, but in carrying out isotonic force-velocity experiments one.secs that at light loads as the velocity of shortening increases so does the Δlmax and alterations in one may provide insight into the functioning of the other.

Another caveat has to be entered that stems from knowledge about fast and slow crossbridges. Our studies described above, have shown that within 2 second of a 10 sec tetanic contraction, the rapid bridges commence slowing. It appears that at about 5 seconds after stimulus onset the overwhelming majority of bridges are slow. Furthermore about 75% of the muscle's isotonic shortening, is completed within 2-3 sec by normally cycling crossbridges which appear to subserve shortening while the slow bridges subserve force development. It is clear from this that if Δlmax is to be studied then the shortening produced within 2 to 3 seconds of the onset of shortening must be measured. Studying isotonic shortening at its plateau value is necessarily restricted to studying the shortening effects of an unknown combination of fast and slow bridges. A plea is made therefore for carrying out such studies at the 2 to 3 second point in contraction.

Studies in our laboratory have shown that in mild hypoxia lmax is reduced (as is V_O) much before P_O. Furthermore while the V_O of the normally cycling bridges is increased that for the slow bridges remains unaltered. In ragweed pollen sensitized airway smooth muscle we have also found that

Δ<u>lmax</u> and V_0 are increased while Po is unaltered (25). Again it is the 2 second crossbridge that demonstrates increased activity while the 10sec is normal (unpublished observations). In vascular smooth muscle from spontaneously hypertensive rats increased Δlmax and V_0 have been detected early in the disease; they preceed changes in Po. As time progresses changes in Po develop, first an increase and then a decrease. All these data strongly support the idea that in attempting to elucidate casual or primary mechanisms early and/or mild disease states must be studied.

Perhaps the only justification for measuring isometric force development is that under some conditions, alterations in Po are accompanied by parallel changes in V_0 and lmax and hence each provides insight into the other. However, as we have shown, changes in Po are relatively late. Secondly the onus is on the investigator to show that in a given smooth muscle for a given set of environmental conditions the force-velocity curve is shifted parallel to the control, because exceptions certainly ext. We have reported (26), for example, that at lower temperatures while Po is unchanged, V_0 drops considerably. Similar results are seen in cardiac muscle (27). In the latter while norpinephrine increases V_0, it does not affect P_0.

Though our initial studies of asthma were conducted in airway smooth muscle from ovalbumen and ragweed pollen sensitized dogs we became aware that many of the changes occurring in asthma, involved small airways. This manifested itself as a change in dynamic pulmonary compliance. It also became apparent that changes in dynamic compliance could just as easily stem from vasoconstriction of small pulmonary blood vessels as from airways. Furthermore the leukotrienes which have been shown to be the most powerful airway agonists known, constrict small blood vessels even more powerfully. This prompted us to study pulmonary smooth muscle from sensitized dogs. The details of the sensitization protocol and of the alterations in mechanical properties of sensitized pulmonary blood vessels have been published by us before (28,29). Figure 10 shows isometric force curves obtained by specific ovalbumen challenge, <u>in vitro</u>, of ovalbumen sensitized dogs. A contractile response (the Schultz - Dale) is seen, that is partially blocked by an H_1 blocker. The curve to the right demonstrates that phentolamine blocks part of the response to the challenge. In sensitized pulmonary vessels the Schultz-Dale response is partially mediated by hisamine and partially by nonadrenaline via α-adrenoceptors. We do not know what the remaining

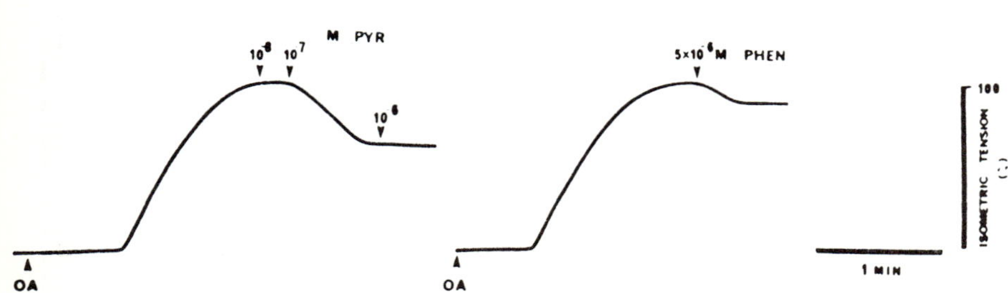

Fig. 10 Isometric force versus time plots of ovalbumen sensitized canine pulmonary artery. The effects of histamine H1 receptor and α- adrenoceptor block are shown.

contractile response (about 40% of the total) is due to, but leukotrienes and PAF-Acether are strong contenders.

Fig 11 shows dose-response curves to histamine. Hyperreactivity (increased efficacy) and hypersensitivity (leftward shift of the curve for the sensitized smooth muscle) are evident. These changes are akin to those seen by us in sensitized tracheal smooth muscle.

Since isometric responses are relatively late indicators of pathophysiology we conducted studies of isotonic shortening

Figure 12 shows force-velocity curves obtained from control and ovalbumen sensitized pulmonary blood vessels (30). It is clear that while Po is unchanged, Vmax (used synonymously with V_0) is considerably increased; Δlmax is also increased.

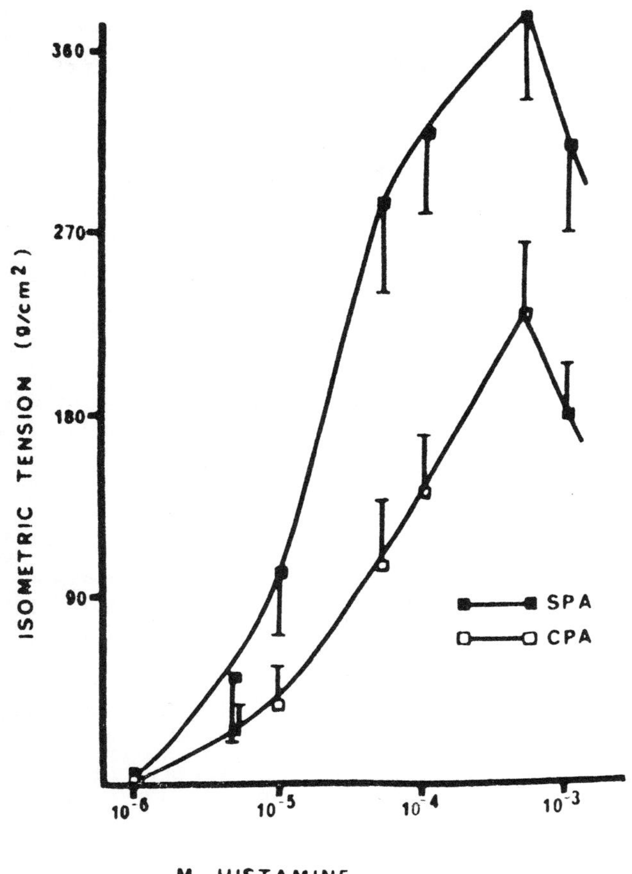

Fig. 11 Histamine dose-response curves of ovalbumen sensitized and littermate control canine pulmonary arteries.

Fig 13 depicts some problems that arise in the interpretation of force-velocity data from smooth muscle. In this figure force-velocity curves for early (2 sec) crossbridges and late (10 sec) crossbridges are seen. The considerable quantitative differences between them have already been pointed out. Conventional force-velocity curves have not taken into

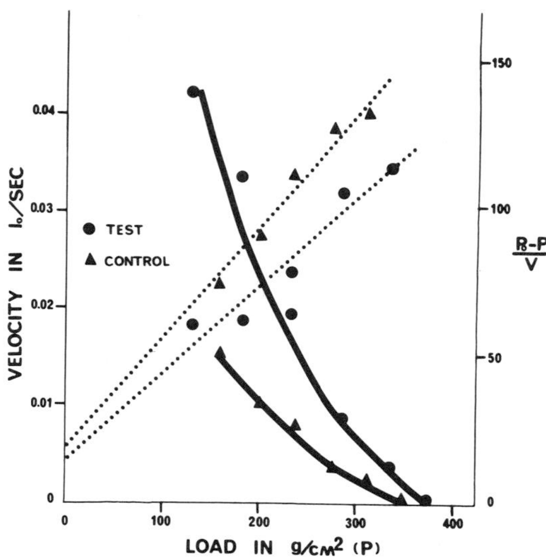

Fig. 12 Typical force-velocity curves elicited in a paired (ovalbumen sensitized and littermate control) experiment. Linearized transforms prove relationships are hyperbolic. From Kong, S.K. and N.L. Stephens. In J. Appl. Physiol.: Respirat. Environ. Exercise Physiol. 55(6): 1669-1673, 1983.

consideration the existence of two types of bridges and their differing machanical properties. In eliciting velocity measurements at light loads the maximum velocity occurs within 1-2 sec of stimulus onset and shortening at that time, in all likelihood, is produced by normally cycling crossbridges. However at loads approaching Po, the muscle spends almost 3 seconds developing isometric force before it can shorten - at this point in time latch bridges are beginning to be recruited. Hence the conventional smooth muscle force-velocity curve is a composite of the activities of the two types of bridges. It is probably for this reason that force-velocity points at heavy loads deviate from a hyperbolic function. In studying smooth muscle shortening therefore force-velocity curves should be carried out early in contraction. This can only be achieved by the load clamp technique.

The above considerations are based on the assumption that two distinct types of crossbridges exist in pulmonary vascular smooth muscle. Since this is the first report of changes in mechanical properties of sensitized

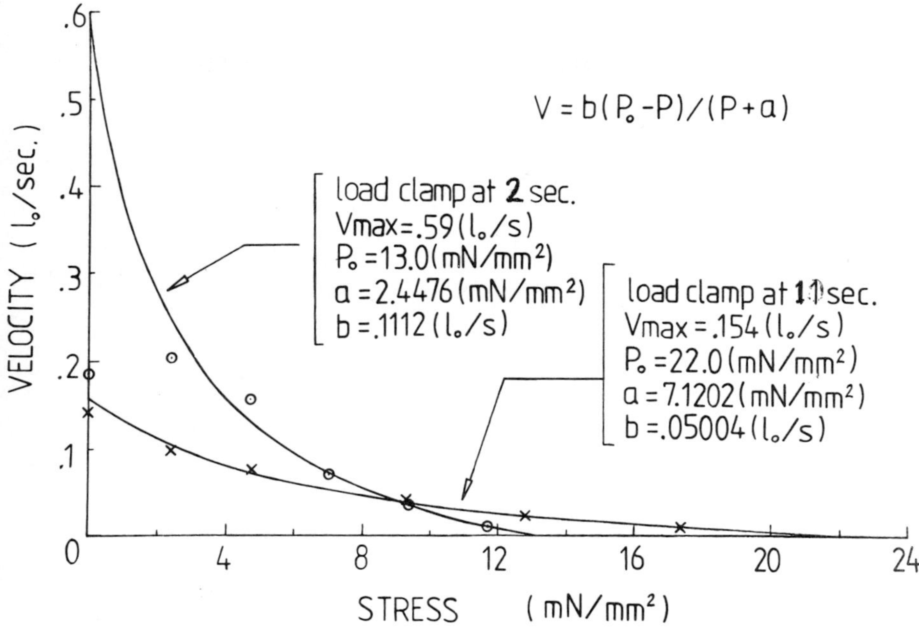

Fig. 13 Force-velocity curves obtained by applying abrupt load clamps at 2 sec and 10 sec during an isotonic contraction.

pulmonary vessels, the determination of whether normally cycling or latch bridges are involved has not yet been considered.

We set out to determine whether the two types of crossbridges exist in pulmonary arterial smooth muscle. Figure 14 which depicts data such as those shown for the tracheali in figure 6, depicts the rapid and slow transient reponses to zero load clamps applied during the course of an isotonic contraction in a strip of canine pulmonary artery. It is clear that Vo diminishes with time thus displaying the behavior seen in the canine trachealis and the hog carotid. Thus two types of crossbridges exist in the pulmonary artery also. We propose in the near future to measure the velocities of crossbridge activity at 4 and 12 seconds in control and sensitized tissues. This will help determine which type of bridge is affected in sensitization. Studies of isotonic shortening (Δlmax) will also

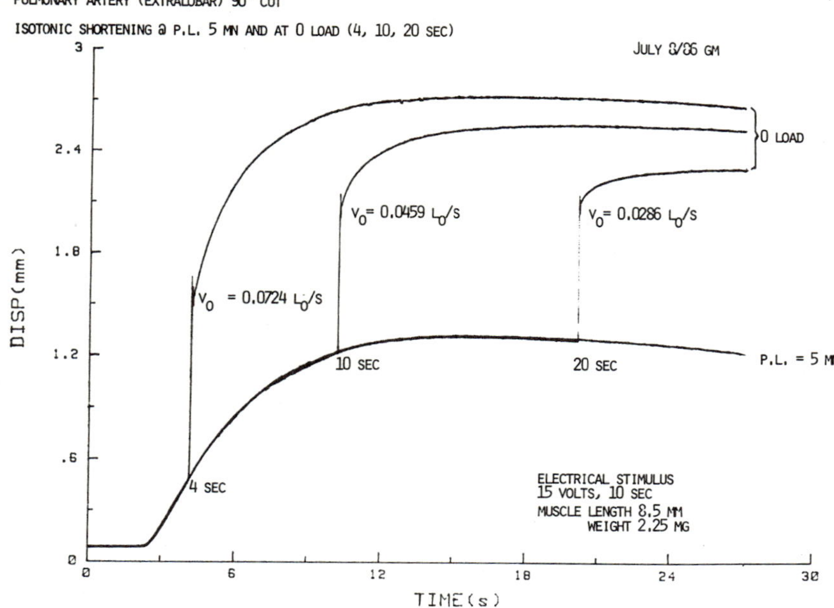

Fig. 14. Displacement (shortening increasing upwards, where 0 represents l_O and 3mm represents $(l_O$-3)mm versus time records from a pulmonary artery strip shortening isotonically. At 4, 10 and 20 sec, zero load clamps were applied. V_O= maximum slope of the slow transient resulting from application of the zero load clamp.

determine whether the sensitized artery has developed an increased capacity for shortening.

CONCLUSIONS

1. In smooth muscle, regulation of cross bridge activity is brought about via phosphorylation of the 20,000 dalton myosin light chain. This process is calcium calmodulin dependent.

2. In smooth muscle contraction the velocity of crossbridge cycling late in contraction is approximately four times slower than in early contraction.

This is quite unlike striated muscle where velocity late in contraction is, if anything slightly faster.

3. Early crossbridges subserve shortening development, while the later subserve tension development.

4. The current consensus is that the latch bridges develop as the result of dephosphorylation of the myosin light chain via the action of specific phosphatases. These bridges are very calcium sensitive. However not all investigators agree that phosphorylation of the chain follows the phasic time course reported by Murphy's group.

5. The existence of slow and fast bridges has been demonstrated in a variety of different mammalism smooth muscles, including systemic and pulmonary blood vessels.

6. In evaluating the role of latch bridges the effects of several other factors - reduced activation due to shortening, development of intracellular acidosis, and fatigue - have to be kept in mind.

7. In altered inotropic states it is now possible to determine which type of crossbridge has been altered in function. In hypoxic airway smooth muscle for example, early crossbridges are slowed, while in antigen sensitization in which velocity of shortening is increased it is the early crossbridge which becomes faster, the late bridge remains normal.

8. Studies of sensitized pulmonary blood vessels have been initiated in our laboratory. The presence of rapid (early) and slow (late) crossbridges has been demonstrated in this tissue also. Studies to determine which of these is altered in function upon antigen sensitization will be carried out in the near future.

Acknowledgements. Thanks are due to Cheryl Toews for excellent typewriting assistance.

BIBLIOGRAPHY

1. Csapo,A. Smooth muscle as a contractile unit. Physiol. Revs. 42, Suppl. 5:7-33, 1962.
2. Gordon, A. Rand, M.J. Siegman. Mechanical properties of smooth muscle. I Length-tension and force-velocity relations. Am. J. Physiol. 1:1243-1249, 1971.
3. Stephens, N.L., E. Kroeger and J.A. Mehta. Force-velocity characteristics of respiratory airway smooth muscle. J. Appl. Physiol. 6: 685-692, 1969.

4.   Halpern, W., M.J. Mulvany, and D.M. Warshaw. Mechanical properties of smooth muscle cells in the walls of arterial resistance vessels. J. Physiol.(Lond.) 275: 85-101, 1978.

5.   Groschel-Stewart U., S. Ceurremans, I. Lehr, and C. Mahlmeister. Production of specific antibodies to contractile prteins and their use in immunofluorescence microscopy. II species specific and species nonspecific antibodies to smooth and striated chicken muscle actin Histochemistry, 50: 271, 1977.

6.   Somlyo, A.V., M. Bond, T.M. Butler, D.F. Berner, F.T. Ashton, H. Holtzen. The contractile apparatus of smooth muscle: an update. In: Smooth Muscle Contraction. Ed. N.L. Stephens, Publ. Marcel Dekker Inc., 1984: 1-20, 1984.

7.   Bozler, E., The heat production of smooth muscle. J. Physiol. (Lond) 119: 442-462, 1930.

8.   Woledge, R.C. The energetics of tortoise muscle. J. Physiol. London 197: 685-707, 1968.

9.   Dillon, P.F., M.O. Aksoy, S.P. Driska and R.A. Murphy. Myosin phosphorylation and the crossbridge cycle in arterial smooth muscle. Science 211: 495-497, 1981.

10. Pato, M.D. and R.S. Adelstein. Dephosphorylation of the 20,000 dalton light chain of myosin by two different phosphatases from smooth muscle. J. Biol. Chem.: 255: 6535-6538, 1980.

11. Siegman, M.J., T.M. Butler, S.U. Mooers, R.E. Davies. Chemical energetics of force development, force maintenance and relaxation in mammalian smooth muscle. J. Gen. Physiol. 76: 609-629. 1980.

12. Stephens, N.L., G. Morgan, C.S. Packer and S.K. Kong. Smooth Muscle Contractility. Effects of Hypoxia: Chest. 885: 223s-229s, 1985 Supplement.

13. Stephens,N.L. Time dependence of shortening velocity in tracheal smooth muscle. Am. J. Physiol. 251 (Cell Physiol. 20): C-C-, 1986.

14. Brutsaert, D.L., V.A. Claes, and E.H. Sonnenblick. Velocity of shortening of unloaded heart muscle and the length-tension relation Circ. Res. 29: 63-75, 1971.

15. Kong, S.K., R. P.C. Shiu and N.L. Stephens. Role of myosin light chain (MLC) phosphorylation in canine tracheal smooth muscle (TSM) contraction. Fed. Proc. 43(3): 427A, 1984.

16. Chatterjee, M., and Murphy, R. Calcium-dependent stress maintenance without myosin phosphorylation in skinned smooth muscle. Science. 221: 464-466, 1983.

17. Stephens, N.L. Airway Smooth Muscle: Physiology, bronchomotor tone, pharmacology and relation to asthma. In Bronchial Asthma. Ed. E.B. Weiss, M.S. Segal and M. Stein; Publ: Little, Brown and Co., Boston. pp. 96-110, 1985.

18. Taylor, S.R. Decreased activation in skeletal muscle fibres at short lengths. In: Physiological Basis of Sterling's Law of the Heart. Eds: R. Porter and D.W. Fitzsimons. Publ: Elsevier/North-Holland, Amsterdam. pp. 93-116, 1974.

19. Siegman, M.J., S. Davidheiser; T.M. Butler and S.U. Mooers. What is the length-tension relation in smooth muscle? Fed. Proc. 44(3): 456A, 1985.

20. Stephens, N.L., M.L. Kagan and C.S. Packer. Time dependence of shortening velocity in tracheal smooth muscle. Am. J. Physiol. 251 C-C-, 1986.

21. Somlyo, A.P. and A.V. Somlyo. Vascular Smooth Muscle I. Normal structure pathology, biochemistry and biophysics. Pharmacol. Rev. 20: 197-272, 1965

22. Paul, R.J., N. Bauer, and W. Pease. Vascular Smooth Muscle: aerobic glycolysis linked to sodium and potassium transport processes. Science: 206: 1414-1416, 1979.

23. Rasmussen,H., and P.O. Barret. Calcium messenger system. An integrated view. Physiol. Revs. 64(3): 938-984, 1984.

24. Anntonissen, L.A., R.W. Mitchell, S.A. Kroeger, N. Kepron, K.S. Tse and N.L. Stephens. Mechanical alterations of airway smooth muscle in a canine asthmatic model. J. Appl. Physiol. Respiration Environ. Exercise Physiol. 46: 681-687, 1979.

25. Mitchell, R.W., L.A. Antonissen, W. Kepron, S.A. Kroeger and N.L. Stephens. Effect of atropine on the hyperresponsiveness of ragweed -sensitized canine tracheal smooth muscle. J. Pharmacol. and Exp. Therap. 236(3): 803-809, 1986.

26. Stephens,N.L., R. Cardinal and B. Simmons. Mechanical properties of tracheal smooth muscle effects of temperature. Am. J. Physiol. 2(2): C92-C98, 1977.

27. Yeatman, L.A. Jr., W.W. Parmley, and E.H. Sonnenblick. Effects of temperature on series elasticity and contractile element motion in heart muscle. Am. J. Physiol. 217: 1030-1034, 1969.

28. Kepron, W., J.M. James, B. Kirk, A.H. Sehon and K.S. Tse. A canine model for reaginic hypersensitivity and allergic bronchoconstriction. J. Allergy Clin. Immunol 59: 64-69, 1977.

29. Kong, S.K. and N.L. Stephens. Pharmacological studies of sensitized canine pulmonary blood vessels. J. Appl. Physiol.:Respirat.Environ. Exercise Physiol. 55(6):1669-1673, 1983.

F. FUNCTIONAL ASPECT OF METABOLISM

23

CONTROL OF GLUCOSE UPTAKE AND UTILIZATION IN THE MYOCARDIUM

I. BIHLER

Department of Pharmacology and Therapeutics, University of
Manitoba, Faculty of Medicine, Winnipeg, Manitoba R3E 0W3
Canada

INTRODUCTION

One still not fully resolved question in cardiac physiology
is how metabolic energy production and work output are orches-
trated in the mammalian heart. A variable proportion of myocardial energy metabolism depends on the utilization of glucose.
This is controlled by feedbacks from various metabolic intermediates and modulation by hormones which interact to control
the activity of individual enzymes and of sarcolemmal glucose
transport.

The rate of glucose utilization in the heart is proportional
to contractile activity at any given moment. It is also governed
by the availability of substrates; fatty acids, ketone bodies and
other non-glucose oxidative substrates are normally preferred to
glucose. Free fatty acids inhibit glucose utilization, an
observation at the base of Randle's concept of the glucose-lipid
cycle (1). Conversely, under anoxic conditions metabolism is
switched to anaerobic glycolysis with increased glucose uptake
and glycogenolysis.

Increased glucose supply inhibits fatty acid metabolism
indirectly, as hyperglycemia normally increases insulin secretion,
causing increased glucose uptake and utilization by the heart
and redirection of metabolism towards enhanced synthesis of
glycogen and triglycerides and decreased lipolysis.

The first step in glucose utilization is its transfer across
the sarcolemma and this process is normally rate limiting for
overall glucose utilization (2). The rate limiting role of the
transport step has often been ignored. Clearly, activation of
intracellular enzymes cannot be effective unless more glucose is
being supplied to the intracellular metabolic machinery.

Not surprisingly, therefore, the various factors affecting glucose utilization in muscle also alter the activity of the membrane transport step. Moreover, there is much evidence that calcium is involved in regulation of the glucose transport step (for reviews, see refs. 3,4,5), giving rise to the hypothesis that alterations in Ca^{2+} binding and/or distribution act as the common mediator of glucose transport regulation.

This communication will be focused on sarcolemmal glucose transport and its regulation in isolated cardiac myocytes. Evidence will be reviewed pointing to calcium as the common mediator of many regulatory influences and as the signal integrating glucose transport with various cellular processes.

MATERIALS AND METHODS

Cardiac myocytes were isolated from adult rat ventricles by collagenase digestion and mechanical disaggregation as described before (6). These cell preparations consist of over 90% noncontracting rod-shaped myocytes with normal morphology, including intact glycocalyx (7). The myocytes are Ca^{2+}-tolerant, survive for 2-3 hours and show normal levels of Na^+, K^+ and ATP and normal responses to electrical and other stimuli. They exhibit all the features of glucose transport and its regulation - including Ca^{2+} dependence (8,9) - which were demonstrated previously in intact cardiac muscle (10).

Sarcolemmal glucose transport was measured by following the uptake of the ^{14}C-labelled nonmetabolized glucose analog 3-_0_-methyl-D-glucose for 0.3 min, a period brief enough to determine initial uptake rates. Incubation was rapidly terminated by dilution with ice-cold stopping solution containing the glucose transport inhibitor cytochalasin B, followed by centrifugation through an inert organic fluid layer. The distribution of $[^3H]$-L-glucose in the same cell samples was used to correct for extracellular space and passive diffusion. Radioactivity was determined by double-label liquid scintillation counting. Details of this procedure have been described (8). Because of variability between cell preparations, all comparisons were performed within a single pool of cells, and data are normalized

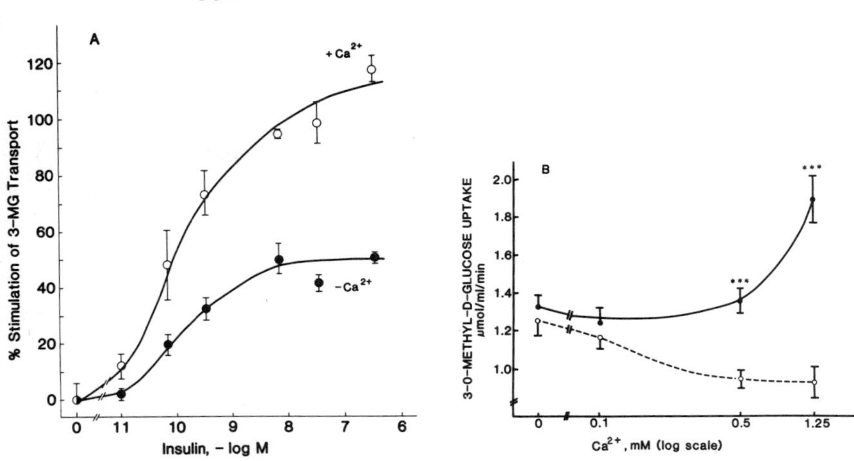

Fig. 1. A - Effect of insulin on 3-methylglucose transport in isolated cardiac myocytes (From (8) by permission). B - Ca^{2+}-dependence of stimulation by insulin.

by expressing them as percent of the basal (unstimulatated) control. The results are presented as means ± S.E. and statistical evaluation was by Student's t-test.

RESULTS

The effect of insulin in this preparation, shown in Fig. 1, exhibits a partial but clearcut Ca^{2+}-dependence, as described in intact cardiac (10) and skeletal (11) muscle. The dose response curves (Fig. 1A) indicate that stimulation of methylglucose transport by insulin reaches a much higher plateau in the presence of 1.25 mM external Ca^{2+} than in its nominal absence. The dependence of these effects on the Ca^{2+} concentration is illustrated in Fig. 1B. As external Ca^{2+} is increased, insulin-stimulated methylglucose uptake rises strikingly. A relatively high concentration of Ca^{2+}, 0.5 mM is required for a significant stimulatory effect. Previous kinetic studies (8) have shown that insulin in the presence of Ca^{2+} causes an almost 5-fold increase in Vmax; in the nominal absence of Ca^{2+} from the incubation medium Vmax increased by about 40%. Changes in Km were not significant.

Apart from insulin there are other factors of physiological significance, as well as many experimental interventions, that affect glucose transport. Table 1 lists several typical effects in cardiac myocytes. These include stimulation by cyanide, serving here as model for anoxia which is technically difficult to achieve in myocyte suspension; inhibition of the Na^+ pump by ouabain or omission of K^+ from the medium; hyperosmolarity; a sodium ionophore, monensin and a Ca^{2+} ionophore, A23187. Most of these stimulatory effects are dependent on the presence of external Ca^{2+}. Under the present conditions only hyperosmolarity was effective in the absence of external Ca^{2+}.

Glucose utilization is also coupled to contractile activity which of course involves the release of Ca^{2+} from the sarcoplasmic reticulum into the cytoplasm. Increased membrane transport of glucose in contracting muscle is well documented. Glucose transport studies in beating myocytes have as yet not been done because of technical difficulties. For this reason, the data in Fig. 2 illustrate earlier experiments (12) in isolated rat left atria. The ouabain dose response curve in resting atria exactly parallels the cellular Na^+ levels determined at the same concentrations of ouabain. The mechanism of this relationship is discussed further below. In atria electrically stimulated to contract at 75 beat/min there is an additional contraction-dependent increment in transport which coincides with the positive inotropic effect of the digitaloid,

Table 1. Stimulation of 3-methylglucose uptake in cardiac
        myocytes

	3-methylglucose uptake, % of control	
Conditions	+ 1.25 mM Ca^{2+}	Ca^{2+}-free
Basal	100.0 ± 4.2 (22)	100.0 ± 6.8 (7)
KCN, 2 mM	136.7 ± 8.2 (7)	100.7 ± 4.4 (10)
K^+-free	130.0 ± 5.7 (17)	100.2 ± 1.6 (11)
Ouabain, 10^{-6} M	169.6 ± 5.9 (13)	89.4 ± 5.2 (9)
Hyperosmolar (+100 mOsm/l)	131.2 ± 4.4 (7)	143.4 ± 5.8 (6)
Monensin, 10^{-8} M	146.0 ± 5.5 (13)	94.7 ± 3.8 (12)
A23187, 2 x 10^{-5} M	157.9 ± 8.5 (7)	97.4 ± 8.3 (4)

Cells were incubated as above for 15 min before transport assay.

Figure 2

Figure 3

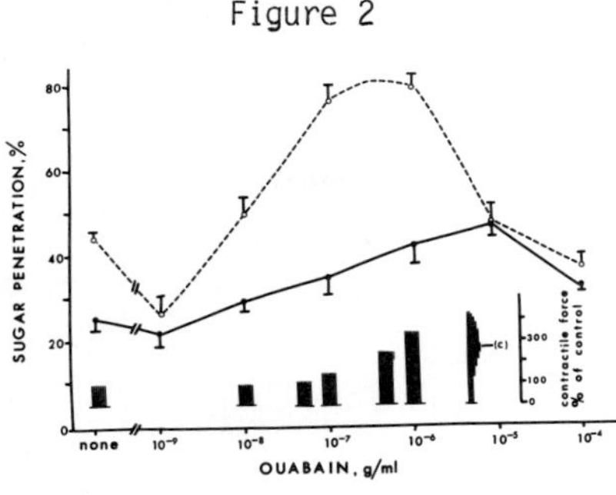

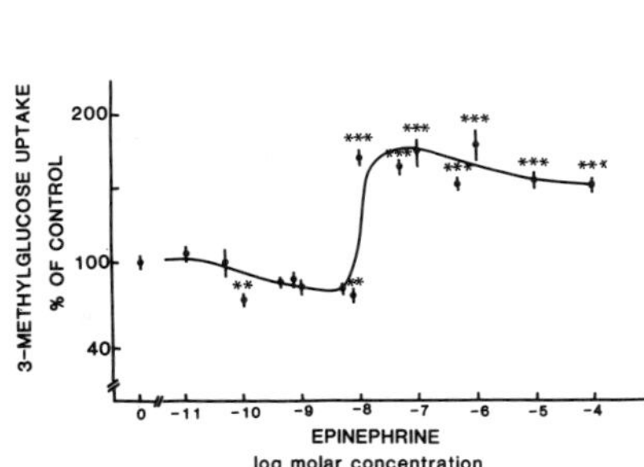

Fig. 2. Effect of ouabain on 3-methylglucose transport and contractile force in perifused guinea pig left atria. Resting (solid line) or electrically stimulated at 75 beat/min (dashed line). (C) indicates contracture. (From (12) by permission).

Fig. 3. Effect of adrenaline on 3-methylglucose transport in isolated cardiac myocytes.

as shown in the contractile force recording (bottom of Fig. 2). The decline in methylglucose transport at very high levels of ouabain coincides with development of contracture.

Stimulation of glucose transport via increased contractile activity is found with many other positive inotropic agents, e.g. adrenergic agonists. In resting muscle it is, however, possible to demonstrate effects of catecholamines which are unrelated to contractile activity. The adrenaline dose-response curve of methylglucose transport in resting cardiac myocytes (Fig. 3) shows inhibition at low and stimulation at higher concentrations of adrenaline. Such a dual effect has been described before (see below).

The nature of adrenergic receptors involved was studied with specific agonists and antagonists as shown in Table 2. In non-contracting cardiac myocytes stimulation of methyl-glucose transport is mediated by both beta and alpha receptor interactions, whereas the inhibitory effect at low concentrations depends purely on beta receptors. Surprisingly, these effects are blocked by specific beta-1 and beta-2, and alpha-1 and alpha-2 inhibitors, respectively. In control experiments methylglucose transport was unaffected by the antagonists at

Table 2. Effects of adrenergic agonists and antagonists in cardiac myocytes.

Additions	3-methylglucose uptake, % of control		
	Adrenaline 10^{-8}M	Adrenaline 10^{-10}M	Phenylephrine 5×10^{-5}M
None (control)	170.0 ± 2.7	70.0 ± 2.5	153.8 ± 6.7
Ca^{2+}-free	97.1 ± 4.5	131.2 ± 2.0	103.8 ± 2.2
D-600, 2 µM	104.4 ± 8.5	94.0 ± 7.0	
TMB-8, 1 µM	110 ± 7.4	94.8 ± 4.9	
propranolol, 0.1, µM	105.0 ± 4.7	107.5 ± 5.4	160.0 ± 4.6
practolol, 40 µM	108.8 ± 9.5	99.5 ± 2.8	
ICI 118, 551[#], 5 ug/ml	127.3 ± 5.5	86.1 ± 5.7	
phentolamine, 50 µM	108.0 ± 3.7	76.7 ± 2.2	108.3 ± 4.3
prazosin, 1 µM	105.5 ± 3.1	76.7 ± 2.9	96.9 ± 18.2
yohimbine, 10 µM	99.6 ± 4.8	76.0 ± 6.8	104.0 ± 5.3

Cells were incubated as above for 15 min before transport assay. Data are means for 6-72 determinations.
[**] p 0.01, [***] p 0.001 for difference from control. # specific beta-2 inhibitor.

the concentrations used here. Both the inhibitory and stimulatory effects are dependent on external Ca^{2+} and are blocked by the calcium channel antagonist, methyoxyverapamil (D600) and by a so-called intracellular Ca^{2+} antagonist, TMB-8[*].

Negative regulation of glucose transport occurs when fatty acids suppress glucose utilization. This cannot be due only to competition for oxidative metabolic pathways because transport of nonmetabolized glucose analogs is also affected. As shown in Fig. 4, insulin-stimulated methylglucose transport in myocytes was depressed by a high but still physiological concentration of added palmitate. This effect was largely reversed by 2-bromostearate, an inhibitor of carnitine acyltransferase which acts to reduce fatty acid oxidation. Another such inhibitor, oxfenicine had the same effect (data not shown). Thus there seems to exist a negative feedback from mitochondrial

---

[*] 3-(N,N-diethylamino)-octyl-3,4,5-trimethoxybenzoate.

fatty acid oxidation to sarcolemmal glucose transport. Earlier
data from intact muscle indicate that stimulation of glucose
transport by contractile activity and other factors is also
antagonized by fatty acid oxidation (13). Basal methylglucose
transport is affected by palmitate only at higher concentrations
where glucose transport was increased, apparently via a mitochondrial uncoupling effect.

The recently developed fluorescent calcium indicator
quin-2 (14) has been used to measure cytosolic Ca^{2+} levels
in various types of cells. In preliminary experiments (Table 3),
stimulation of sarcolemmal glucose transport by insulin and
other factors was antagonized in a dose dependent manner in
cardiac myocytes loaded with quin-2. This inhibitory effect
is most probably due to its powerful intracellular calcium
chelating ability; it makes quin-2 unsuited for the intended
purpose. The exact intracellular concentration of quin-2 in
the myocytes has not yet been determined but the external
concentrations of quin-2/AM used to load the myocytes were
within the range used by other researchers.

DISCUSSION

The above results serve to illustrate the relationships
between hormonal influences, pattern of metabolism and contractile activity on the one hand and glucose utilization and

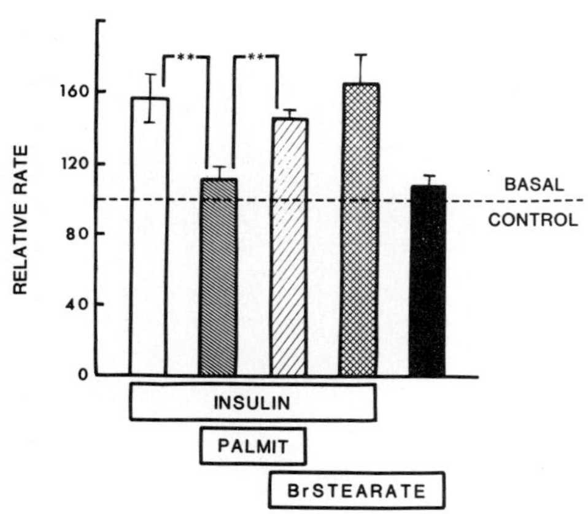

Fig. 4. Effects of 1.5 mM
palmitate and 4 mM
2-bromostearate on
3-methylglucose transport
in isolated cardiac myo-
cytes. Insulin, 5 munit/ml,
albumin, 3.25%. (From (13)
by permission).

Table 3. Effects of loading with quin-2 on 3-methylglucose
transport in cardiac myocytes.

Conditions	3-methylglucose uptake	
	% of control	% inhibition
Insulin, 50 mu/ml	197.1 ± 3.8 (24)	
+ quin-2, 10 μM		11.1
20 μM		18.0
40 μM		25.4
80 μM		43.4
120 μM		44.5
Hyperosmolar	135.4 ± 1.4 (4)	
+ quin-2, 80 μM		40.2
Ouabain, 10^{-6}M	155.1 ± 9.1 (6)	
+ quin-2, 80 μM		32.6
Monensin, 10^{-8}M	146.0 ± 5.4 (4)	
+ quin-2, 80 μM		50.5
Low-Na^{+} medium (85 mM)	148.1 ± 6.0 (9)	
+ quin-2, 40 μM		25.0
80 μM		43.9

Cells were incubated as above for 15 min before transport
assay.

its rate controlling step, transport across the sarcolemma,
on the other. The data indicate that Ca^{2+}-dependent regulation
of transport occurs in association with several major functional
and metabolic changes in the myocardia cell. By the multiplicity
of its regulatory effects on a wide variety of enzymes, transport
systems and receptors, Ca^{2+} appears well suited to integrate
various cellular functions, carrying signals from changes in
cell activity, metabolism or hormones to the sarcolemmal
glucose transport step. In addition, Ca^{2+} has concerted
effects on a number of enzymes involved in glucose utilization.

Studies in intact cardiac and skeletal muscle (3,4,5,15)
have shown that glucose transport stimulation in muscle is
associated with increased Ca^{2+} efflux (suggesting elevation of
cytosolic Ca^{2+}) and with increased Ca^{2+} influx and/or with Ca^{2+}
release from intracellular storage sites. It was therefore

proposed (3,4,5) that the common signal for glucose transport activation by a variety of modulating factors may be the increased availability of Ca^{2+} for binding to an intracellular regulatory site.

In this context, the effects of Na^+ pump inhibition, the sodium ionophore and, (in part) of hyperosmolarity and anoxia may be attributed to increased internal Na^+ levels leading to greater Ca^{2+} influx via sarcolemmal Na^+-Ca^{2+} exchange. The reverse happens when the Na^+ pump is stimulated, and methyl-glucose transport with very low concentrations of ouabain and adrenaline is decreased. This explanation is consistent with measurements with ^{45}Ca. The calcium ionophore, A23187 increases sarcolemmal Ca^{2+} permeability directly. The effects of anoxia and of hyperosmolarity may in part be due also to Ca^{2+} release from the mitochondria when oxidative metabolism is inhibited or when mitochondrial Na^+-Ca^{2+} exchange is stimulated. We have demonstrated a decrease in Ca^{2+} content of mitochondria isolated from skeletal and heart muscle after exposure to these conditions (16).

The dual effect of adrenergic agents in the absence of muscular contraction was previously described in intact diaphragm (17), isolated left atria (18) and very recently also in isolated cardiac myocytes (19). The decrease in methyl-glucose transport at low concentrations may be linked to the known stimulation of the Na^+ pump by catecholamines; at higher adrenaline concentrations this effect seems to be overshadowed by a stimulatory effect linked to the massive hormone-stimulated influx of Ca^{2+}. Thus, adrenergic stimulation of the Na^+ pump would seem to occur at agonist concentrations insufficient to activate Ca^{2+} influx. The adrenergic effects on glucose transport involve Ca^{2+}. In cardiac myocytes both sarcolemmal Ca^{2+} influx and its release from intracellular sites play a role, as was previously shown in isolated left atria (10) and skeletal muscle (17). These earlier studies indicated that the effects in skeletal muscle and in isolated left atria are mediated by beta-receptors. An effect of alpha-adrenergic agonists on glucose utilization in ventricular myocardium has,

however, been demonstrated (20). What remains unexplained at
present is that both beta-1 and beta-2 and alpha-1 and alpha-2
receptors seem to be involved in cardiac myocytes. Nonspecific
effects of the antagonists are unlikely but have not been completely excluded.

Studies in skeletal muscle (21), intact heart (22) and
isolated atria (23), have shown that the increase in glucose
utilization with muscular exercise is also expressed at the
level of sarcolemmal glucose transport. It was suggested (21)
that Ca^{2+} release from the sarcoplasmic reticulum may be the
signal causing increased glucose transport. Evidence that
changes in cellular ATP levels serve as the signal is equivocal;
recent NMR measurements (24) indicate no change in ATP, ADP
and CrP levels when cardiac work output is varied. Even when
ATP levels do change, e.g. in anoxia, any effects on glucose
transport may be mediated by consequent alterations in Ca^{2+}
fluxes and distribution.

Data in skeletal muscle (21) and isolated atria (23)
also show that glucose transport remains elevated long after
contraction had ceased. This suggests that glucose transport
does not depend directly on the rapidly changing cytosolic Ca^{2+}
concentration but more likely on the availability of Ca^{2+} to
another site or pool, turning over more slowly. Dependence of
glucose transport stimulation on contraction frequency (23)
and work load (22) also suggests that the time-averaged level
of Ca^{2+} availability may be the operant factor.

The main negative control over glucose transport comes
from the oxidation of alternative non-glucose oxidative
substrates, such as fatty acids. The evidence for such a
mechanism in skeletal and cardiac muscle has been reviewed
recently (13). This negative feedback is highly useful for
the sparing of glucose in starvation (and possibly also during
intense muscle exercise) but it may become misdirected under
pathological conditions. It has been suggested that stress-
induced elevation of adrenergic tone leading to enhanced
lipolysis may act in this manner, decreasing glucose
tolerance or exacerbating existing diabetes (13). It is also

conceivable that it may in part explain the peripheral "insulin
resistance" in non-insulin dependent diabetes where the concentrations and the oxidation rates of fatty acids are abnormally
high. This possibility is at present under study.

Two likely mechanisms of this negative feedback are now
being investigated. Mitochondrial Ca^{2+} accumulation may increase
during rapid oxidation and thus cause an intracellular redistribution of Ca^{2+} away from the hypothetical transport
regulating site. This would be the reverse of the Ca^{2+}
release occuring in anoxia. Alternatively, long-chain
acylcarnitines accumulate in diabetes (25), and presumably in
other situation where fatty acid oxidation may be overloaded
and inhibit Ca^{2+} fluxes associated with excitation contraction
coupling (26). Ca^{2+} fluxes associated with glucose transport
regulation could be similarly affected. Other data (27) also
suggest that long-chain acylcarnitines may be closely related
to suppression of glucose utilization.

The present data show that insulin-induced stimulation
of methylglucose transport in isolated cardiac myocytes is
partially dependent on external Ca^{2+}, as shown earlier
in intact heart (10) and in skeletal muscle (11), where Sr^{2+}
could replace Ca^{2+} (28). Other evidence favouring a role of
Ca^{2+} in the effect of insulin on glucose transport includes
increased Ca^{2+} influx in skeletal muscle (16) and in muscle
cells in tissue culture (29), inhibition by Ca^{2+}-antagonistic
heavy metals in isolated atria (30), enhancement of muscular
contraction in skeletal muscle (31), and the correlation of
increased glucose transport with inhibition of the plasma-
lemmal Ca^{2+} pump (Ca^{2+}-ATPase) in adipocytes (32). On the
other hand, Ca^{2+}-independent effects of insulin have been
described in skeletal muscle (33) and in isolated cardiac
myocytes (34). Some of these contradictions may be resolved
if insulin acts by releasing Ca^{2+} from one type of sites making
it available for binding to the hypothetical glucose transport
regulating site, without major perturbations in mean cytosolic
Ca^{2+} levels.

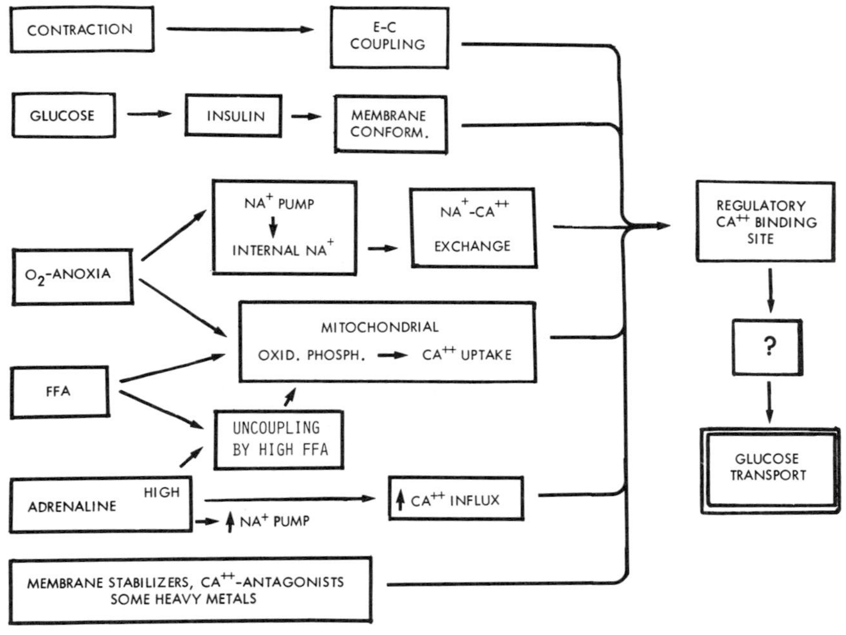

Fig. 5. Overview of Ca^{2+}-dependent stimulatory effects on glucose transport in heart muscle.

The evidence on the role of Ca^{2+} in glucose transport regulation in heart and other muscles is up to now circumstantial, and a more direct data on levels of cytosolic Ca^{2+} in vivo would be highly desirable. The recently developed intracellular fluorescent Ca^{2+} indicator, quin-2 (14) is unsuitable because it inhibits glucose transport stimulation by insulin and other factors (Table 3), presumably because of its Ca^{2+} chelating effect. Similar results have recently also been reported for adipocytes (35). Newer fluorescent calcium indicators, such as fura-2 (26) are unlikely to cause such interference and may be better suited. However, as indicated above, activation of glucose transport need not necessarily be associated with a large rise is cytosolic Ca^{2+}.

It is uncertain if sugar transport activation by the various modulating factors occurs by a single or multiple mechanisms. Insulin may act by a different molecular mechanism than muscular contraction or anoxia, for example. One may, however, design the simplest scheme consistent with evidence currently available. Fig. 5 depicts the mechanisms whereby major physiological modulating factors may affect sarcolemma glucose transport via a Ca^{2+}-dependent step.

Among many possible mechanisms whereby Ca^{2+} may affect glucose transport, two stand out. Ca^{2+} may act on the translocation of glucose transporters from intracellular sites to the sarcolemma (37,38) which is currently thought to explain glucose transport activation by insulin and perhaps other factors. Translocation is essentially an exocytotic process, and exocytosis is invariably Ca^{2+} dependent. Alternatively, Ca^{2+} may act on regulatory phosphorylation-dephosphorylation which is often Ca^{2+}-dependent. Transport regulation via these two processes need not be mutually exclusive. Both may occur simultaneously or translocation may occur with some modulating factors and activation of carriers in situ with others.

ACKNOWLEDGEMENTS

This work was supported by grants from the Medical Research Council of Canada, the Manitoba Heart Foundation and the Canadian Diabetes Association. The author is a Career Investigator of the MRC.

REFERENCES

1. Randle, P.J., Garland, P.B., Hales, C.N. and Newsholme, E.A. Lancet (1): 790-791, 1963.

2. Morgan, H.E., Henderson, M.J., Regen, D.M. and Park, C.R. J. Biol. Chem, 236: 253-261, 1961.

3. Elbrink, J. and Bihler, I. Science 188: 1177-1184, 1975.

4. Clausen, T. Curr. Topics Membr. Transp. 6: 169-226, 1975.

5. Clausen, T. Cell Calcium 1: 311-325, 1980.

6. Bihler, I., Ho, T.K. and Sawh, P.C. Can. J. Physiol. Pharmacol. 62: 581-588, 1984.

7. Bihler, I., Thomas, T.P. and Singal, P.K. Can. J. Cardiol. in press, 1986

8. Bihler, I., McNevin, S.R. and Sawh, P.C. Biochim. Biophys. Acta 844: 9-18, 1984.

9. Bihler, I., McNevin, S.R. and Sawh, P.C. Biochim. Biophys. Acta 846: 208-215, 1985.

10. Bihler, I. and Sawh, P.C. Mol. Cell. Endocrinol. 19: 93-100, 1980.

11. Bihler, I. In: The role of membranes in metabolic regulation (Eds. Mehlman, M.A. and Hanson, R.W.). Academic Press, New York, 1972, pp. 411-422.

12. Bihler, I., Sawh, P.C. J. Mol. Cell Cardiol. 11: 407-141, 1979.

13. Bihler, I. and Sawh, P.C. In: Pathogenesis of stress-induced heart disease (Eds. Beamish, R.E. Panagia, V. and Dhalla, N.S.) Martinus Nijhof, Boston, 1985, pp. 416-428.

14. Tsien, R.Y. Nature 290: 527-528, 1981.

15. Sorensen, S.S., Christensen, I. and Clausen, T. Biochim. Biophys. Acta 602: 433-445, 1980.

16. Bigornia, L. and Bihler, I. Biochim. Biophys. Acta 816: 197-207, 1985.

17. Bihler, I., Sawh, P.C. and Sloan, I.G. Biochim. Biophys. Acta 510: 349-360, 1978.

18. Bihler, I. and Sawh, P.C. Can. J. Physiol. Pharmacol. 54: 714-718, 1976.

19. Shanahan, M.F., Edwards, B.M. and Ruoho, A.E. Fed. Proc. 45: 900, 1986.

20. Clark, M.G., Patten, G.S., Fulsell, O.H., Repucci, D. and Leopardi, S.W. Biochem. Biophys. Res. Comm. 108: 124-131, 1982.

21. Holloszy, J.O. and Narahara, H.T. J. Gen. Physiol. 50: 551-562, 1967.

22. Neely, J., Bowman, R.H. and Morgan, H.E. Am. J. Physiol. 216: 804-811, 1969.

23. Bihler, I. and Sawh, P.C. J. Mol. Cell Cardiol. 7: 345-355, 1975.

24. Balaban, R.S., Kantor, H.L., Katz, L.A. and Briggs, R.W. Science 232: 1121-1123, 1986.

25. Lopaschuk, G.D., Katz, S. and McNeill, J.H. Can. J. Physiol. Pharmcol. 61: 439-448, 1983.

26. Lopaschuk, G.D., Tahiliani, A.G., Vadlamudi, R.V.S.V., Katz, S. and McNeill, J.H. Am. J. Physiol. 245: H969-H976, 1983.

27. Werner, J.C., Schuler, H.G., Rannels, A. and Whitman, V. Fed. Proc. 42: 1257, 1983.

28. Bihler, I., Charles, P. and Sawh, P.C. Can. J. Physiol. Pharmacol. 64: 176-179, 1986.

29. Schudt, C., Gaertner, U. and Pette, D. Eur. J. Biochem. 68: 103-111, 1976.

30. Bihler, I., Hoeschen, L.E. and Sawh, P.C. Can. J. Physiol. Pharmacol. 58: 1184-1188, 1980.

31. Clausen, T., Elbrink, J. and Dahl-Hansen, A.B. Biochim. Biophys. Acta 375: 292-308, 1975.

32. Pershadsingh, H.A. and McDonald, J.M. Cell Calcium 5: 111-130, 1984.

33. Yu, K.T. and Gould, M.K. Diabetologia 21: 482-488, 1981.

34. Eckel, J., Pandalis, G. and Reinauer, H. Biochem. J. 212: 385-392, 1983.

35. Pershadsingh, H.A. Shade, D.L., Delfert, D.M. and McDonald, J.M. Fed. Proc. 45: 1722, 1986.

36. Grynkiewicz, G., Poenie, M. and Tsien, R.Y. J. Biol. Chem. 260: 3440-3450, 1985.

37. Cushman, S.W. and Wardzala, L.J. J. Biol. Chem. 255: 4758-4762.

38. Suzuki, K. and Kono, T. Proc. Nat. Acad. Sci. USA 77: 2542-2545, 1980.

24

BLOCKADE OF SUGAR TRANSPORT DECREASES CONTRACTILITY OF
AORTIC SMOOTH MUSCLE

PETER E. DRESEL

Department of Pharmacology, Faculty of Medicine, Dalhousie
University, Halifax, N.S., Canada

We recently described (1) the activity of phloretin and
of Cytochalasin B, two agents which share the ability to
block the transport of glucose into cells, to block the
cardiac positive inotropic effect of Compound BAY 8644 K, a
compound which combines with the calcium channel in cardiac
and smooth muscle and increases the "open time" of this
channel (2). It seemed of interest to determine whether
these agents also affected the operation of the calcium
channel in smooth muscle. We report here that both grossly
interfere with smooth muscle function.

METHODS

Aortic strips obtained from rabbit of either sex which
had been killed by cervical dislocation were mounted in
10-15 ml organ baths in Krebs-Henseleit solution containing
145 mM Na^+, 4.0 mM K^+, 1.18 mM Mg^{++}, 1.8 mM Ca^{++}, 26.2 mM
HCO_3^-, 125.6 mM Cl^-, 1.18 mM SO_4^{--} and $H_2PO_4^-$, and 11 mM
glucose, bubbled with 5% CO_2-95% O_2. Resting tension was
adjusted to 1 g and the tissues equilibrated for a minimum
of 1 hr at 37°C. Calcium was removed from the medium in
certain experiments, with or without further addition of
EGTA, as described in Results. Noradrenaline and histamine
were dissolved (1 mg/ml) as the bitartrate and chloride
respectively and kept in the cold for periods less than
two weeks, dilutions from the stock solutions being made
fresh daily. Tension was recorded with Grass FT03 transducers using a Grass P7 polygraph.

RESULTS

Our first observation was that both phloretin and
Cytochalasin B blocked the effect of calcium entering the
cell through voltage dependent channels. The normal
Krebs-Henseleit medium was replaced with one containing only
0.06 mM Ca^{++} for 10-30 min. The tissue was then depolarized
partially by increasing the potassium concentration to 40 mM.
mM. Calcium was then added to the medium to achieve graded
concentrations up to 3.6 mM. Fig. 1A shows the effect of
Cytochalasin A and Fig. 1B that of phloretin. Blockade was
virtually complete with Cytochalasin B (20 microM) and
phloretin (100 microM). Lower concentrations of phloretin
have not been tested. A 2-fold reduction in the concentration of Cytochalasin B caused only approximately 50%
blockade, and 1.0 microM Cytochalasin B had no significant
effect.

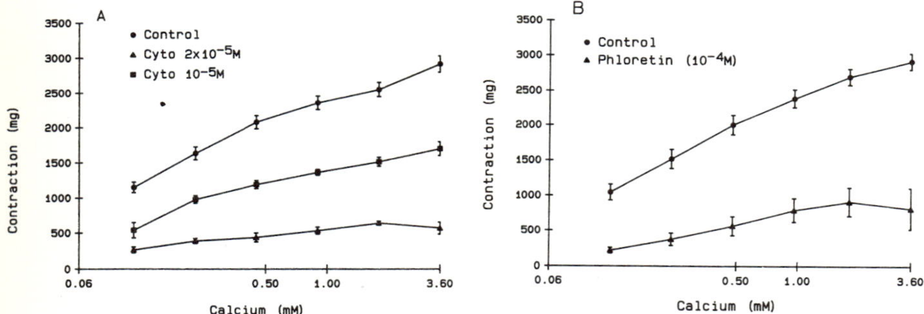

Figure 1: Blockade of contractions due to graded
concentrations of Ca^{++} in rabbit aortic strips depolarized
with 40 mM K^+. A. ● Control; and in presence of ■ 10 and
▲ 20 micromolar Cytochalasin B.

Both compounds also blocked, in what appeared to be a
non-competitive manner, the contractions produced by noradrenaline and histamine in tissues exposed to these drugs
in normal Krebs-Henseleit medium. Figs 2 and 3 show the
dose- response curves to these agonists. Although I show
responses to only one of the antagonists for each of the

agonists, blockade of the maximal response amounted to
approximately 30-50% with both agonists and both antag-
onists.No attempt has been made to test higher concentrations of the antagonists because of the non-specific
effects which one would expect. However, time of exposure
to phloretin seems important. Short exposures (10 min)
before beginning the noradrenaline or histamine dose-
response curves caused less blockade than the 90 min
exposure shown in Figure 3.

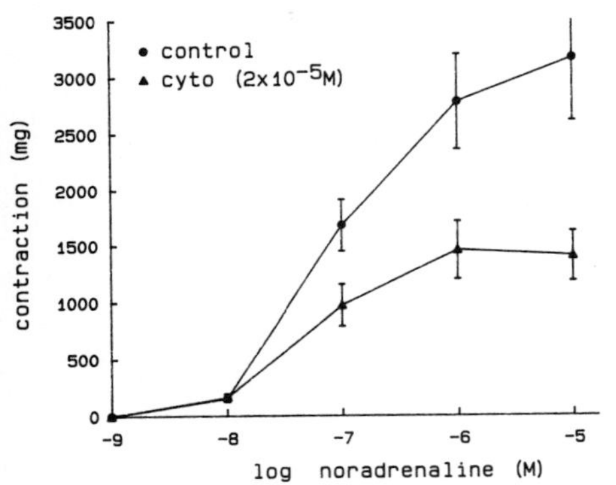

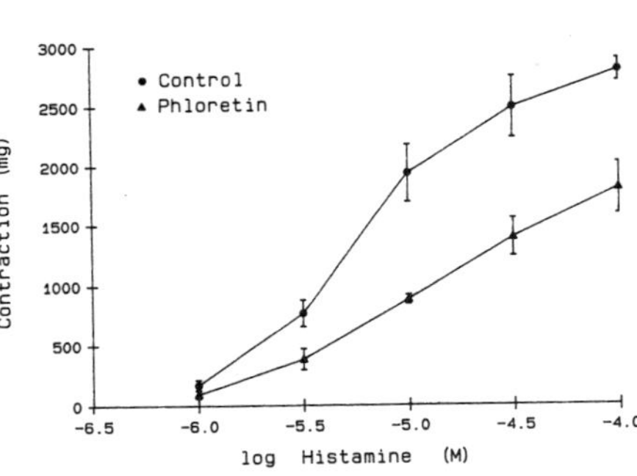

Figure 2:
Effect of Cytochalasin B on
the responses of aortic
strips to noradrenaline. The
calcium concentration in the
medium was 1.8 mM. ● Control ▲ in
the presence of 2x10⁻⁵M Cytochalasin B.

Figure 3:
Dose-response curves for
histamine in control tissues
(●) and in the presence of
phloretin 10⁻⁴M (▲).

Both noradrenaline and histamine are known to release
calcium from internal stores. Phloretin and Cytochalasin B
interfere with the contractions caused by this release. The
tissues were equilibrated in normal Krebs-Henseleit solution
and then exposed to a 0-calcium solution containing 0.2 mM
EGTA. Responses to high concentrations were then elicited.
Only a single response was measured in an individual
tissue. The results are seen in Fig. 4. Again, the
blocking agents caused more than a 50% decrease in the
responses. We confirmed these results in one experiment
with four aortic strips in which a control response to nor-

adrenaline was obtained in 0-calcium-EGTA after which the tissue was re-equilibrated with 1.8 mM calcium for 90 min before being tested in 0-calcium-EGTA to which phloretin had been added.

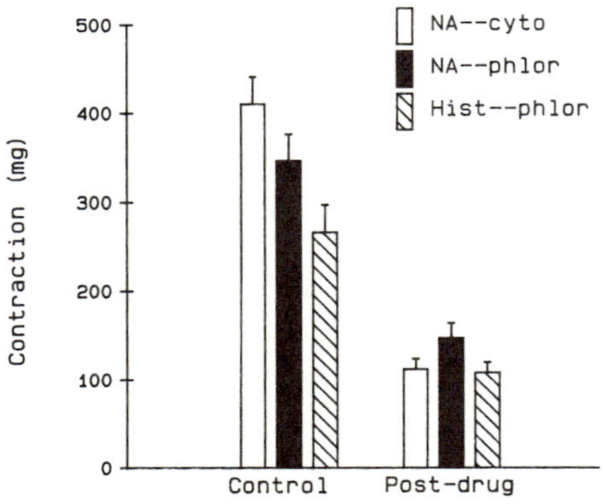

<u>Figure 4:</u>
Contractions produced by noradrenaline (NA 10^{-5} M) and by histamine (10^{-4} M) in aortic strips in zero-calcium-0.2 mM EGTA medium in the presence and absence of Cytochalasin B or phloretin.

DISCUSSION

Phloretin and cytochalasin B prevent contraction of aortic strips independent of the mechanism used to elicit it. We have shown in cardiac muscle that neither compound has a direct effect on contractile force but that both block the positive inotropic effect of Compound BAY 8644K, an agent specific for the calcium channel. This led us to consider the possibility that an effect at the level of the channel was involved. The results presented here show that calcium entry through voltage activated channels is blocked but the effect of the same ion entering through receptor activated channels or released from internal stores is also decreased. The fact that the effect of both the voltage regulated and the receptor operated entry of calcium into the cell are blocked would indicate that the antagonists are not specific for a particular calcium channel although this conclusion should be tested in a tissue such as tracheal smooth muscle in which the two types of channel are more clearly differentiated. I believe, however, that the lack of any specificity speaks for a mechanism of action which is post-receptor or post-channel in nature.

Phloretin at the concentration used here is considered to have a fair degree of specificity for the sugar transport system in intact preparations although it has been shown to have many effects in dispersed systems (3). One of these is blockade of the Na^+,K^+-activated ATPase which would secondarily affect sodium-calcium exchange. Cytochalasin B has two major mechanisms of action.   The first, blockade of sugar transport by direct combination with the transporter molecule (4), occurs at concentrations lower than those utilized for the present experiments. The other, inter-ference with the formation of actin microfilaments, occurs at the concentrations used in our experiments.   There is considerable evidence, however, that cytochalasin B does not interfere with the actin associated with the contractile apparatus (5).

Although there is no direct evidence for a causal relationship, blockade of sugar transport may be the primary explanation for our results. Unlike cardiac muscle, smooth muscle obtains much of its energy for initial contraction from aerobic glycolysis (6,7). This energy source appears to be required for a change in contractile tension, much less so for the maintenance of the increased contractile tone. It has been shown that glucose is an optimal sub-strate for the contractile effect of several agonists, but these experiments were performed in substrate depleted preparations (8). The inhibition of glucose entry under the conditions of the present experiments would be expected to be close to complete. It would appear possible therefore that anearobic glycolysis is a requirement for contraction in tissues which have not been depleted of endogenous substrate.

This explanation is facile but probably not sufficient.It does not provide an explanation for the

relatively greater blockade of the calcium effect in
depolarized preparations compared to the effects of added
drugs, especially of histamine which does not activate
adenyl cyclase. It is also difficult to understand why the
lower concentration of cytochalasin B which remain well
within the range required to depress sugar transport, were
ineffective in blocking the contractions. Finally, we have
confirmed that simple omission of glucose from the medium
does not prevent calcium induced contractions in depolarized
aorta.

It is hoped that the observations reported here will
provide an additional method of examining the mechanism of
contraction of smooth muscle.

ACKNOWLEDGEMENT: I thank Mrs. Gwen Dawe for excellent
technical assistance. This work was supported by grants
from the Medical Research Council of Canada and the Nova
Scotia Heart Foundation.

REFERENCES
1. Dresel, P.E.,and Ogbaghebriel,A., Proc.Canad. Fed. Biol.
   Soc. 29:85, 1986.
2. Kokubun,S., and Reuter,H., Proc.Natl.Acad.Sc.USA,
   81:4824-4827, 1984.
3. Crane, R.K., In: Handbook of Physiology, Sect. 6,
   Vol III, Amer. Physiol. Soc., Washington, D.C.,
   pp 1323-1352
4. Lin,S.,and Spudich, J.A.,J.Biol.Chem.,249:5778-5783,1974.
5. Croop,J.,and Holzer, H., J. Cell Biol. 65:271-285, 1975.
6. Lundholm,L., Anderson, R.G.G., and Mohme-Lundholm,E., In:
   The Biochemistry of Smooth Muscle (Ed. N.L.Stephens)
   University Park Press, Baltimore, pp 127-159.
7. Coe,J.,Detar,R.,and Bohr,D.F., Am. J. Physiol.
   214:245-250, 1968.
8. Furchgott, R.F., Bull. N.Y.Acad.Med. 42:996-1006,1966.

25

CONTROL OF ENERGY TRANSPORT IN CARDIAC MUSCLE

Dissociation of ATP levels from contractile function; cardiac failure due to phosphocreatine deficiency.

V.A.Saks, V.I.Kapelko, V.V.Kupriyanov, Z.A.Khuchua, V.L.Lakomkin, N.A.Novikova, E.K.Ruuge, V.G.Sharov, A.Ya.Steinschneider, M.Yu.Zueva.

USSR Research Center for Cardiology, 3 Cherepkovskaya 15 A, Moscow 121552, USSR.

INTRODUCTION

The research of the mechanism of energy supply for contraction has reached a stage when the importance of coupled creatine kinase (CK) reactions in energy transport (1, 2) is studied in vivo by using ^{31}P-NMR technique (3–6). Especially decisive may be a combination of this method with depletion of phosphocreatine and creatine stores by feeding experimental animals with guanidinopropionate, an analog of creatine which is not used rapidly in the creatine kinase reaction (1–4). By now, however, the use of these approaches has caused only confusion: several groups have reached a conclusion of the nonimportance of the coupled creatine kinase reactions (3, 4), in spite of abundant biochemical and physiological evidence (1, 2) and in contrast with other groups who have found good evidence for phosphocreatine shuttle by using a ^{31}P-NMR technique (5, 6). This has even led Bessman to conclude that "the discrepancies above indicate the serious technical problems that beset NMR measurements to date" (2). Obviously, in this situation very careful performance and critical analysis of the ^{31}P-NMR experiments under various conditions of heart function by several independent groups of investigators is vitally important to establish the true course of events in heart cells. In the current work we describe the results obtained in our laboratories in ^{31}P-NMR studies of the effect of ATP and phosphocreatine depletion on heart function, and also analyse the important question of the influence of physiological ion composition of solution on the coupled CK reaction in mitochondria.

METHODS

1. Mitochondria and mitoplasts were isolated in two different media: 1) 0.3 M sucrose, 10 mM Tris-HCl pH 7.4, 0.2 mM EDTA. 2) physiological salt solution (PSS) with composition most closely simulating the intracellular medium: 20 mM imidazole, pH 7.4, 20 mM taurine, 130 mM K^+, 30 mM Cl^-, 15 mM creatine, 15 mM PCr, 5 mM PO_4^{2-}, 3 mM glutamate, 3 mM malate, 0.5 mM dithiothreitol, 10 mg/ml BSA. Creatine kinase activity and oxidative phosphorylation were assesed as described earlier (7).

2. Mitochondrial creatine kinase (CK_{mit}) was isolated and purified from rat hearts according to the method of Blum (8). Antibodies against this CK_{mit} were produced in chicken and purified by an affinity chromatography method.

3. ^{31}P-NMR studies were carried out as described (5) on Langendorff-perfused rat hearts. Hearts were perfused with Krebs-Henseleit solution.

To deplete cytoplasmic ATP, hearts were perfused with 2-deoxyglucose (DG) (8-13 mM) for 1 hour followed by 1 hour of DG washout. From the beginning of experiment 5 mM pyruvate was present to support mitochondrial oxidative metabolism.

To deplete phosphocreatine in rat hearts, Wistar line rats were fed during 6-8 weeks with regular diet containing 1% of guanidinopropionate. Both in control group and GPA group the amount of food was limited to avoid the difference in growth. In experiments on rats' hearts with guanidinopropionic acid (GPA) the perfusion by Langendorff method in NMR instrument was performed using 11 mM glucose as a substrate.

4. Perfusion of the working hearts according to Neely (9) was performed at 37°C by a Krebs solution containing 11 mM glucose, 5 mM pyruvate and insulin (10 IU/l). Initial filling pressure was 15 cm H_2O, aortic resistance - 80 cm H_2O. Three types of load were applied after 30 min of perfusion: 1) volume load by increasing filling pressure stepwise from 5 to 20 cm H_2O at constant aortic resistance of 80 cm H_2O; 2) at fixed filling pressure of 20 cm H_2O aortic resistance was increased stepwise (each step - 3 min) to 100, 120 cm H_2O and then the

outflow of perfusate from aortic chamber was completely closed (cardiac output was equal to coronary flow); 3) after subsequent perfusion for 15 min at 80 cm H_2O the heart rate was increased by electrical stimulation to 7 Hz, each period was not less than 30 sec. Cardiac output was determined by Carolina Medical Electronics flowmeter, aortic pressure and left ventricular pressure (by using needle introduced into the cavity of the left ventricle) – by Gould Statham 23 Gb electromanometers.

RESULTS

I. _The mitochondrial creatine kinase reaction in solution with physiologycal ion composition and ionic strength._

Studies with isolated mitochondria have shown that CK_{mit} is bound to cardiolipin domain in the inner mitochondrial membrane which also contains adenine nucleotide translocase (ANT), and as a consequence the functional coupling between CK_{mit} and ANT ensures very efficient aerobic phosphocreatine (PCr) synthesis from mitochondrial ATP with PCr/O~3 (1, 2, 7, 10). In these coupled reactions adenine nucleotides turn over in almost closed cycle and energy is carried into cytoplasm by PCr (1, 2, 7). However, the doubt has recently been expressed (11) whether this enzyme (CK_{mit}) stays at the membrane also under physiological conditions since 120 mM KCl was shown to remove enzyme from the membrane. Therefore, it is necessary to understand the influence of the composition of solution close to the intracellular medium on the binding of CK_{mit} to the membrane.

Fig.1 shows that mitochondria isolated in the PSS medium perfectly preserve their ultrastructure. After removal of the outer membrane by a digitonine procedure, the mitoplasts contained unchanged creatine kinase activity and showed good respiratory characteristics.

Table 1 shows that CK_{mit} is not extracted from mitoplasts in PSS, but is extracted in 125 mM KCl; however, in the latter case this extraction is completely inhibited by addition of 10 mM borate which in fact further increases the ion strength. Therefore, the latter cannot be considered as an important factor determining the binding of CK_{mit} to the membrane. What seems to be important is the ion composition of solution.

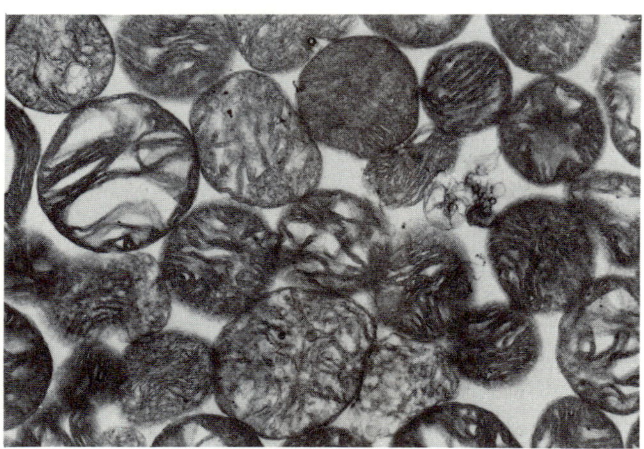

Fig. 1. Electron micrograph of mitochondrial preparation isolated in PSS. Magnification 30000x.

Table 1.

INFLUENCE OF ION COMPOSITION OF SOLUTION ON THE ASSOCIATION OF CK_{mit} WITH THE MITOPLASTS MEMBRANE.

Incubation medium	Ionic strength, mM	CK_{mit} activity of mitoplasts suspension (0.5 mg/ml)		% of CK_{mit} extraction
		before centrifugation IU/ml	after centrifugation in supernatant, IU/ml	
Sucrose	15	2.85±0.16	0.48±0.09	16.8
PSS	180	2.45±0.10	0.3±0.02	12.3
KCl, 125 mM	125	2.62±0.22	1.55±0.17	59.2
KCl, 125 mM + borate 10mM	155	2.61±0.2	0.3±0.03	11.5
KCl, 125 mM + ADP, 20 mM	215	2.56±0.2	2.49±0.30	97.3

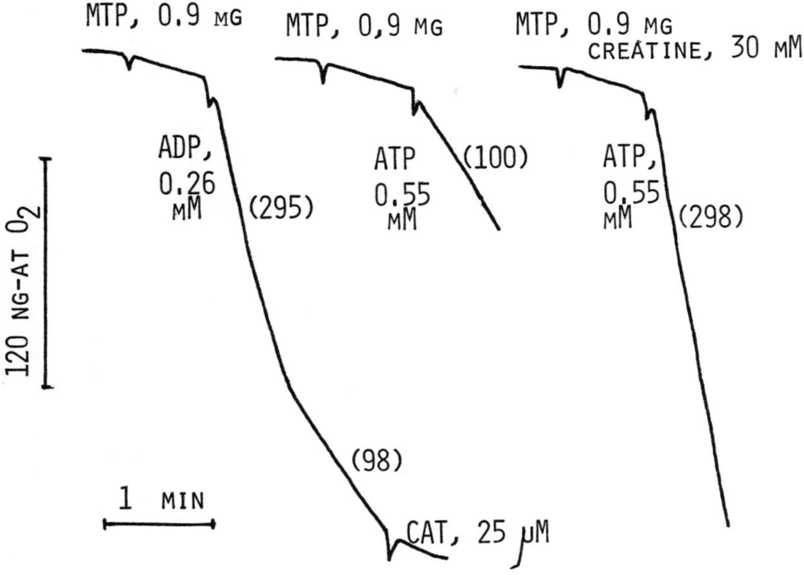

Fig. 2. Oxygraph traces of recordings of respiration of mitoplast preparation isolated in PSS. Reaction rates were determinated at 30ºC in 3 ml of PSS from which ATP, creatine and PCr were omitted. MTP – mitoplasts; CAT – carboxyatractyloside.

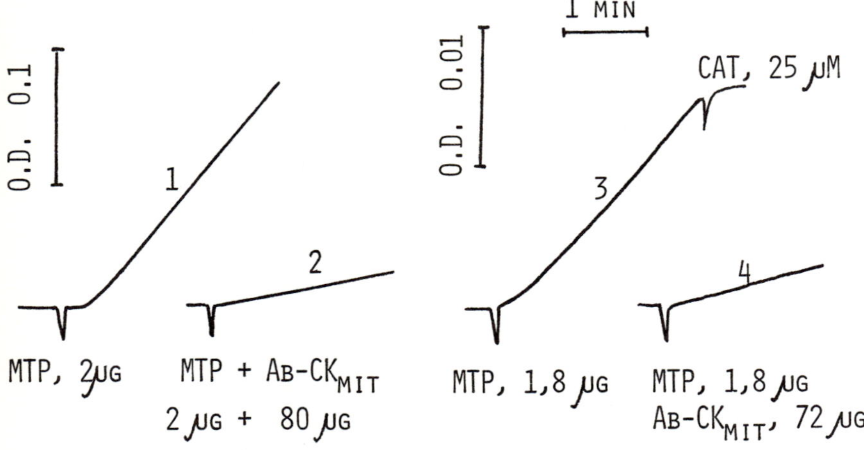

Fig.3.   Inhibition of CK activity (curves 1 and 2)   and ATP
production from extramitochondrial ADP (curves 3 and 4)
by antibodies against mitochondrial creatine kinase (Ab-
CKmit) in mitoplasts in PSS.
Reaction rates were recorded in CK and oxygraph media
discribed in (7   ). 1 and 2 — recordings of the rate
of CK reaction. The volume of mixture was 1 ml. 1 —
control; 2 — activity of CK in the presence of Ab-CKmit.
Mitoplasts (0.125 mg/ml) were incubated with Ab-CKmit (5
mg/ml) in 0.2 M borate, pH 8.0 with 1 mg/ml bovine serum
albumin, for 20min at 30°C and aliquats were taken for
assessment of CK activity (1,2) and ATP production rate
from ADP (50 uM). In control (1,3) incubation was carried
out in the same way without Ab-CKmit.

383

Fig.2 shows that CK$_{mit}$ which is bound to the mitoplast membrane completely controls the reaction of mitochondrial oxidative phosphorylation in the PSS.

Fig.3 demonstrates that in the PSS antibodies against mitochondrial creatine kinase, Ab-CK$_{mit}$, inhibit in the same extent the CK activity and the rate of oxidative phosphorylation - exactly as it has been shown for sucrose medium (12). In conclusion, these results show that there is the specific binding of CK$_{mit}$ to the inner mitochondrial membrane in PSS and its close spatial relation to the ANT (Fig.4) remains to be the basis for active functioning of the mitochondrial cycle of phosphocreatine pathway for intracellular energy transport under physiological conditions (1, 7, 12).

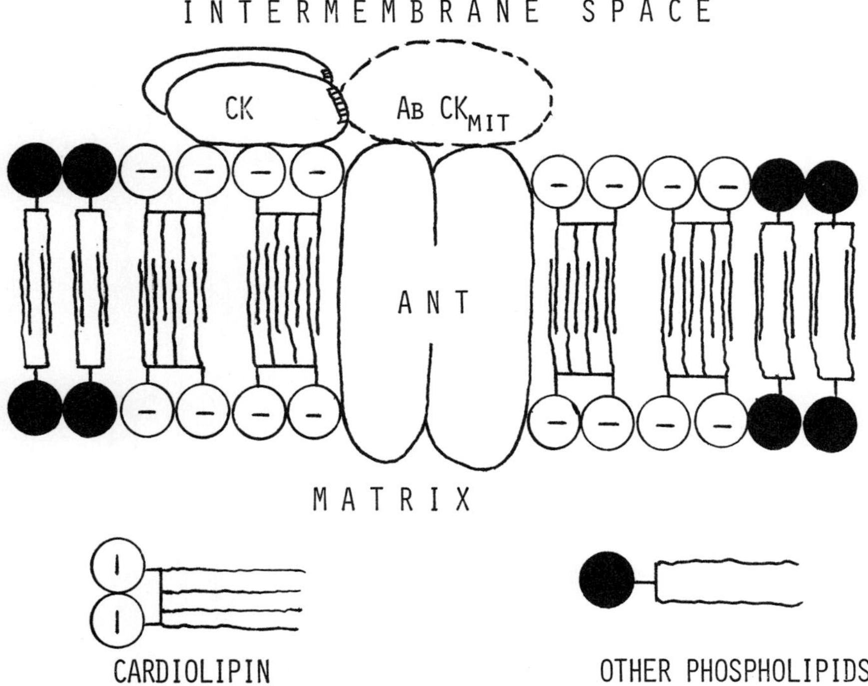

Fig.4. Association of CKmit with inner mitochondrial membrane. Ab-CKmit bind to antigenic determinations in CKmit near active site and block ANT due to spatial relationship between CKmit and ANT.

II. <u>Dissociation of tissue ATP levels and contractile function of the heart.</u>

Phosphocreatine pathway for energy transport is related to compartmentation of adenine nucleotides, mostly ATP, in cardiac cells (1, 2, 5, 7). In studies of the ischemic myocardium it has been found that the contractile force decreases to zero at almost unchanged ATP levels (9). The results demonstrated below show that under aerobic condition when oxidative energy metabolism is supported by pyruvate oxidation, the reversed situation is observed: ATP levels can be decreased significantly (by ~ 70%) by perfusion of the hearts with deoxyglucose (DG) without significant changes in the contractile force. These results are demonstrated on Fig.5 and 6. The ^{31}P-NMR spectra in Fig.5 show that perfusion of the hearts with DG results in significant decrease of the ATP content and appearence of DG-6P peak (simultaneously we observed the appearance of high amount of inosine in perfusate due to adenine nucleotides degradation), but during reperfusion PCr peak can be almost completely restored (it is also decreased during perfusion with DG). It is most remarkable that the contractile force under those conditions is not significantly decreased. Moreover, these hearts with decreased ATP content were perfectly and very reproducibly resistant to the ischemic period of 25 min and did not develop the

contracture at reperfusion. Fig.6 shows the correlation between ATP and PCr contents and cardiac work after DG treatment. ATP levels could be decreased to 30-40% of initial value without any changes in the contractile force which correlated better with the PCr content. This result is completely in accordance with those of Neely and Groythyohann (13). During DG perfusion, ATP in cytoplasm which is available the hexokinase is used to accumulate DG-6P. The latter is not metabolized and traps phosphate and a rise in ADP gives start to its degradation into adenosine and inosine which leave the heart. The remaining 30% of ATP is most probaly localized in mitochondria and in myofibrils which are apparently not impaired by DG. This compartmentalized ATP supports coupled CK

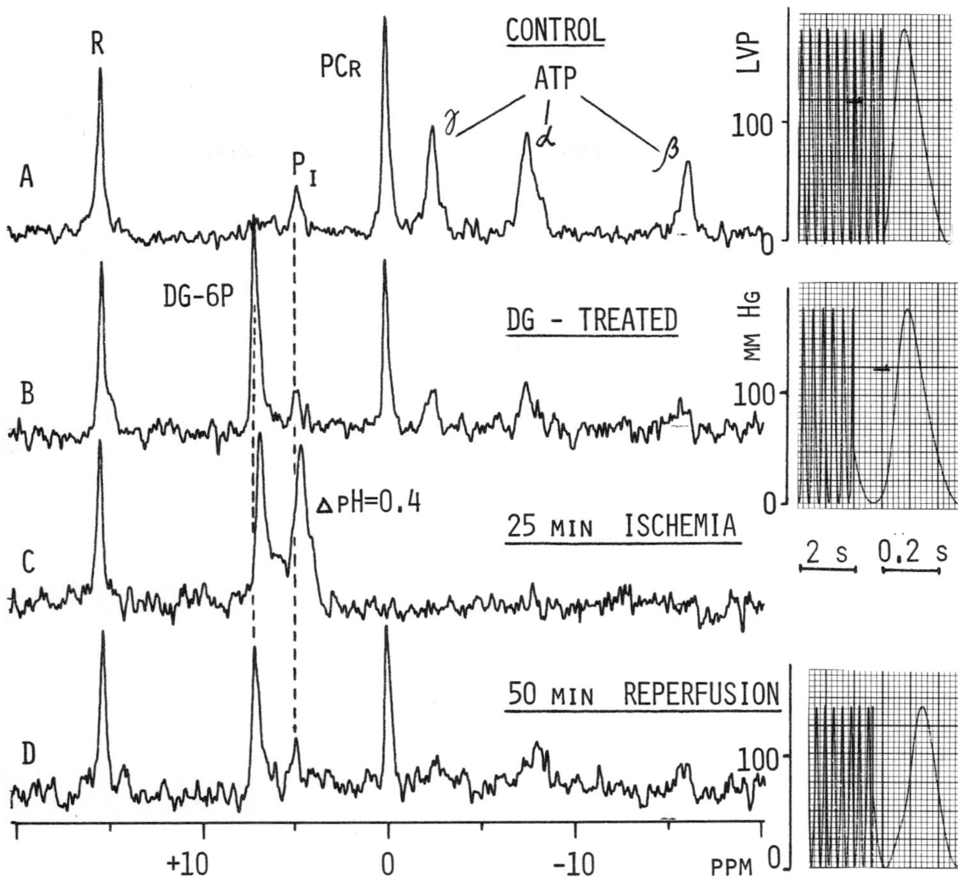

Fig.5.   The effects of 2-DG treatment (B) and subsequent ishemia (C) and reperfusion (D) on ^{31}P-NMR spectra and contraction of Langendorf-perfused rat hearts. LVP - left ventricle pressure. Peaks assigment: R - reference, 1 - methyl-1-amino-methylenediphosphonate; DG-6P, 2-deoxyglucose-6-phosphate; Pi, inorganic phosphate; PCr - phosphocreatine; PGPA, phospho- -guanidinepropionate; ATP, α, β γ respective phosphates of ATP.

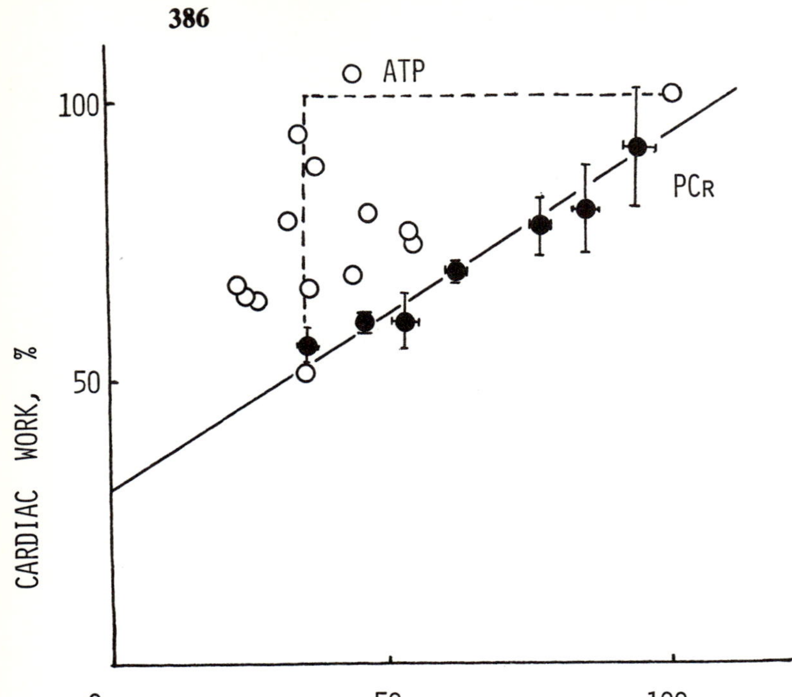

Fig.6.   Relationship   between   cardiac   work   and   ATP   and   PCr
contents after treatment of isovolumic rat hearts with DG
in   aerobic   conditions   in the presence of 5mM   pyruvate
(see Fig.5.).

cycles and PCr pathway and therefore maintains the contractile
function completely at least in isovolumic Langendorff perfused
hearts.   In   fact,   data   in   Table 2 show that   energy   fluxes
through CK   determined by saturation transfer ^{31}P-NMR   remain
high.

III.   <u>Contractile function of the hearts depleted of PCr by GPA</u>
       <u>diet.</u>

Rats kept on diet with 1% of GPA developed PCr   deficiency
due to the inhibition of Cr uptake and replacement of Cr pool
by GPA.   Instead,   GPA and PGPA, which has been shown not to be
used in beat to beat contraction accumulated in the hearts.
This PCr depletion is clearly seen in ^{31}P-spectra shown in
Fig.7. This Figure shows an extreme case of PCr depletion which

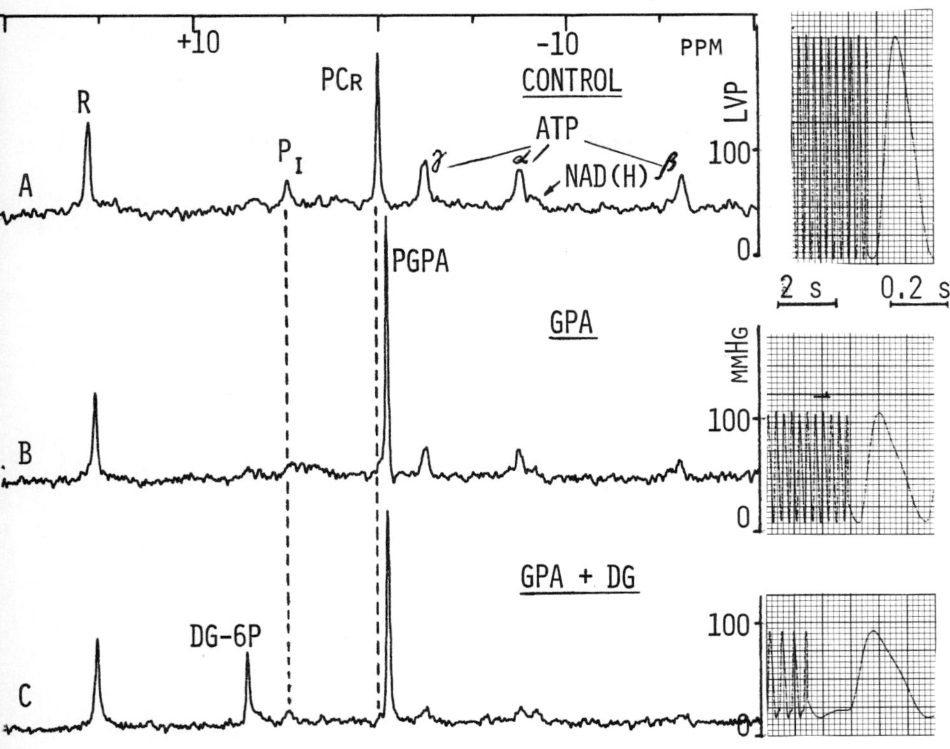

Fig.7. Changes in ^{31}P-NMR spectra and contractile activity of
the langendorff-perfused rat hearts induced by GPA-diet
(B) and following 2-DG administration (C). Assignmemt of
peaks as described in the legend to Fig.5.

content was decreased from approx. 28 μmoles/g.dw. to approx. 2
μmole/g.dw. in this experiment and could be seen only as a
shoulder at the P-GPA peak. On the right of Fig.7 the
recordings of the contractile cycles of isovolumic Langendorff
perfused rat hearts are shown. The contractile force is
decreased by ~60% after PCr depletion, and also the rate of
both tension development and relaxation are decreased. Rate

Table 2.

THE EFFECT OF 2-DEOXYGLUCOSE TREATMENT ON CREATINE KINASE FLUX IN THE RAT HEARTS.

Conditions	N	Cardiac work, mm Hg/min ($\times 10^3$)	Rate constant, s^{-1}	Flux PCr->ATP, umol/min per gramm dry wt.	ATP	PCr
1. Control	3	0.0	0.22 ± 0.04	531 ± 76	18.2 ± 2.7	40.1 ± 2.6
	3	32.5 ± 0.06	$0.42\pm.003$	846 ± 42	21.0 ± 3.9	33.8 ± 1.43
2. DG-treated hearts	4	0.0	0.20 ± 0.02	375 ± 60 (70%)	5.1 ± 1.0	35.0 ± 3.0
	5	21.0 ± 1.5	$0.26\pm.026$	545 ± 50 (64%)	8.8 ± 1.3	32.8 ± 5.2

	ATP	PCr
		umol/gramm dry wt.

pressure work was decreased from 46×10^3 to 19×10^3 mm Hg/min in this experiment. Usually, ~80% depletion of Cr and ~90%of PCr pools did not change ATP content (see Table 3) but the depletion of PCr below ~10% of initial level always was associated with decrease in the cardiac work index. In the extreme case of PCr depletion shown in Fig. 7 ATP content was decreased by about 40% but it follows from Fig.6 that this is not important for contraction. Further decrease of ATP by DG treatment (lower recording in Fig.7) in fact decreased the contractile force further. Therefore, it seems that under conditions of severe energy (PCr) deficiency depletion of ATP has more profound effect on the contractile force than in the presence of high amount of PCr. Table 3 shows that the energy fluxes through CK in direction of ATP -) PCr are decreased not more than by 50% and still exceed the rate of ATP turnover significantly, in contrast with data of Radda's group (3).

To describe the effect of PCr depletion on cardiac function, isolated perfused working heart preparation was studied under various conditions of cardiac workload. The results of these studies clearly showed development of cardiac failure in the hearts depleted of phosphocreatine. These

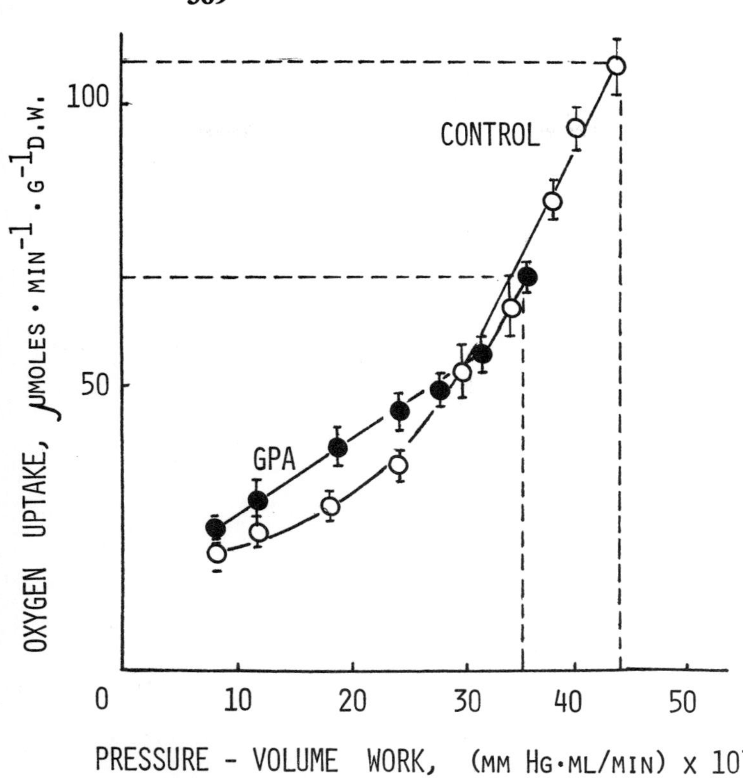

OXYGEN UPTAKE, μMOLES $\cdot$ MIN^{-1} $\cdot$ G^{-1} D.W.

PRESSURE - VOLUME WORK, (MM HG$\cdot$ML/MIN) x 10^{-2}

Fig.8.   Relationship   between   pressure-volume   work   and   oxygen
         uptake   rates in isolated working heart   preparations   in
         control   and   GPA   groups.   The values were   observed   in
         separate series of experiments.   Both groups contained   6
         hearts.

results are summarised in Table 4 and show that depletion of
PCr (by ~70-80% in average) in lesser extent influences heart
work in volume load studies, but very remarkably decreases the
maximal work capacity in resistance load studies: the maximal
value of the volume-pressure work that shows the external work

Table 3.

HIGH ENERGY PHOSPHATES (μmoles/g d.w.) AND CK FLUXES (μmoles/min per g d.w.) IN CONTROL AND GPA-FED RAT HEARTS.

Parameter	Control	GPA-group
Number of experiments	18	9
ATP	19.2 ± 0.87	18.3 ± 1.15
PCr	23.2 ± 1.35	2.72 ± 0.5
Total Cr	37.1 ± 1.5	8.2 ± 0.8
P-GPA	0	26.6 ± 2.28
Total GPA	0	48.1 ± 4.5
Flux ATP -> PCr a) restig	654 ± 78	314 ± 51
b) rate x pressure work mm Hg/min V_{ATP}=230 μmoles/min·g dr.w.	800 ± 126	400 ± 102

Mean values and standard deviation are given.

perfomance which could be reached by heart in experiments was decreased in resistance load group by 38% and in rate load group by 50%. When in the group with resistance load the aortic outflow was completely closed, the maximal left ventricular systolic pressure in the control reached the value of 177±5 (n=8) mm Hg, but in the GPA group was not elevated above 133 ±6 (n=7) mm Hg. The character of dependences between oxygen consumption and heart work was not influenced but the oxygen uptake rates maximally observed were decreased in accordance with the work capacity reduction by about 30-40% (Figs.8 and 9). This effect is predictable on the basis of PCr pathway for energy transport and shows the limitation of energy supply via this system if creatine and PCr concentration are lowered significantly. One interesting effect of GPA is several-fold increase in the end-diastolic LV pressure (fig.10A) and related to it increase of LV stiffness (Fig.10B). At constant filling pressure an increase in LV stiffness decreases diastolic filling of the heart and therefore the cardiac output is dimished, that resulting in a decrease of volume-pressure work.

All these data show that severe PCr (and Cr) deficiency

leads to clearly significant heart failure. That could be observed mostly at high levels of the workload. Probably, those were not high enough in the work of Shoubridge et al. (3) who failed to show the effect of GPA on cardiac function. Also,

Table 4.

EFFECT OF GPA DIET ON PHYSIOLOGICAL FUNCTION OF WORKING ISOLATED PERFUSED RAT HEART PREPARATION.

Parameter	Volume load		Resistance load		Heart rate increase	
	control (19)	GPA (14)	control (13)	GPA (10)	control (8)	GPA (7)
Heart rate min^{-1}	251±5	241±8	247±6	230±10	420±0	369±17**
Cardiac output, ml/min	41±2	37±3	28±2	20±2*	37±4	20±4*
Coronary flow, ml/min	15±1	14±1	28±2	20±2*	16±1	11±1**
Aortic flow, ml/min	26±1	23±3	0	0	21±2	9±2**
Volume-pressure work index (mm Hg x ml/min)	2625 ±118	2203 ±236	3586 ±398	2233 ±328*	2201 ±266	1112 ±313*
Rate-pressure work index (mm Hg/min x 10^{-3})	16.10 ±0.72	14.01 ±0.92	31.64 ±1.64	25.09 ±1.85*	27.29 ±0.24*	22.73 ±1.75*

* p <0.05; ** <0.01.

very low flux through creatine kinase observed in their work (150 μmoles/min g d.w. versus 400 in our work) seems to be underestimated due to measurements of changes of very small peak of PCr. In our study the flux in reverse direction was determined using high peaks of ATP.

The neccessity to use high loads to detect the influence of PCr depletion on the physiological function of GPA fed rat hearts shows that the phosphocreatine pathway for energy supply is in fact very effective and can operate with significant rate at PCr concentrations as low as about 1-2 mM inside the cells. That value in fact is still close to the K_m for PCr in the myofibrillar CK reaction (1.6 mM (14)) and due to high activity of myofibrillar CK the net rate of the reaction may perfectly meet the energy requirements of heart muscle contraction at low

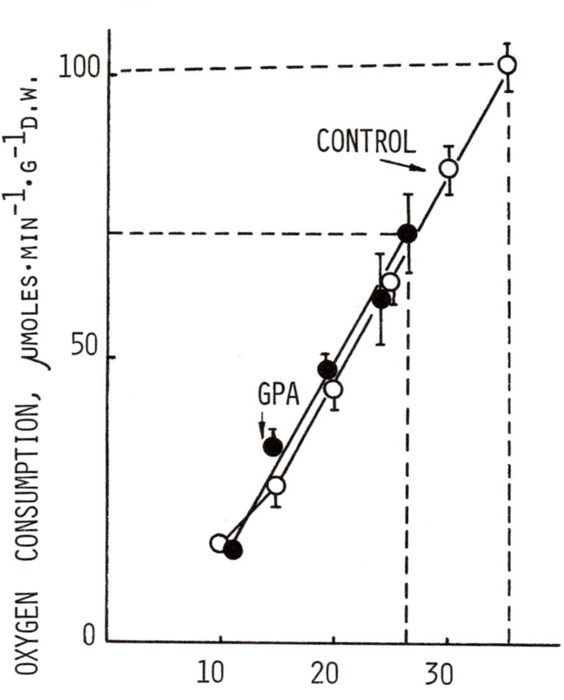

Fig.9.   Relationship   between   pressure — rate   work   and   oxygen
consumption   rates   in   isolated   working   rat   hearts   series
of 6 hearts.

workloads   but   not   at high load when   energy   supply   becomes
limiting due to its decreased transport rate.

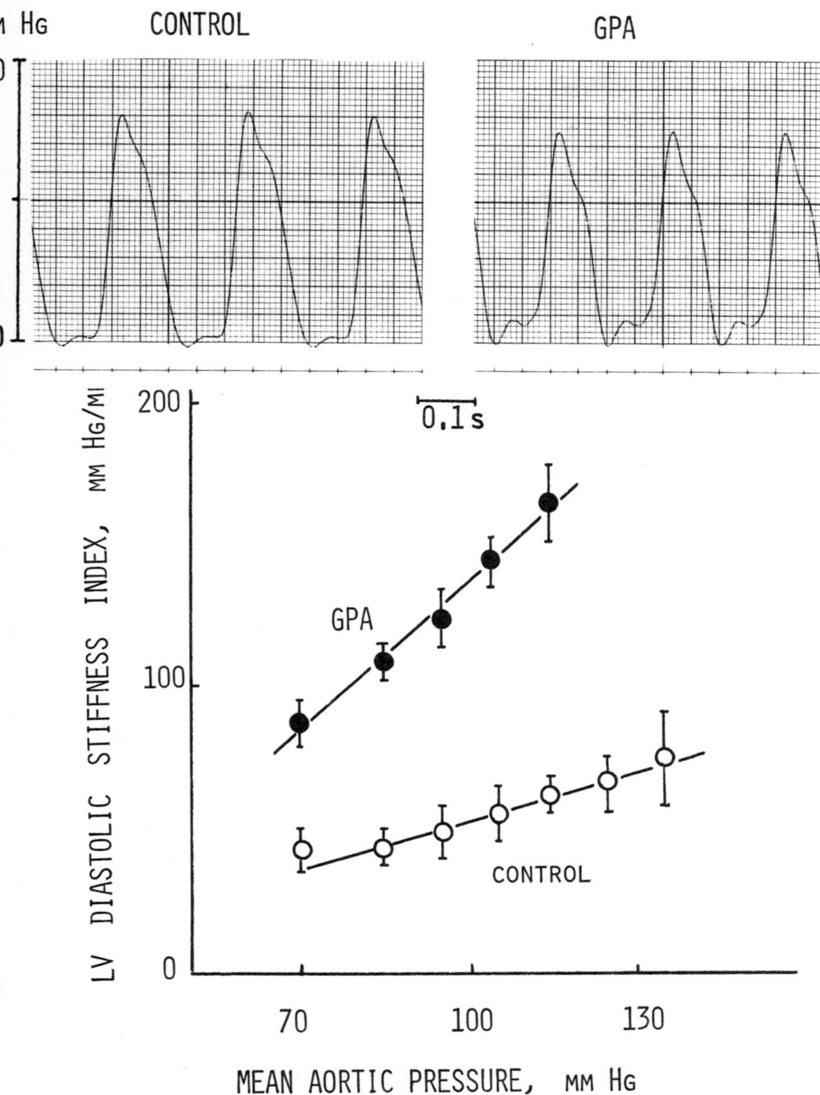

Fig.10. A. Recordings of the contractile cycles of isolated perfused working heart preparations in control and GPA groups under normal load condition.

B. LV diastolic stiffness index calculated as ratio of rise in diastolic pressure and diastolic volume as function of aortic pressure in control and GPA groups.

394

SUMMARY

In the physiological salt solution with ionic strength 180 mM mitochondrial creatine kinase stays firmly attached to the outer side of the inner mitochondrial membrane and coupled to the to the adenine nucleotide translocase.

In ^{31}P-NMR studies with isolated isovolumic Langendorff-perfused rat hearts depletion of ~70% of ATP by perfusion with deoxyglucose did not change contraction significantly. ATP depleted hearts showed good recovery of function after 25 min period of ishemia. Depletion of phosphocreatine (PCr) by feeding rats with guanidino propionate resulted in severe cardiac insufficieany. All these data are consistent with the concept of PCr pathway for intracellular energy transport.

ACKOWLEDGEMENTS

The authors thank G.Elizarova and L.Makhotina for their skillful assistance in preparing the manuscript of this work.

REFERENCES

1. Jacobus W.E. Ann. Rev. Physiol. 47, 707-725, 1985.

2. Bessman S.P., Carpenter C.L. Ann. Rev. Biochem. 54, 831-862, 1982.

3. Shoubridge E.A., Jeffry F.M.M., Keogh J.M., Radda G.K., Seymour A.-M.L. Biochim. Biophys. Acta 847, 25-32, 1985.

4. Degani H., Laughlin M., Campbell S., Shulman R.G. Biochemistry 24, 5510-5516, 1985.

5. Kupriyanov V.V., Steinschneider A.Ya., Ruuge E.K., Kapelko V.I., Zueva M.Yu., Lakomkin V.L., Smirnov V.N., Saks V.A., Biochim. Biophys. Acta, 805, 319-331, 1984.

6. Bittle J.A., Ingwall J.S. J.Biol. Chem. 260, 3512-3520, 1985.

7. Saks V.A., Kuznetsov A.V., Kupriyanov V.V. Miceli M.V., Jacobus W.E. J.Biol. Chem.

8. Blum H.E., Deus B., Gerok W., J Biochem. 94, 1247-1257, 1983.

9. Neely J.R., Rovetto M.J., Whitmer J.T., Morgan H.E., Am.J.Physiol., 225, 651-658. ...

10. Muller M., Moser R.D., Cheneral , E.Carafoli, J.Biol. Chem. 260, 3839-3843, 1985.

11. Wenger W.C., Murphy M.P., Brierly G.P., Altschuld R.A. J.Bioenerg. Biomembranes 17, 295-303, 1985.

12. Saks V.A., Chernousova G.B., Lyulina N.V., Khuchua Z.A., Preobrazhenskiy A.N. and Ventura-Clapier R., in " Celulular and Molecular Aspects of the Regulation of the Heart" (Eds. L.Will-Shahab, E.G. Krause, W.Schulze) Academia Verlag, Berlin 1984, p.41-48.

13. Neely J.R., Grotyohann L.W., Circulation Res. 55, 816-824, 1984.

14. Saks V.A., Ventura-Clapier R., Khuchua Z.A., Preobrazhensky A.N., Emelin I.V. Biochim. Biophysic Acta 803, 254-264, 1984.

26

CREATINE KINASE AND MECHANICAL PROPERTIES OF RAT VENTRICULAR
MUSCLE

R. VENTURA-CLAPIER ; H. MEKHFI ; V. SAKS* and G. VASSORT
Laboratoire de Physiologie Cellulaire Cardiaque, INSERM U-241
Université Paris-Sud, Bât. 443 F-91405 Orsay, Cedex, France
* Laboratory of Cardiac Bioenergetic, Cardiology Research Center,
Moscow USSR.

INTRODUCTION

Creatine kinase is an abundant enzyme in muscle cells. It
exchanges energy -rich phosphate between MgADP and MgATP (the
Lohmann reaction : MgADP + PCr + H$^+$ MgATP + Cr). In the heart,
its total activity represents 2400 IU/g dry weight. Three
isoenzymes are found: MM, MB and mitochondrial, but all display
the same enzymatic activity. The difference in these isoenzymes
results from differences in their subcellular localization. The
mitochondrial type is bound to the outside of the inner membrane
of mitochondria (1) ; it represents $\approx$ 20-30 % of total creatine
kinase activity in rat heart (2).The MB form is mainly cytosolic
while the MM form is found in the cytosol and bound to myofibrils
and membranes such as sarcoplasmic reticulum and sarcolemmal
membrane (1).The MM-creatine kinase has also been identified as a
constituant of the M band in the sarcomere of skeletal and heart
muscle. The activity of this M-band bound creatine kinase is 4-5
% of total activity in skeletal muscle and is able to
rephosphorylate MgADP produced during activation of the
actomyosin ATPase (3).

The role of creatine kinase in cardiac function is still
under question. Does it play the role of an efficient sink for
energy-rich compounds (4) or does it also constitute a dynamic
process for production and utilization of energy in heart cells ?
The relations between cardiac contraction and level of
phosphocreatine (15-20 mM) have been known for a long time, and a
compartmentation of adenine nucleotides has often been evoked to
account for the stability of the adenine nucleotide pools during
contractile failure (5). From these observations and from studies
on the mitochondrial creatine kinase it has been proposed that
creatine phosphate will be a sort of energy transport molecule

398

(or a shuttle) between mitochondria and myofibrils. To account
for these effects two mechanisms have been described: either a
compartmentation of substrates between inner and outer membranes
of mitochondria at one site and inside myofibrils at the other
(6), or a functional enzymatic coupling between translocase and
creatine kinase in mitochondria, and actomyosin ATPase and
creatine kinase in myofibrils (7,8). A third possibility is that
the high amounts of soluble creatine kinase and phosphocreatine
in the cytosol will behave as a device of "facilitated diffusion"
of MgATP (9).The role of creatine kinase in heart cell is not
clear although the answer to this question constitutes an
important key for the regulation of heart function and
metabolism.

RESULTS AND DISCUSSION

Information on the role of creatine kinase in cardiac
contraction can be obtained using skinned cardiac fibre
preparations. This technique appears very useful since it allows
one to alter selectively the numerous parameters involved in
cardiac contraction. Specially, it appears necessary to control
the Ca fluxes when studying contraction. In skinned cardiac
ventricular muscle, creatine kinase is present in high
concentration (2 IV/mg Prot).This enzyme slowly detaches from the
fibres (14% in 30 min). A muscle in which creatine kinase
activity has been inhibited by fluorodinitrobenzen (FDNB)
recovers high creatine kinase activity in less than 10min after
incubation with a solution containing soluble creatine kinase.
The calculated Km of rebinding is about 2 μM.These observations
seem to indicate that bound creatine kinase is in equilibrium
with cytosolic MM-creatine kinase (10).Savabi et al (11) using
glycerinated cardiac fibres have been able to show that, when
phosphocreatine was added to allow rapid rephosphosylation of
MgADP, cardiac contraction was stronger and quicker than when
MgATP was present and that P_i from phosphocreatine appeared
more efficiently used by actomyosin ATPase than P_i from MgATP.
Mc Clellan et al (12), Veksler and Kapelko (13) and Ventura-
Clapier and Vassort (14) showed that MgATP formed by the
rephosphorylation of MgADP by creatine kinase was more efficient

than MgATP in relaxing rigor tension . This efficiency is evidenced by a 40-fold shift of the pMgATP tension relationship towards lower MgATP concentration (Fig.1A).

When phosphocreatine was present, the half maximal relaxing effect of MgATP was shifted from 209 µM to 6.6 µM. .However, it was important to ensure that the diffusion gradient of MgATP inside our preparations was not the limiting step of ATPase activity (9,15). To test this, we studied the relaxing effect of MgATP in the presence and absence of creatine phosphate on four preparations of different diameter taken from the same heart (Fig. 1B). It can be seen that for a $\approx$ 10 fold change in fibre

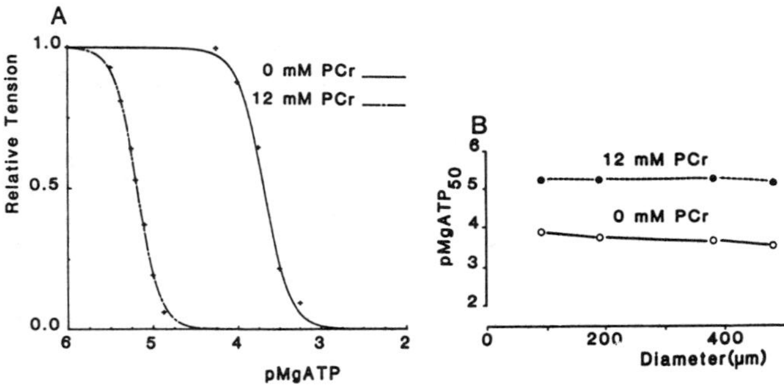

Fig. 1. a) pMgATP/tension relationship of a Triton X100 treated ventricular fibre of rat. Diameter of the preparation : 100 µm ; Maximal tension at pCa 4.5 : 67 mg ; resting tension : 11 mg ; sarcomere length : 2.1 µm. The fibre was skinned in a relaxing solution containing pCa 9, pMg 2.5, pMgATP 2.5, PCr 12 mM, pH 7.1, ionic strength 0.16 M adjusted with potassium acetate, EGTA 10 mM, imidazol 30 mM, Na 30 mM (see 14) Solutions were calculated in order to keep pMg, pH, ionic strength, EGTA, imidazol and pMgATP or pCa constant. Muscles were bathed in stirred solutions of increasing pMgATP in the presence (interrupted line) or in the absence (continuous line) of 12 mM phosphocreatine. Tension has been normalized to maximal rigor tension in each experiment. Lines represent the linearization of the Hill equation $T = (S)^{n_H}/K + (S)^{n_H}$ where T is relative tension; S, the substrate concentration; n_H the Hill coefficient and K an association constant ; the pS to obtained half maximal effect ,pS_{50} ,is given as $pS = (-Log_{10}K)/n_H$. $pMgATP_{50}$ and n_H were respectively 3.68 and 2.82 without phosphocreatine and 5.18 and 3.3 with phosphocreatine added.
b)Four fibres of different diameters were taken from the same heart and pMgATP /relationship has been obtained in the absence ( ) or presence ( ) of 12mM phosphocreatine. $pMgATP_{50}$ have been calculated and are reported as a function of diameter. Sarcomere length has been adjusted to 2.1 µm for each fibre.

diameter only a slight change is observed in the pMgATP needed for half maximal relaxation with or without phosphocreatine and the effect of addition of phosphocreatine is present whatever the diameter. In a recent paper, Krause and Jacobus (16) reported that on isolated rat heart myofibrils, a shift of the apparent Km of actomyosin ATPase was obtained when phosphocreatine was added to myofibrils; the shift was comparable to what we obtained on skinned fibres whatever their diameter.

The second type of argument for a unique role of creatine kinase in promoting myosin ATPase activity arises from alterations in the release of MgADP by phosphocreatine in isolated myofibrils and skinned preparations . On isolated myofibrils, creatine kinase and its substrates appeared more efficient than a soluble MgATP regenerating system to rephosphorylate MgADP produced by actomyosin ATPase.This led to the concept of functionally coupled enzyme system between MgATPase and creatine kinase (8).

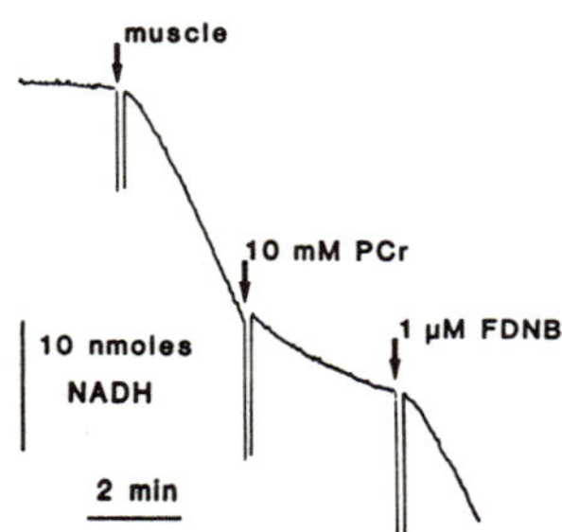

Fig. 2. MgADP release from a skinned rat ventricular fibre (87 μg prot) was determined fluorometrically by a coupled pyruvate kinase lactate dehydrogenase enzyme system in a solution containing 3 mM MgATP, 0.05 mM NADH, 2mM phosphoenolpyruvate, 2 IV of both pyruvate kinase and lactate dehydrogenase per ml, 10 mM EGTA, p Ca 4.5, pMg 2.5; ionic strength was adjusted to 0,16M with K acetate, pH was 7.1 with 30 mM imidazol and T°30°C. The arrows show the addition of the muscle in the cuvette and the recording of MgADP release by the activation of actomyosin ATPase in the presence of saturating Ca concentration ; then the addition of phosphocreatine (10 mM) activates creatine kinase and inhibits MgADP release in the incubation medium . After inhibition of creatine kinase by 1 μM FDNB, MgADP is released at the same velocity into the incubation medium as before adding phosphocreatine.

A similar effect of creatine kinase can also be observed on a skinned preparation (Fig. 2) where the release of MgADP in the incubation medium was inhibited by the addition of phosphocreatine. Furthermore, the figure also shows that this inhibition was overcome when creatine kinase was inhibited by 1 µM FDNB. Thus, both from the shift in the apparent Km of the actomyosin ATPase or of the $pMgATP_{50}$ and from the inhibition of MgADP release, it seems very probable that the role of myofibrillar creatine kinase is mainly related to functional coupling between MgATPase and creatine kinase.

We have been dealing so far with the role of creatine kinase on contraction in conditions of low activation of actomyosin ATPase (low Ca concentration).Of more physiological importance might be the role of creatine kinase during Ca-activated contraction.

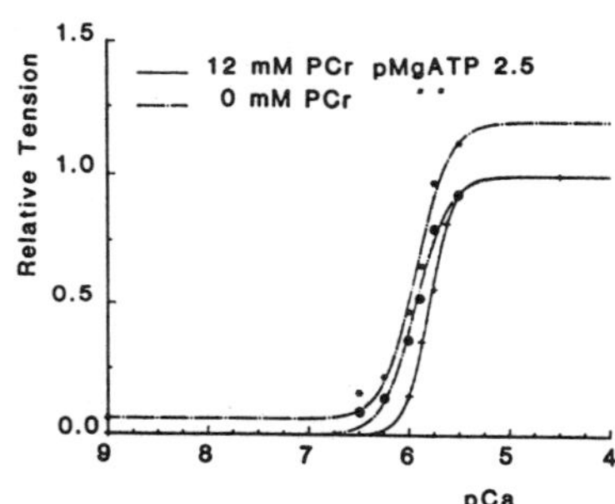

Fig. 3. pCa/tension relationship of a Triton X100 treated rat ventricular fibre in the presence (continuous line) and in the absence (interrupted line) of 12 mM phosphocreatine. Intermediate pCa have been obtained by mixing two solutions of pCa (9 and 4.5) (see legend Fig. 1.). In the presence of 12 mM PCr and pMg ATP 2.5 (+, continuous line), pCa for half maximal activation (pCa_{50}) was 5.8 and Hill coefficient (n_H) 3.7. When phosphocreatine was withdrawn ,resting tension for this fibre increased by 5% of maximal Ca-activated tension while maximal tension increased to 120 % (*, interrupted line) ; when the curve was normalized to 0 % at pCa 9 and 100 % at pCA 4.5 (, interrupted line) the pCa was shifted to 5.93 and Hill coefficient decreased to 2.66. Fibre diameter 100 µm; maximal tension : 32 mg ; resting tension:7.2 mg; sarcomere length:2.1 µm.

Phosphocreatine withdrawal in the presence of MgATP (3.16 mM) induced several alterations of the pCa/tension relationship. A slight increase in resting tension was generally observed as well as an increase in maximal tension at pCa 4.5. These changes were accompanied by an increase in apparent sensitivity of contraction to Ca and by a decrease in the slope coefficient of the pCa/tension relationship (Fig. 3). All these changes have also been observed when MgATP was decreased in skeletal and heart muscle (17, 18) and may be attributed to the influence of substrates on the actomyosin ATPase. Of significance is also the observation of a decrease in the maximum velocity of shortening in skinned skeletal muscle (15, 19) as well as in skinned heart muscle (20), when phosphocreatine concentration was decreased.

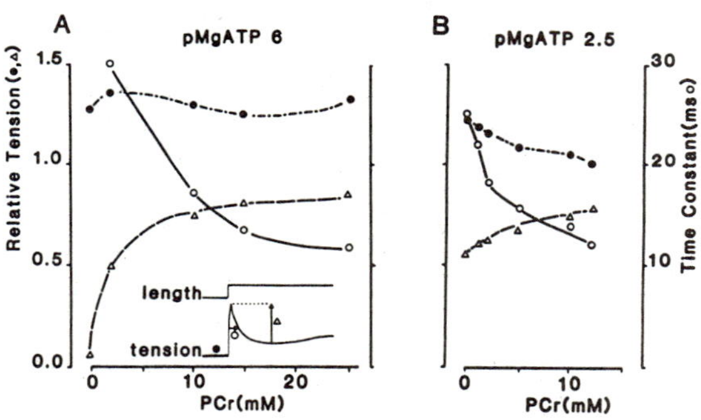

Fig. 4. Contractile parameters of Triton X100 treated cardiac fibres at different phosphocreatine concentrations.
Fibres were mounted between an AME transducer (Horten, Norway) and a vibrator GW1 (Gearing Watson, Eastbourne, England) which permitted length changes within 2 msec. Both were coupled to a Gould digital storage oscilloscope (GOULD OS 4020) connected to a computer HP85. Length changes were measured and controlled by a position detector (Hamamatsu Photonics K.K., Japan). Muscles were fully activated at pCa 4.5 and phosphocreatine concentration was varied at either pMgATP 6(A) or pMgATP 2.5 (B). Maximal tension was measured ( ) and quick stretches were applied to the muscle. Tension responses were recorded and analyzed. Extent of tension recovery ( ) was calculated and averaged for 5 to 7 stretches ; statistical variation was smaller than the symbols. A time constant of recovery ( ) was estimated as the time for an e-fold change in tension. It has been calculated between two points taken at 63 % (T63 %) and 90 % (T90 %) recovery using the equation T = (T90 %-T63 %)/ln 3.7. 5 to 7 measures were averaged for each reported value. A. Fibre diameter:230 µm ; maximal tension: 563 mg; resting tension 38 mg ; sarcomere length 2.1 µm. B. Fibre diameter:140 µm ; resting tension 5 mg ; maximal tension 75 mg ; sarcomere length:2.1 µm.

The influence of phosphocreatine on the speed of development of isometric contraction may be studied by using the quick length changes technique applied to skinned heart muscle preparations. Indeed in skeletal muscle, the tension responses are present when the cross bridges are able to cycle in the presence of Ca and substrate (high concentration of MgATP) and are absent in the absence of MgATP. Furthermore, it was shown that the time constant of tension recovery is proportionnal to the speed of contraction (21).Using this technique on thin papillary muscles or small ventricular preparations, the influence of phosphocreatine on the speed of development of isometric contraction was investigated.

Following a quick stretch, tension increaseu in phase with length change. The spontaneous tension recovery which followed can be characterized by two terms: the extent of the tension recovery which is an approach to the amount of Ca activated tension the muscle is able to develop and the time constant of the recovery process which could be related to the speed of development of isometric contraction at constant Ca concentration. The results show (Fig. 4A) that while maximum tension at pCa 4.5 is slightly increased when phosphocreatine is decreased below 10 mM, the part of tension due to active contraction (cycling cross bridges) decreases drastically below 5 mM phosphocreatine while the time constant for redevelopment of tension is increased. Comparison of figure 4A and 4B shows that the same effects are present in high MgATP (pMgATP 2.5) although less pronounced. A decrease in phosphocreatine below 5-10 mM thus results in an increase in rigor tension, a decrease in Ca activated tension and a decrease in the velocity of contraction. All these effects are enhanced when MgADP is added (22). The role of myofibrillar bound creatine kinase may be to decrease MgADP concentration and increase MgATP concentration at the vicinity of the myosin ATPase, thus increasing its efficiency. These observations may be correlated to what is observed during hypoxia. It is well known that soon after the onset of hypoxia or ischemia in the perfused heart, twitch tension decreases within one or two minutes. The underlying reason for this fall in heart function is not yet completely understood. A modification in beat-to-beat Ca regulation does not seem to be involved since the

Ca current is not modified during tension decrease (23) and no
changes in the peak of aequorin signal has been recorded during
cyanide poisoning (24). A slight acidification has been proposed
since a decrease in pH has been shown to decrease Ca induced Ca
release by the sarcoplasmic reticulum as well as to shift the
pCa/tension relationship of skinned heart cells towards higher Ca
concentrations (25). However, a carefull study of the time
dependent changes in both pH and twitch tension show that a
possible implication of acidification will take place later than
the sharp tension decrease ; moreover, using a different
metabolic inhibitor, Na amobarbital, it can be seen with 31P-NMR
technique that cardiac contraction is depressed without any
acidification (26). It has also been known for a long time, using
either biochemical analysis of freeze clamped hearts or 31P-NMR
technique, that ATP concentration does not vary during tension
decrease. This observation has led to the concept of
compartmentation of adenine nucleotides in heart cells. Two
factors, P_i and phosphocreatine, vary quickly and
significantly.In skinned heart preparations, P_i which increases
as a result of phosphocreatine breakdown, has been shown to
depress tension (27) as well as to decrease Ca
sensitivity(28).These changes are important enough to depress
contractility during hypoxia. In addition to P_i, phosphocreatine
decrease may also participate in the depression of contractility.
First, because it decreases the extent of Ca-activated tension
and second because it slows the development of contraction. As a
consequence, hypoxic muscle will develop less force even though
the Ca transient is similar in normal and hypoxic heart.

Creatine kinase system is highly organized in cardiac cells.
It has been found in many structures involved in excitation -
contraction coupling. Among these structures, mitochondria and
myofibrils, represent the two main sites for production and
utilization of energy in the metabolic regulation of heart cells.
Extensive studies have provided evidence for enzymatic coupling
between creatine kinase and ATP-ADP translocase in mitochondria.
Enzymatic coupling between myofibrillar MgATPase and bound
creatine kinase has been shown in heart and skeletal muscle
(3,8,11) and evidence has been given here of the implication of
creatine kinase in cardiac function. A clear role of facilitated

diffusion of metabolites in the cytosol of large muscle cells can be attributed to cytosolic creatine kinase (9). 31P-NMR studies are actively developing to study the dynamic exchanges between MgATP and phosphocreatine and conflicting interpretations have been given so far (29,30). Interest for the role of creatine kinase in regulation of cardiac function however has been growing in the last decade, and is under intensive investigation.

1. Sharov, V.G., Saks, V.A., Smirnov, V.N., and Chazov, E.I. Biochim. Biophys.Acta 468: 495-501, 1977.

2. Scholte, H.R. Biochim. Biophys. Acta 305: 413-427, 1973.

3. Walliman, T.H. and Eppenberger, H. In: Cell and Muscle Motility, (Ed. J.W. Shay), Plenum Publishing Corp. Vol. 6, 1985, pp. 239-285.

4. Cain, O.F. and Davis, R.E. Biochemical and Biophysical Research Communications 8: 361-366, 1962.

5. Gudbjarnason, S., Mathes, P. and Ravens, K.G. J. Mol. Cell. Cardiol. 1: 325-339, 1970.

6. Bessman, S.P., Carpenter, C.L. Ann. Rev. Biochem. 54: 831-862, 1985.

7. Saks, V.A., Kuznetsov, A.V., Kupriyanov, V.V., Miceli, M.V. and Jacobus, W.E. J. Biol. Chem. 260: 7757-7764, 1985.

8. Saks, V.A., Ventura-Clapier, R., Huchua, Z.A., Preobrazhensky, A.N. and Emelin, I.V. Biochim. Biophys.Acta 803: 254-264, 1984.

9. Meyer, R.A., Sweeney, H.L., Kushmerick, M.J. Am. J.Physiol. 246: C365-C377, 1984.

10. Saks, V.A., Vassort, G. and Ventura-Clapier, R. J. Physiol. (Lond.) Proceeding UCL Meeting, marsh 86 (in press).

11. Savabi, F., Geiger, P.J. and Bessman, S.P. Am. J. Physiol. 247: C424-C432, 1984.

12. McClellan, G., Weisberg, G.A. and Winegrad, S. Am. J. Physiol. 245: 423-427, 1983.

13. Veksler, V.I. and Kapelko, V.I. Biochim. Biophys. Acta 803: 265-270, 1984.

14. Ventura-Clapier, R. and Vassort, G. Pflügers Arch. 404: 157-161, 1985.

15. Cooke, R. and Pate, E. Biophys. J. 48, 789-798, 1985.

16. Krause, S.M. and Jacobus, W.E. Biophys. J. *49*: 248 a, 1986.

17. Brandt, P.W., Cox, R.N., Kawai, M. and Robinson, T. J. Gen. Physiol. *79*: 997-1016, 1982.

18. Fabiato, A. and Fabiato, F. J. Physiol. (Lond) *249*: 497-517, 1975.

19. Ferenczi, M.A., Goldman, Y.E. and Simmons, R.M. J. Physiol.(Lond) *350*: 519-544.

20. Maughan, D.W., Low, E.S. and Alpert, N.R. J. Gen. Physiol. *71*: 431-451, 1978.

21. Heinl, P., Kuhn, H.J. and Ruegg, J.C. J. Physiol. (Lond.) *237*: 243-258, 1974.

22. Vassort, G. and Ventura-Clapier, R. J. Physiol. (Lond). *369*: 76P, 1985.

23. Ventura-Clapier, R. and Vassort, G. J. Mus. Res. Cell. Motility *1*: 429-444, 1980.

24. Allen, D.G. and Orchard, C.H. J. Physiol. (Lond.) *329*: 107-122, 1983.

25. Fabiato, A. and Fabiato, F. J. Physiol. (Lond.) *276*: 233-256, 1978 c.

26. Hoerter, J.A., Lauer, C., Ventura-Clapier, R. and Guéron, M. J. Mol. and Cell. Cardiol. Abstract of the 8th Annual Meeting ISHR, American section.

27. Herzig, J.W., Peterson, J.W., Petterson, J.W., Ruegg, J.C. and Solaro, R.J. Biochim. Biophys. Acta *672*: 191-196, 1981.

28. Kentish, J.C. J. Physiol. (Lond.) *370*: 585-604, 1986.

29. Shoubridge, E.A., Jeffry, F.M.H., Keogh, J.M., Radda, G.K. and Seymour, A.M.L. Biochim. Biophys. Acta. *847*: 25-32, 1985.

30. Kupriyanov, V.V., Steinschneider, A.Y., Ruuge, E.K., Kapel'ko, V.I., Zueva, M.Y.U., Lakomkin, V.L., Smirnov, V.N. and Saks, V.A. Biochim. Biophys. Acta. *805*: 319-331, 1984.

27

HEMODYNAMIC PERFORMANCE OF CREATINE-DEPLETED RAT HEART IN ISOLATED
BLOOD-PERFUSED WORKING PREPARATION

Y. BRANDEJS-BARRY, B. KORECKY

Department of Physiology, University of Ottawa, Ottawa, Ontario, Canada.

INTRODUCTION

It is well known that adenosine triphosphate (ATP) is the immediate
substrate supplying energy for muscular contraction (1). The largest
portion of the energy generated by ATP is used for contraction and
relaxation. Creatine phosphate (CP) has also been considered to play a
role in energy provision but has always been postulated to be either a
buffer or a secondary store of energy used primarily to replenish ATP.
More recently it has been hypothesized that CP acts as an energy
intermediate by transferring or shuttling the high energy phosphates
from the mitochondria to the myofibrils and other sites of intracellular
ATP utilization (2-4). This creatine shuttle hypothesis is based in
part on the observation that subcellular structures such as the
mitochondria (5,6), the myofibrils (7,8) and sarcoplasm (3) contain
specific isozymes of creatine kinase (CK). In addition to the above,
kinetic studies on isolated myocytes (9,10) and isolated frog atria and
ventricles (11,12) also support this hypothesis and demonstrate the
positive effects of CP on contractile force and action potentials of
hypodynamic frog heart.

The role of CP in muscle contraction has been investigated after
the depletion of creatine by feeding structural analogs of creatine to
animals (13-15). The most effective and competitive analog used for
inhibiting creatine entry into skeletal muscle has been β-guanadinopro-
pionate (GPA). GPA is absorbed well through the gastrointestinal tract
and competes with creatine for entry into the cell at the uptake sites
on the sarcolemmal membrane. It is a poor substrate for CK producing a
Vmax 0.3% of that produced by creatine under optimal conditions.
Maximal depletion of creatine that can be obtained in skeletal muscle is
about 95% (15-17) and 80-90% in cardiac tissue (19,21). The
substitution of creatine with analogs such as GPA has little effect on

skeletal muscle steady-state performance and endurance _in vitro_ (17,18).
In the myocardium, the role of the creatine shuttle has been
investigated in the isolated non-working (19-21) and working heart
preparation in normal and creatine depleted rats (21-23). At the
present time there is no general agreement on the biological
significance of the role of creatine shuttle. While some studies
support its existence (20,22), others do not (19,21).

The principal objective of this study was to further clarify the
role of the creatine shuttle in the myocardium and to determine if
indeed the shuttle is important in the transfer of CP from the
mitochondria to other compartments in the beating heart under
normoxemia. If this is the case then severe depletion of creatine and
creatine phosphate should lead to the reduction of the maximum cardiac
output and/or shortening of the duration of the steady state performance
at high levels of cardiac output in the isolated working heart
preparation, provided that an adequate oxygen supply is available.

Although working heart models have been used to test the role of
the creatine shuttle, all have utilized oxygenated electrolyte
solutions. Under these conditions, coronary flow reaches values well
above the physiological range. However, this does not eliminate the
possibility of myocardial hypoxia which may become a limiting factor.
To overcome this potential problem, a method utilizing reconstituted
blood, consisting of washed red blood cells (RBC) suspended in an
electrolyte solution and bovine albumin, has been developed (24). The
hemodynamic performance obtained with this RBC enriched perfusate
approaches that observed in an intact animal (25). We therefore decided
to use this model since it has the capacity to provide adequate oxygen
supply to the myocardium even at high workloads.

In order to deplete the heart of creatine we used two compounds in
the previously tested GPA as well as the more recently used creatine
analog, β-guanidinobutyrate (GBA), (16). It has been shown that GBA
depletes creatine in the myocardium to a greater extent that GPA (16),
is practically not used as a substrate for creatine kinase, and it does
not inhibit the enzyme's activity. Also, no signs of toxicity or
histopathological changes have been observed in skeletal muscles of rats
fed with GBA for 4-6 weeks (26) but some ultrastructural changes have
been observed in GBA-fed Cornish chicks (27). Since our study involved

long term feeding with these analogs we examined myocardium of treated
rats for possible ultrastructural alterations as well.

MATERIALS AND METHODS
<u>Treatment of Animals</u>.

Male Sprague-Dawley rats (Charles River Canada Inc., 250-300 g)
were randomly divided into three groups. Group I was the control (C)
and received normal diet (Purina powdered rat chow); group II received
the above diet and 2% GBA. GBA was synthesized from β-amino butyric
acid and cyanamide according to Rowley et al. (28) with minor
modifications. Group III received the normal diet supplemented with 1%
GPA (Sigma) for seven or ten weeks at which time the rats weighed
350-400 g. To minimize the differences in caloric intake the groups
were pair-fed as suggested by Mainwood et al. (29).

The concentration of total creatine, GBA and GPA was determined as
follows: the hearts were rapidly frozen between aluminum blocks cooled
in liquid nitrogen and then extracted in cold perchloric acid (29).
Total creatine, was measured by the method of Ennor and Stockten (30)
and GBA and GPA by the Sakaguchi reaction as described by Bonas et al.
(31). Negligible amounts of both guanidino-compounds gave some positive
reaction with creatine assay reagents. Correction for the falsely
elevated creatine levels was performed (38). ATP, adenosine and CP
concentrations were determined in rats that were fed for 10 weeks by
high pressure liquid chromatography.
<u>Electron Microscopy</u>.

Rats fed for 7 weeks were anaesthetized with Somnotol (46 mg/kg),
heparinized (200 IU) and perfused through the carotid artery with
fixative-containing cacodylate buffer (45 mM, 1.5% gluteraldehyde, pH
7.4). Upon fixation, the hearts were excised and cut into 2 mm pieces.
The individual pieces of ventricle were fixed for 2 hours with 150 mM
cacodylate buffer containing 2% osmic acid, and then embedded in
Araldite (520) for 2 days. Semi-thin and thin sections were cut with a
diamond knife, stained with uranyl acetate (saturated in 50% methanol pH
4.4), counter stained with lead citrate (pH 12.0), and examined in a
Philips Elu-300 electron microscope.
<u>Isolated Heart Preparation</u>

Rats after 7 or 10 weeks of feeding were anaesthetized with ether

and injected intravenously with sodium heparin (200 IU). A laparotomy
was performed, and the abdominal aorta was transected. This was
followed by a thoracotomy and the superior and inferior venae cavae were
isolated, ligated and cut. The heart was quickly excised and dropped
into a beaker with ice-cold saline. The aortic stump was attached to a
cannula and the heart was retrogradely perfused with an oxygenated
Krebs-Henseleit bicarbonate buffer from a reservoir at 100 cm H_2O
pressure. The pulmonary artery was cannulated to allow for the
collection of coronary sinus effluent. The left atrium was then
cannulated with a curved cannula through one of the pulmonary veins and
the heart was switched from the non-working to the working mode as the
left atrial cannula was attached to a reservoir containing red blood
cell (RBC) enriched perfusate. A needle (22 gauge) attached to a
pressure transducer (Statham P23) was pushed through the left
ventricular wall to measure intracavitary pressure and its first
derivative (dP/dt). Maximal cardiac output in each heart was obtained
by gradually increasing the left atrial filling pressure to the values
ranging between 18 cm H_2O and 23 cm H_2O while the heart pumped against a
set aortic pressure of 110 cm H_2O. Once the maximum cardiac output was
obtained, the left atrial filling pressure was decreased in order to
reduce the cardiac output (CO) to 75-80% which was considered as the
submaximum steady-state cardiac output.

The perfusate contained human RBC suspended in a Krebs-Henseleit
solution consisting of: NaCl (120 mM), KCl (4.7 mM), $CaCl_2$ (2.0 mM),
$MgSO_4$ (1.2 mM), K_2PO_4 (1.2 mM), sodium pyruvate (2.0 mM), $NaHCO_2$ (30.0
mMO and glucose (11.0 mM). Bovine serum albumin (fraction V) was added
for a final concentration of 15 mg/ml and the hematocrit was adjusted to
27%. The perfusate was warmed to 37°C in a waterbath and its
homogeneity was maintained by a magnetic stirrer. The perfusate was
continuously pumped through a Bently infusion filter (PFF 100) and was
oxygenated by continuous passage through the hollow fibers of an
artificial kidney (Cordis Dow C-Dak 1.8D) while a gas mixture (95% O_2/5%
CO_2) was flushed through the outer compartment in a countercurrent
manner. The recirculation system was adapted from Duvelleroy et al.
(34) and consisted of a K-H buffer reservoir, thermostated RBC perfusate
and atrial reservoir, peristaltic pump, filter, gas oxygenator, aortic
flowmeter and aortic, ventricular, and atrial pressure transducers.

411

Samples of RBC perfusate from the aortic outflow track and coronary sinus effluent were taken every 15 minutes in the 7 week fed hearts and every 10 minutes in the 10 week fed hearts. Measurements of partial pressures of O_2 and CO_2, and of pH were performed using an IL 813 pH/Blood Gas analyzer and oxygen content was determined using a IL 282 CO-Oximeter. Myocardial oxygen consumption (MVO2) was calculated as a product of coronary flow times the arteriovenous O_2 difference. Cardiac efficiency was derived from the ratio of total external cardiac work produced to total energy expended. Total external cardiac work was calculated from its pressure [Wp] and kinetic [Wk] components.

<u>Statistical Analysis</u>.

All data were expressed as means and standard errors of the mean, and were analyzed using analysis of variance. Any significant differences among the treatment groups were identified with the Scheffe test. Calculations of percent survival of the hearts on the isolated system were done using modified Life Tables (32) and any differences obtained among the groups were identified using the Chi-square analysis.

RESULTS

Table 1 presents the body weight, left ventricular weight and the percentage of left ventricular weight of body weight. After 10 weeks on the diet, the mean body weight of the GBA group was significantly lower (p<0.01) than in control and GPA group even though an attempt was made to maintain similar caloric intake in all three groups. A decrease in left ventricular weight in the GBA group was observed after 10 weeks but the difference was not statistically significant when compared to the control or the GPA group. The relative weight remained almost identical indicating that the heart weight to body weight relationship remained undisturbed.

	BODY WEIGHT (g)		LEFT VENTRICULAR WEIGHT (g)		LEFT VENTRICULAR WEIGHT (%)	
	7 WK	10 WK	7 WK	10 WK	7 WK	10 WK
C	387 ± 6	418 ± 5	0.80 ± 0.06	1.00 ± 0.05	0.21 ± 0.02	0.24 ± 0.01
GBA	378 ± 7	380 ± 10*	0.86 ± 0.06	0.86 ± 0.06	0.20 ± 0.02	0.22 ± 0.01
GPA	383 ± 7	408 ± 7	0.89 ± 0.04	0.94 ± 0.08	0.23 ± 0.0±	0.23 ± 0.02

Table 1: Body weight, absolute ventricular weight (left ventricle and septum) and relative ventricular weight (% of left ventricular weight of body weight) of C, GBA and GPA rats fed for 7 and 10 weeks. Number of animals was 9 at 7 weeks, and 7 at 10 weeks. Statistical significance between control and experimental groups (p<0.05), no statistical differences between experimental groups were found.

The concentrations of myocardial total creatine, GBA and GPA of rats fed for 7 and 10 weeks are presented in Table 2. After 7 weeks, total creatine levels were reduced by 75% in the hearts of the GBA group (hGBA) and in the hearts GPA group (hGPA). After 10 weeks, the depletion became maximal both in hGBA (90%) and in hGPA (85%) and did not change thereafter. Maximal accumulation of GBA and GPA after 10 weeks was 6.8 ± 0.6 and 14.3 ± 1.9 µM/g of wet weight, respectively. Although the accumulation of GPA was significantly greater it did not result in greater depletion of creatine than with GBA.

	CREATINE		GBA		GPA	
	7 WK	10 WK	7 WK	10 WK	7 WK	10 WK
C	13.8 ± 1.8	14.8 ± 1.8	0.05 ± 0.01	0.03 ± 0.02	0.04 ± 0.02	0.04 ± 0.01
GBA	$3.5 \pm 0.8*$	$1.5 \pm 0.4*$	$5.5 \pm 1.2*$	$6.8 \pm 0.6*$	-	-
GPA	$3.6 \pm 0.5*$	$2.4 \pm 0.6*$	-	-	$11.1 \pm 1.0*$	$14.3 \pm 1.9*$

Table 2: Total creatine, GBA and GPA concentrations in hearts of Control, GBA and GPA rats fed for 7 and 10 weeks. Number of animals was 9 at 7 weeks and 7 at 10 weeks. Concentrations are expressed as mol/g of wet weight of the left ventricle (free wall and septum). *Statistical significance between controls and experimental groups ($*p<0.01$), no significant differences were found between GBA and GPA groups.

Figure 1 shows the myocardial ultrastructure of a control rat. Myofibrils and columns of mitochondria with well defined cristae are clearly visible. Transverse tubules are dilated and well defined, and granules of glycogen can be observed in this longitudinal midwall section. The ultrastructure of the myocardium of GPA and GBA groups after 7 weeks are shown in Figures 2 and 3 respectively. Although the myocardium in both GBA and GPA groups was generally similar to that of the control, some focal changes did take place as seen in Figure 2. In this micrograph of the longitudinal midwall section of GPA-fed rat myocardium some loss of myofilaments has occurred and many of the remaining myofilaments are compacted and arranged in disorganized strips. Also, dilated mitochondria with lamellar cristae and transluscent matrix are present in the affected areas. Figure 3 depicts similar focal ultrastructural changes in this longitudinal midwall section of the myocardium of GBA-fed rat. The mitochondria have dilated matrices and have lost some of the cristae. Myofibrilar lysis with the presence of disorganized strip formation is also evident. Some

dilatation of sarcoplasmic reticulum was noted in both Figures 2 and 3.
The observed ultrastructural changes were rare, extremely focal and
cannot be taken as definitive signs of degeneration which is usually
manifested by a high number of lipofusion granules. Apart from the
above, the myocardium of the analog-fed rats appeared normal.

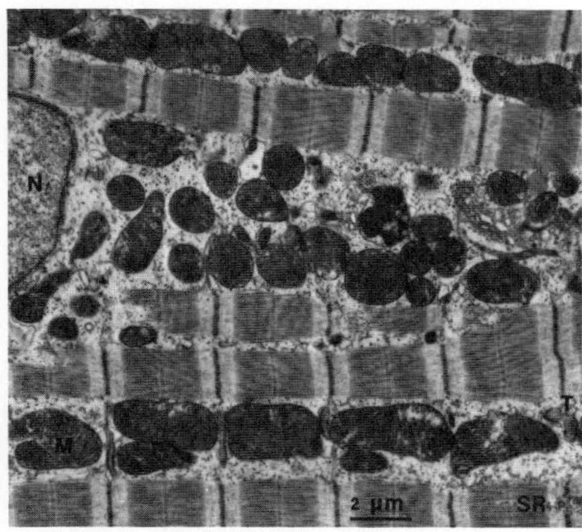

Figure 1: Transmission electron micrograph of the left ventricular myocardium from a control rat. (M) mitochondria, (T) transverse tubules, (SR) sarcoplasmic reticulum, (N) nucleus (uranyl acetate and lead citrate-stained sections).

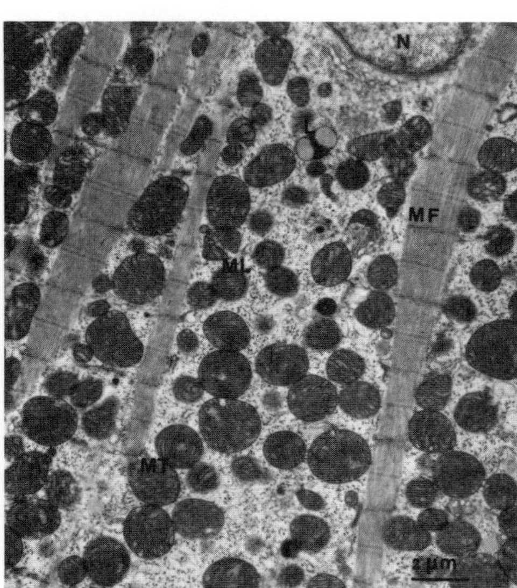

Figure 2: Transmission electron micrograph of the left ventricular myocardium from a rat fed GPA for seven weeks. (ML) mitochondria with deranged lamellar cristae, (MT) mitochondria with translusent matrix, (MF) myofilaments that are compacted into disorganized strips, (L) lipofusin granules, (N) nucleus (uranyl acetate and lead citrate -stained sections).

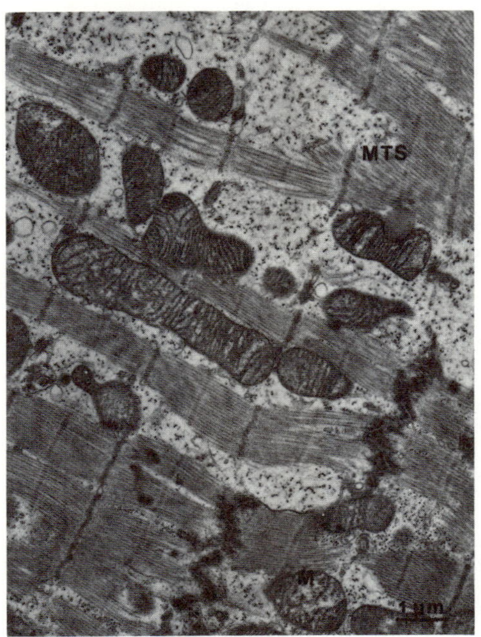

Figure 3. Transmission electron micrograph of the left ventricular myocardium from a rat fed GBA for seven weeks. (MTS) myofibrilar strips, (M) dilated mitochondria at different stages of degeneration (uranyl acetate, lead citrate-stained sections).

Cardiac performance was evaluated after 7 and 10 weeks of creatine depletion using the isolated working heart preparation. When we compared the hemodynamic data of the corresponding control and experimental hearts between 7 and 10 week groups we could not see any significant differences. This was also the case when we compared the performance of control and experimental hearts within either the 7 or 10 week groups (Table 3).

Among the recorded hemodynamic parameters, the cardiac output was the most consistant indicator of the time dependent performance of control and the experimental groups. Figure 4 (top graph) shows that after 7 weeks on the diet all of the hearts were able to maintain the initial submaximum steady-state cardiac output (as defined in the method section) for 60 minutes. During the second hour the cardiac output began to decline in all hearts and some of them ultimately failed (failure was defined as CO less than 10% of the initial submaximum

steady state CO). The rate of decline of CO in the hGBA and hGPA was
much faster in comparison to the hearts of control (hC). By 75 minutes,
the CO decreased to 50% in the hGBA, and to 66% in hGPA which was
significantly lower (p<0.05) from the CO of the control group. The
hearts of the control group (hC) at 75 minutes maintained CO at 89%. By
120 minutes, the hearts of both GBA and GPA groups had CO less than 20%
while the CO of control hearts was at 54% of the initial submaximum
steady-state. No significant differences were obtained between the
hearts of the GBA and the GPA groups.

	C	GBA	GPA
n	15	15	16
Hematocrit %	27 ± 1	27 ± 1	26 ± 1
pH a	7.42 ± 0.03	7.41 ± 0.04	7.43 ± 0.02
pH c.s.	7.34 ± 0.02	7.31 ± 0.01	7.33 ± 0.02
PO_{2a} mmHg	305 ± 72	291 ± 50	344 ± 68
PO_{2cs} mmHg	31 ± 3	39 ± 5	32 ± 3
PCO_{2a} mmHg	40 ± 7	36 ± 9	39.6 ± 2
PCO_{2cs} mmHg	46 ± 2	41.9 ± 6	46 ± 4
$C\,O_{2a}$ ml O_2/dl	13.1 ± 1.3	14.1 ± 1.1	14.1 ± 1.6
$C\,O_{2cs}$ ml O_2/dl	9.2 ± 0.9	9.1 ± 2.0	9.8 ± 1.5
Hb g%	8.6 ± 0.9	9.7 ± 0.7	9.7 ± 0.4
Heart Rate/min	290 ± 15	305 ± 20	275 ± 30
Aortic Flow ml/min/g	55 ± 6	51 ± 7.1	54 ± 5.1
Coronary Flow ml/min/g	6.6 ± 1.1	6.7 ± 0.9	5.2 ± 1.3
Myocardial Oxygen Consumption ml/min/g	0.32 ± 0.11	0.30 ± 0.13	0.27 ± 0.12
Power Input mW/g	117 ± 14	106 ± 19	104 ± 13
Total External Power mW/g	10.8 ± 1.8	10.1 ± 1.6	9.7 ± 1.1
Efficiency %	9 ± 1	10 ± 2	10 ± 2
LVP mmHg	125 ± 6	120 ± 10	119 ± 2
LVEDP mmHg	8.8 ± 1.5	11.8 ± 1.2	11.5 ± 1.6
+dP/dt mmHg/sec	3558 ± 105	3616 ± 350	3296 ± 193
-dP/dt mmHg/sec	3265 ± 286	2944 ± 241	3116 ± 207

Table 3: Hemodynamic data (means and SEM) of isolated working rat hearts of
control, GBA-fed and GPA-fed rats, perfused with red blood cell enriched
perfusate. a = aortic, c.s. = coronary sinus, PO_2, PCO_2 = partial pressure
of oxygen, carbon dioxide, $C\,O_2$ = total oxygen content, Hb = hemoglobin, LVP
= peak left ventricular pressure, LVEDP = left ventricular end-diastolic
pressure. Data were expressed per gram of left ventricular wet weight (free
wall and septum).

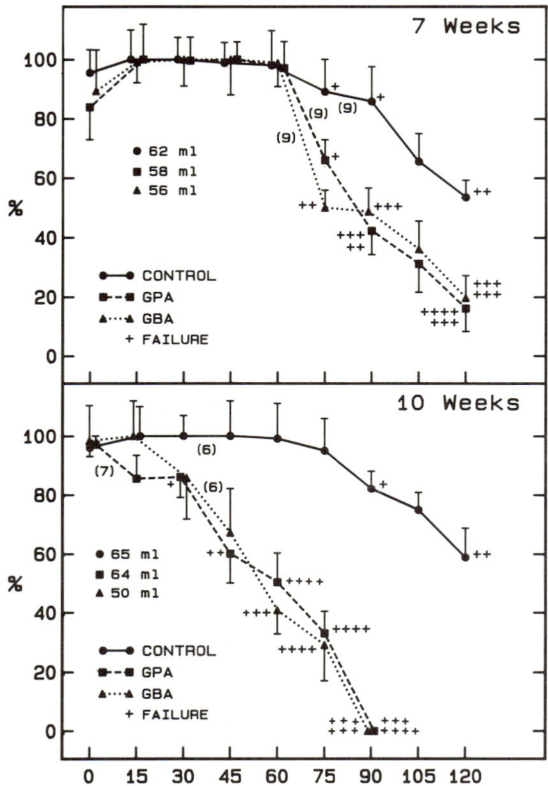

Figure 4: Mean values ± SEM of cardiac output with the time were
expressed as percentage of the submaximum steady-state cardiac output of
Control, GBA and GPA rats fed for 7 and 10 weeks. This cardiac output
was achieved within 15 minutes of stabilization, which were taken as
100%. The numbers in brackets represent initial numbers of hearts in
each group. + sign indicates one heart whose cardiac output fell below
10%. The mean value then represents the average cardiac output of the
surviving hearts.

After 10 weeks on the diet, the maximum and consequently the
submaximum steady-state CO in all three groups were similar to those of
7 week fed rats. However, the onset of decline in the hearts of the GBA
and GPA groups occurred sooner as seen in Figure 4 (bottom graph). By
45 minutes the CO declined to 67% of the initial maximum steady-state
and to 60% in hGPA while the hC maintained their initial maximum
steady-state CO. Cardiac output in hGBA and hGPA at 45 minutes was

significantly lower (p<0.05) than the CO of the control group but no
significant differences were observed in CO between the two creatine
depleted groups. By 90 minutes, all of the hearts in the GBA and GPA
groups failed while the control group maintained 82% of the initial CO.

Cardiac output of the GBA and GPA groups began to decrease earlier,
and the hearts failed sooner than in the control group and consequently
the number of surviving hearts (CO of more than 10% of the initial
steady-state CO) decreased faster (Fig. 5). In the 7 week fed rats, all
of the hearts survived in the first hour, but by 90 minutes only 56% of
the hGBA and hPGA survived while 89% of all hearts in the control group
survived (p<0.05). By 120 minutes only 23% of hGBA and 32% of hGPA
survived while 78% of the hearts in the control group survived (p<0.01).
After 10 weeks only 50% of hGBA and 40% of hGPA survived at 60 minutes
while the control group showed 100% survival. At 90 minutes 70% of the
hearts of the control group survived while there were no surviving
hearts from the creatine depleted groups (p<0.01).

Left ventricular end-diastolic pressure (LVEDP) was compared among
the three groups at 15, 90 and 105 minutes in the surviving hearts of 7
week fed rats and 15, 45 and 75 minutes in surviving hearts of 10 week
fed rats as shown in Table 4. The LVEDP in the rats fed for 7 weeks
increased significantly in hGBA when compared to hC and hGPA at 90 and
105 minutes (p<0.01). After 10 weeks increase in LVEDP was observed in
both hGBA and hGPA when compared to hC at 75 minutes, however
statistical analysis was not possible due to the low number of surviving
hearts in the GBA and GPA groups at that time. When we compared
myocardial oxygen consumption, heart rate, work input and output,
efficiency, or stroke volume we found no significant differences among
control, GBA and GPA groups throughout the time-course of the
experiment.

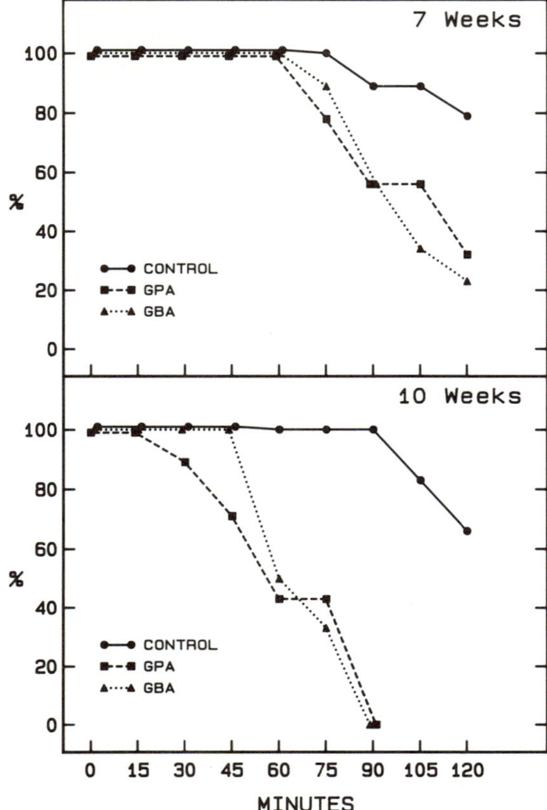

Figure 5: Percentage of surviving hearts of Control, GBA and GPA rats fed
for 7 and 10 weeks, whose cardiac output remained above 10% of the initial
value. The number of hearts as indicated for each group in Figure 1 was
taken as 100%.

7 WEEK	15 min	90 min	105 min
Control	9.7 ± 1.7(9)	10.5 ± 1.6(9)	12.3 ± 1.7(9)
GBA	13.8 ± 1.2(9)	17.6 ± 1.7(6)*	21.4 ± 2.7(6)*
GPA	10.7 ± 1.9(9)	12.7 ± 2.0(4)	12.8 ± 2.2(4)
n		9	

10 WEEK	15 min	45 min	75 min
Control	7.9 ± 1.0(6)	8.0 ± 1.0(6)	11.8 ± 1.4(6)
GBA	9.7 ± 0.8(6)	9.7 ± 0.3(6)	14.7 ± 1.9(2)
GPA	10.3 ± 1.2(7)	12.0 ± 1.8(5)	18.3 ± 2.3(2)

Table 4: Left ventricular end-diastolic pressure (mmHg) of Control, GBA- and
GPA-fed hearts for 7 and 10 weeks. Numbers in brackets represent the numbers
of surviving hearts. Statistical significance between control and
experimental groups (*p<0.01).

In rats fed Control, GBA and GPA diet for 10 weeks, CP, ATP and adenosine concentrations were measured in frozen tissue from the isolated blood-perfused hearts at three different time points: at 15 min in hearts that maintained 100% submaximum steady-state CO; at 45 min in hGBA and hGPA that attained 60% of the submaximum steady-state CO and in control that maintained 100% of the submaximum steady-state CO; at 90 minutes in hGBA and hGPA that failed and in hC that maintained 80% of the submaximum steady-state. The concentrations of CP, ATP and adenosine in the control group at 15 minutes were taken as a reference and all subsequent measurements were compared to these levels, since submaximum steady-state CO was obtained at that time (Figure 4). In the hGBA and hGPA the CP levels at 15 minutes were decreased by 76%, and were significantly lower ($p < 0.05$) than those of the control group as shown in Table 5. In spite of that, ATP concentrations and cardiac performance (Figure 4) remained similar to that of the control hearts. By 90 minutes, the CP levels in hGBA and hGPA decreased by 96% ($p < 0.05$) when compared to the levels in the control group at 15 minutes. The concentrations of ATP at 90 minutes were also significantly decreased by 70% ($p < 0.05$) from control levels at 15 minutes however, at 90 minutes, the adenosine levels in hGBA and hGPA were significantly increased by 250% ($p < 0.05$), when compared to levels obtained in the control group at 15 minutes. Cardiac failure was observed in all of the creatine deple- ted hearts at 90 minutes while hC still maintained 80% of submaximum steady-state CO. Concentration of total creatine (C and CP) at 90 minutes decreased by 6 μmol/g in hC, 2.2 μmol/g in hGBA and by 1.8 μmol/g in hGPA when compared to concentrations obtained at 15 minutes.

	Total Creatine	Creatine	Creatine Phosphate	ATP	Adenosine
15 min					
C	66.6 ± 1.5	51.0 ± 0.7	15.6 ± 2.1	9.1 ± 0.7	3.6 ± 1.0
GBA	9.9 ± 1.0*	6.2 ± 1.1*	3.7 ± 0.1*	7.9 ± 0.8	3.7 ± 0.4
GPA	10.4 ± 0.6*	7.3 ± 1.8*	3.1 ± 0.1*	8.6 ± 1.3	3.3 ± 1.0
45 min					
C	58.7 ± 0.8	54.3 ± 0.6	4.4 ± 1.8	6.4 ± 0.2	12.6 ± 1.5
GBA	8.4 ± 0.7*+	7.1 ± 1.2*+	1.3 ± 0.1*+	4.0 ± 0.5*+	9.5 ± 2.0+
GPA	8.5 ± 1.1*+	7.4 ± 1.2*+	1.1 ± 0.3*+	5.0 ± 0.4*+	13.8 ± 1.8+
90 min					
C	59.8 ± 1.6	56.9 ± 2.6	2.9 ± 0.5	3.5 ± 0.4	5.9 ± 0.3
GBA	7.6 ± 1.2*+	7.0 ± 1.6*+	0.6 ± 0.4*+	2.3 ± 1.0+	9.1 ± 1.1*+
GPA	8.6 ± 1.9*+	7.7 ± 2.3*+	0.9 ± 0.4*+	2.8 ± 2.3+	7.4 ± 0.2*+
n	3	3	3	3	3

Table 5: Myocardial concentrations of creatine, CP, ATP and adenosine in the isolated blood perfused rat heart at 15, 45 and 90 minutes in Control, GBA and GPA rats fed for 10 weeks. Units are mol/g dry weight, dry wt/wet wt = 0.20. Statistical significance between control and experimental groups, (*p< 0.05). Statistical significance between control at 15 minutes and experimental at 45 or 90 minutes (+p<0.05).

DISCUSSION

By feeding rats with structural analogs of creatine we obtained a 90% decrease in total myocardial creatine concentration which is in agreement with data obtained by others (16,18,21). However, while some laboratories attained a 90% decrease in total creatine in 4-6 weeks (16) we achieved a comparable decrease only after 10 weeks of feeding only, since our animals were older at the start of the feeding trail. We chose older and heavier animals for these studies to obtain hearts of adequate size for the isolated heart preparation. We found that the accumulation of GBA in the myocardium was significantly lower than that of GPA. In fact, the latter analog appeared to accumulate reciprocally to the concentration of creatine. A similar pattern of accumulation has also been observed in skeletal muscle (16). However, in the skeletal muscle, analogs accumulated to a much higher concentration (15 µM/g of wet weight in the GBA-fed rats and 30 µM/g of wet weight in GPA-fed rat) than in the myocardium.

Most studies report a 5-10% decline in body weight after feeding with the creatine analogs (16,18,29). Pair-feeding done in this study and by others (18,29), did not prevent a modest (10%) weight loss in the GBA group. The decrease in body weight may have been due to minor metabolic effects since some focal changes in myocardial ultrastructure were observed. These changes in ultrastructure were similar to but not so extensive as those observed in Cornish chicks fed 2% GBA for 6 weeks (27). Interestingly, the ultrastructural alterations observed in these chicks were reversed when 6% creatine was included in the diet.

The isolated working heart perfused with RBC enriched K-H perfusate is considerably more complex and difficult to set up and maintain than an isolated heart preparation perfused with an electrolyte solution only. However, the use of a perfusate containing red blood cells ensures better oxygen delivery. In our preparation, maximum cardiac output, total work output and myocardial oxygen consumption were higher, while the coronary flow was lower, when compared to hearts perfused with K-H only (33,34). The hemodynamic values that we obtained in this study are in agreement with those of Duvelleroy et al. (24) who also used RBC enriched perfusate. It is generally accepted that <u>in vivo</u>, the fraction of coronary flow is approximately 5% of cardiac output, in our blood-perfused hearts it was 7%, while in hearts perfused with an electrolyte solution it is 26% (33). Low dry weight to wet weight ratio (0.15) observed usually in hearts perfused with electrolyte solutions containing albumin indicates considerable edema. In our experiments, where hearts were perfused with RBC enriched perfusates containing albumin, the dry weight to wet weight ratio was 0.20 indicating that considerably less edema developed in these hearts. The use of the RBC perfusate in the isolated working heart is therefore preferable since it is more physiological and provides for better oxygenation at high cardiac output levels.

Our experiments indicate that in the analog treated groups the creatine levels decreased , the duration of steady state performance of the isolated working hearts declined faster and the number of surviving hearts decreased earlier when compared to the control hearts. The concentration of CP in all three groups by 90 minutes was only one fifth of the levels obtained at 15 minutes. The concentration of ATP was similar in the three groups at 15 minutes and decreased to one-third in all three groups by 90 minutes. Cardiac performance at 90 minutes in the hC was relatively unchanged from 15 minutes, while in GBA and GPA groups, all hearts had failed. It appears therefore, that CP concentrations are more important to sustain a long-term cardiac performance than ATP concentrations and that the levels of CP can decrease quite considerably before cardiac function is impaired. The lowest levels to which CP can fall while ATP concentrations remain relatively high are most probably between 1.5-2.5 mol/g of dry weight (Table 4). When CP falls below this concentration, ATP levels decline and cardiac performance deteriorates. The decline of CP concentration in our experiments during the 90 minutes perfusion may have resulted from some washout of creatine and inorganic phosphate or due to loss of functioning of some mitochondria which would decrease the supply of high energy phosphate bonds.

The concentrations of CP and ATP measured in our experiments by HPLC were lower than those obtained by others (35,36). It is possible that some hydrolysis of CP and ATP occurred during the freezing process since the heart weighed about 1 gram. This large tissue may take several seconds to freeze and substantial hydrolysis of CP has been reported even during one second of freezing (37). Nonetheless, the relative decreases in concentrations of CP and ATP in creatine depleted rats are in agreement with other data (19).

Left ventricular end-diastolic pressure (LVEDP) kept increasing in all three groups from start of the experiment to the end. However, LVEDP in the creatine-depleted groups was significantly higher when compared to the control group by the end of the experiment. Direct measurement of the left ventricular volume was not done in our experiment thus we can only speculate why LVEDP rose more significantly in the creatine depleted groups. It may have been because of a higher end-diastolic volume in the hearts of the creatine depleted rats or because the ventricles were stiffer. Since decreased ATP concentrations were observed in all three groups (Table 4) by the end of the experiment this could have caused a fall of the ATP/ADP ratio, which may be associated with an increase in cytosolic levels of Ca^{++}. A fall in the ATP/ADP ratio will decrease G ATP which is a critical parameter controlling the release and uptake of Ca^{++} from the terminal cysternae of the sarcoplasmic reticulum. Therefore, a decrease in ATP/ADP ratio, will limit the uptake of Ca^{++} from the cytosol back into SR (38) and slow the relaxation of myocardium (29,38), and thus increase the resistance to filling. In the creatine depleted hearts the CP

concentration decreased to very low levels and this could have
contributed to incomplete relaxation and explain the higher LVEDP. In
the presence of incomplete myocardial relaxation, given filling pressure
will not distend the myocardial fibers adequately leading to a reduction
of end-diastolic volume and impairment of cardiac performance.

The initial concept of the creatine shuttle was based on
experiments leading to regional cardiac ischemia in vivo in which it was
shown that myocardial contractile function ceased when CP levels
decreased by 75% and ATP levels declined by 25% (39). In our
experiments contractile function was maintained in hearts depleted of
creatine and CP by 85-90% of the initial resting CP levels yet
myocardial function was unaffected. However, once the CP levels
declined below some critical level, ATP levels declined and cardiac
performance deteriorated. Therefore, CP may play an important role in
the maintenance of normal myocardial function, but normal levels of CP
are not essential to steady-state cardiac function under normoxemic
conditions.

SUMMARY

We investigated the effects of reduction of myocardial
concentration of creatine and creatine phosphate on hemodynamic
performance of rat hearts under normoxemia. Rats were fed a diet
containing structural analogs of creatine (β-guanidinobutyric acid and
β-guanidinopropionic acid) which led to 75-90% reduction in total
myocardial creatine after seven to ten weeks of feeding. We found that
in isolated blood-perfused working heart preparation the maximum cardiac
output at constant arterial pressure (110 cm H_2O) and consequently the
steady-state cardiac output (75% of the maximum) were not affected by
creatine depletion. However, the length of time during which the
creatine depleted hearts were able to maintain this steady-state (75%)
cardiac output decreased with decreasing levels of myocardial creatine.
The survival time of the creatine depleted hearts under the above
experimental conditions was significantly shorter when compared to
control hearts. The onset of failure could be related to decreasing
levels of myocardial CP and ATP. A significant increase in LVEDP was
observed in creatine depleted isolated hearts with time as compared to
normal control hearts. In spite of the fact that short term maximum

cardiac volume work remained unaffected after creatine depletion, there
was a significant shortening of time during which submaximal volume work
could be sustained.

ACKNOWLEDGMENTS

This work was supported by Heart and Stroke Foundation of Ontario.
The authors of this study thank Mrs. Linda Jui and Mrs. Marika Masika
for their skillful technical assistance.

REFERENCES

1. Cain, D.F., Davis, R.E. Biochem. Z. 281: 361-366, 1962.
2. Gerken, G., Schlette, H. Experientia 24: 17-19, 1968.
3. Saks, V.A., Rosenshtraukh, L.V., Smirnov, V.N., Chazov, E.I. Can.
    J. Physiol. Pharmacol. 56: 691-706, 1978.
4. Bessman, S., Geiger, P.J. Science 211: 448-452, 1981.
5. Jacobs, H., Heldt, H.W., Klingenberg, M. Biochem. Biophys. Res.
    Commun. 16: 516-521, 1964.
6. Sobel, B., Shell, W.E., Kelin, M.S. J. Mol. Cell. Cardiol. 37:
    1079-1085, 1972.
7. Scholte, H.R., Weijers, P.J., Wit-Peters, E.M. Biochim. Biophys.
    Acta. 291: 764-773, 1973.
8. Turner, D.C., Walliman, T., Eppenberger, H.M. Proc. Natl. Acad.
    Sci. U.S.A. 70: 702-705, 1973.
9. Bessman, S., Fonyo, A. Biochem. Biophys. Res. Comm. 8: 361-366,
    1966.
10. Jacobus, W.E., Lehninger, A.L. J. Biol. Chem. 248: 4803-4810,
    1972.
11. Saks, V.A., Rosenshtraukh, L.V., Undrovinas, A., Smirnov, V.N.,
    Chazov, E.I. Biochem. Med. 16: 21-36, 1976.
12. Rosenshtraukh, L.V., Saks, V.A., Yuriavichus, I.A., Nesterenko,
    V.V., Undrovinas, A.I., Smirnov, V.N., Chazov, E.I. Biochem.
    Med. 21: 1-15, 1978.
13. Fitch, C.D., Shields, R.P., Payne, W.F., Dacus, J.M. J. Biol.
    Chem. 243: 2024-2027, 1968.
14. Fitch, C.D., Jellinek, M., Mueller, E.J. J. Biol. Chem. 249:
    1060-1063, 1974.
15. Fitch, C.D., Jellinek, M., Fitts, R.H., Bladwin, K.M., Hossoszy,
    J.O. Am. J. Physiol. 22i: 1123-1125, 1975.
16. Fitch, D.C., Chevli, R. Metabolism, 29: 686-690, 1980.
17. Petrofsky, J.S., Fitch, C.D. Pflugers Arch. 384: 123-129, 1980.
18. Mainwood, G.W., Alward, M., Eiselt, B. Can. J. Physiol. Pharmacol.
    60: 120-127, 1982.
19. Meyer, R.A., Brown, R.T., Kushmerick, M.J. Biophys. J. 45: 91,
    1984.
20. Bittl, J.A., Ingwall, J.S. Biol. Chem. 260: 3312-3517, 1985.
21. Shoubride, E.A., Jeffry, F.M.H., Keogh, J.M., Radda, G.K.,
    Seymour, M.L. Biochim. Piophys. Acta. 847: 25-32, 1985.
22. Mathews, P.M., Bland, J.L., Gadian, D.G., Radda, G.K. Biochim.
    Biophys. Acta. 721: 312-320, 1982.

23. Ingwall, J.S., Kobayashi, K., Bittl, J.A. Biomed. J. 41: 1a, 1983.
24. Duvelleroy, M.A., Duruble, M., Martin, J.L., Teisseire, B.,
    Droulez, J., Cain, M., J. Appl. Physiol. 41: 603-607, 1976.
25. Dowell, R.T., Cutilletta, A.F., Sodt, P.C. J. Appl. Physiol.
    39: 1043-1047, 1975.
26. Shields, R.P., Whitehair, C.K., Carrow, R.E., Heusner, W.W., Van
    Huss, W.D. Lab. Inves. 33: 151-158, 1975.
27. Laskowski, M.B., Chevli, R., Fitch, C.D. Metabolism 30: 1080-1085,
    1981.
28. Rowley, G.L., Greenleaf, G.L. J. Amer. Chem. Soc. 93: 5542-5551,
    1971.
29. Mainwood, G.W., Totosy De Zepetnek, J. Nerve Muscle 8: 774-782,
    1985.
30. Ennor, A.H., Stocken, L.A., Biochem. J. 42: 557-563, 1984.
31. Bonas, J.E., Cohen, B.D., Natelson, S. Microchem. J. 7: 63-77,
    1963.
32. Fleiss, J.L., Dunner, D.L., Stallone, F., Fiene, R.R. Arch. Gen.
    Psych. 33: 189-196, 1976.
33. Neely, J.R., Liebermeister, H., Battersby, E.J., Morgan, H.E.
    Amer. J. Phys. 212(4): 804-814, 1967.
34. Opie, L.J., Mansford, R.L., Owen, P. Biochem. J. 124: 475-490,
    1971.
35. Fossel, E.T., Morgan, H.E., Ingwall, J.S. Proc. Natl. Acad. Sci.
    USA 77: 3654-3658, 1980.
36. Saks, V.A., Kupriyanov, V.N., Smirnov, V.N. Proc. Int. Union
    Physiol. Sci. 16: 66, 1986.
37. Kushmerick, M.J., Meyer, R.A. Amer. J. Physiol. 245: C542-C549,
    1985.
38. Hasselbach, W., Oetliker, H. Ann. Rev. Physiol. 45: 325-339, 1983.
39. Gudbjarnason, S., Mathes, P., Ravens, K.G. J. Mol. Cell. Cardiol.
    1: 325-339, 1970.

28

LOCALIZATION OF GLUCOSE-6-PHOSPHATASE (G-6-PASE)
IN THE RAT HEART MUSCLE CELLS

Han Yu-Sheng, *Jung Yeh-Chih

Department of Biophysics, Shanghai Second Medical University,
*Department of Internal Medicine, Hsin-Hua Hospital, Shanghai
Second Medical University,
Shanghai, CHINA

INTRODUCTION

Glucose-6-phosphatase (G-6-Pase) activity has been studied cytochemically and regarded as a marker enzyme of endoplasmic reticulum in many tissues as liver, kidney, intestine et al[1]. But the G-6-Pase was seldom studied in heart muscle cells. The purpose of the present paper is to study G-6-Pase reaction cytochemically in the sarcoplasmic reticulum of rat heart muscle cells and its distribution in the myocardial cells.

METHODS

The experiment has been undertaken in our laboratory to study G-6-Pase reaction cytochemically and localization in the rat myocardial cells. The experiment was done for five times in the five wistar rats with the controls to be carried out. The experimental rat hearts were fixed by retrograde perfusion[2] of the coronary arteries with 1.5% glutaraldehyde solution in 0.1 M sodium cacodylate buffer (pH 7.2) less than five minutes, then the free wall of the left ventricle was finely cut into small blocks. The tissue blocks were then immediately washed with cacodylate buffer solution, and cut into 75 microns thin sections using a Solvall TC-2 machine (Du Pont Instruments).

The speciments were divided into two groups, one group was the experimental, and the other one was the control.

1) The group I (experimental group):

The G-6-Pase incubation solution was prepared according to the Teutsh's method[3]. The incubation solution medium composed of:

0.1 M d-glucose-6-phosphate mono-sodium	1 ml
0.2 M Tris-Maleate (pH 6.5)	2 ml
Distilled water	3 ml
36 mM lead nitrate	1 ml
1 M sucrose	3 ml

Sections were incubated in the above solution for 60 min at 37°C.

Then the sections were washed in 0.1 M sodium cacodylate buffer, and postfixed in 1.5% potassium ferrocyamide-1% reduced osmium tetroxide[4] for 1 hr at 4°C, dehydrated and embedded in Epon. Ultrathin sections were stained with lead citrate and studied in the Hitachi-500 electron microscope operated 75 Kv.

2) The group II (control group):

Sections in these control groups were incubated in solutions not containing the substrate, the other steps were all the same.

RESULTS

G-6-Pase reaction was shown clearly to be localized throughout the sarcotubular system including the sarcoplasmic reticulum tubule and cisternae in the myocardial cells of the rat ventricle. The experiment was done for five times in 5 rats, all with the same results. But the G-6-Pase activity was negative in all the controls.

The sarcoplasmic reticulum could be seen with the different appearance at various sections. In the longitudinal sections of the myocardial cell, the G-6-Pase reaction was found in the SR between myofibrils, of diads and trids, and nuclear membrane (Fig.1). The reactive products appeared to be more strong in front of A-band of myofibrils, and weaker in front of I-band of myofibrils. In the section taken parallel to the myofibrilar surfaces, the deposition just covering the myofibrils was shown as an extensive network of SR extending along the myofibrilar surface. Especially fa-

cing A-band, the deposition was appeared to form as a meshwork of anastomotic tubules and crowded together, while in
the adjacent areas facing I-band, the deposition appeared
to form the large polygonal meshes and to be more sparse
(Fig.2,3).

At the Z line, there was significant deposition of G-
6-Pase reaction in SR. Some of SR formed the distended sacs,
that ran parallel on one or both sides of the T tubules,
such sacs were connected with each other by short bridging
tubular cistenae above or below the T tubules (Fig.4). In
the space of SR network, a great deal of glycogen granules
could be seen.

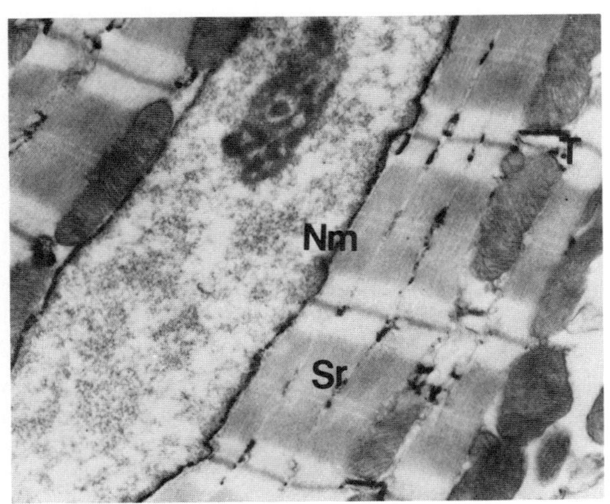

FIG.1 - Longitudinal section of rat myocardium, relaxed,
showing deposition of G-6-Pase reaction in SR(Sr) between
myofibrills, of diads (T) and nuclear membrane (Nm)(x16,000).

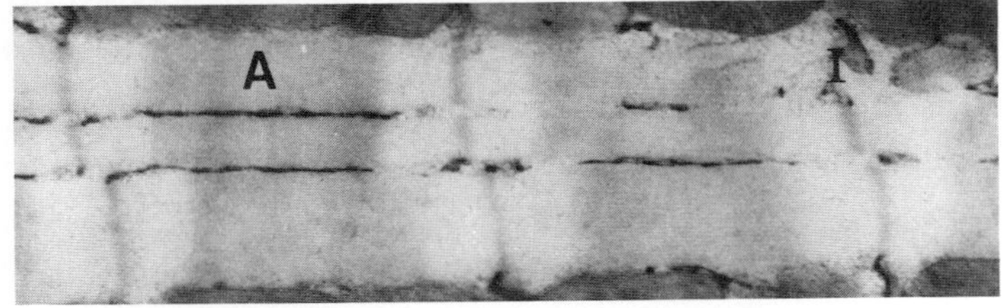

FIG.2 - Longitudinal section of rat myocardium, relaxed, showing more strong G-6-Pase reaction in SR at the A-band (A),
and weaker at the I-band (I)(x17,500).

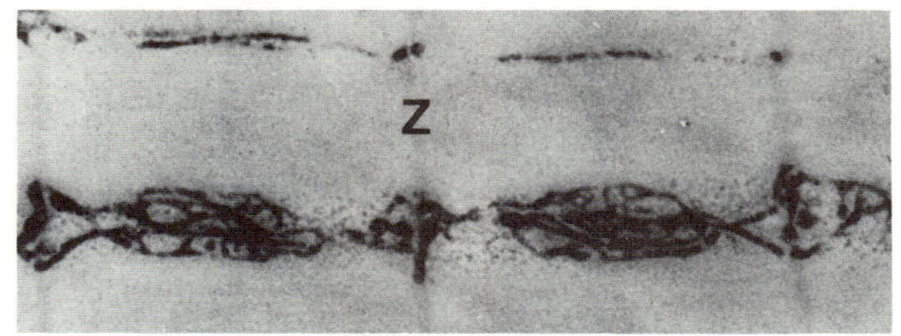

FIG.3 - The section taken parallel to the myofibrilar surface, contracted, showing two sarcomeres and facing A-band,
the deposition appeared to form as a meshwork of anastomotic tubules. At the Z line, there was significant deposition
of G-6-Pase reaction in SR(x35,000).

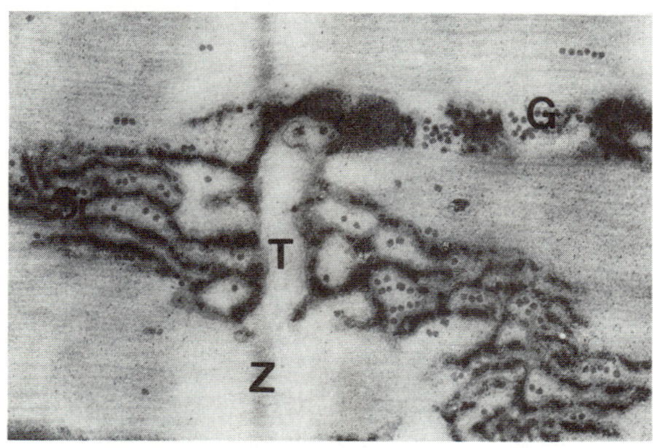

FIG.4 - The T tubule (T) just covering the Z-line (Z). It
is shown between SR(Sr) and T tubule (T) cytochemically.
In the space of SR network glycogen granules (G) were shown
(x40,000).

DISCUSSION

G-6-Pase activity has been studied cytochemically and
found in the endoplasmic reticulum as a marker enzyme in many tissues, but the G-6-Pase was seldom studied in the heart
muscle cells. Borgers[5] has shown the G-6-Pase reaction in
myocardial cells with the cytochemical method, but Lewis[1]
indicated that there was lack of G-6-Pase activity in the
muscle cells. In Forbes[6] study, It has been reported that
the enzymatic reaction in SR was difficult and tedious to be
studied. Thus, G-6-Pase activity was investigated in our la-

boratory. The results of the present investigation is more or less the same as Borgers observation. It has been shown that G-6-Pase activity is existed in the SR of myocardium. Tice[7] supposed that this particular distribution of G-6-Pase is plausible and it is assumed that the endoplasmic reticulum is an intracellular transport system concerned with the transport of glucose from glucogen-containing sites.

We think that several points are crucial to study G-6-Pase cytochemically. G-6-P enzyme is so sensitive that only a few minutes contact when the heart was fixed by perfusion can be tolerated, in our experiments the heart was fixed by a retrograde perfusion with 1.5% glutaraldehyde solution in 0.1 M sodium cacodylate buffer less than 5 minutes. Borgers suppored that G-6-Pase was totally inhibited when perfusion fixation time exceeded 10 minutes. The results may be also related to the thickness of the sections, and also the incubation medium[8].

Earlier studies on the structural organization of the SR in myocardial cell have only demonstrated the transverse and longitudinal continuty of this intracytoplasmic membranous system throughout the muscle fibers. These studies have not stressed the differences in its distribution at the level of the A-band and I-band or the SR cistenae in detail. In the present study, the G-6-Pase reaction was found clearly at SR between myofibrils, and shown that SR between myofibrils were selectively distributed, the network appeared to be distributed as a curtain, i.e. the network appeared to be more crowded in front of A-band, and more sparse in front of I-band. It could be related to the adaption of this organelles, the SR network, to the selectivel shortening of the myofibrils at the I-band during contraction[9].

REFERENCES

1. Lewis PR et al: Staining methods for sectioned material. In "Practical method in electron microscopy". Ed. by Glauert AM; Amsterdam, North-Holland, Vol.5, p.137, 1977
2. Singal PK et al: Morphological methods for studing

cardiac membranes. In "Methods in studing cardiac membranes", Ed. by Dhalla NS, CRC Press, Florida, Vol.II p.3, 1984
3. Teutsh HF : Histochemistry 57:107, 1978
4. Karnovsky MJ : Use of ferrocyanide-reduced osmium tetroxide in electron microscopy. Proc. 11th Am. Soc. Cell Biol., New Orleans, Louisiana, Abstract 284, p.146, 1971
5. Borgers M et al: J Histochem Cytochem 19:528, 1971
6. Forbes MS et al: J Ultrastruct Res 60:306, 1977
7. Tice et al: J Histochem Cytochem 10:754, 1962
8. Han Yu-Sheng et al: Chinese J Cell Biol 4:44, 1982
9. Segratain D et al: Anat Rec 200:139, 1981